NEUROPHARMACOLOGY
Clinical Applications

RM
315
.N472
1982

NEUROPHARMACOLOGY
Clinical Applications

Edited by

Walter B. Essman, M.D., Ph.D.
Queens College of the City University
 of New York
Flushing, New York

Luigi Valzelli, M.D.
Mario Negri Institute for Pharmacological
 Research
Milan, Italy

SP MEDICAL & SCIENTIFIC BOOKS
a division of Spectrum Publications, Inc.
New York

Copyright © 1982 Spectrum Publications

All rights reserved. No part of this book may be reproduced in any form, by photostat, microform, retrieval system, or any other means without prior written permission of the copyright holder or his licensee.

SPECTRUM PUBLICATIONS, INC.
175-20 Wexford Terrace, Jamaica, N.Y. 11432

Library of Congress Cataloging in Publication Date
Main entry under title:

Clinical applications of neuropharmacology.

   Includes index.
   1. Neuropharmacology. 2. Neuropsychopharmacology.
I. Essman, Walter B. II. Valzelli, Luigi, 1927-
[DNLM: 1. Mental disorders—Drug therapy. 2. Nervous system diseases—Drug therapy. 3. Psychotropic drugs.
QV 77 C6401]
RM315.C546   615′.78   81-8574
ISBN 0-089335-154-7   AACR2

Contents

Chapter	Page
1. Neuronal-Glial Metabolic Interactions in Stress .... 1 *Leonid Pevzner*	
2. Somatosensory Affectional Deprivation (SAD) Theory of Drug and Alcholic Behaviors .... 19 *James W. Prescott*	
3. Neurotransmitter and Neuropeptide Correlates of Cigarette Smoking.. 41 *Athan Karras*	
4. Nicotine and the Regulation of Smoking Behavior .... 67 *R. Kumar and M. Lader*	
5. Pharmacological Concepts in Learning and Memory Dysfunction .... 105 *Walter B. Essman*	
6. Neuropharmacological Perspectives in the Amnestic and Dysmnestic Syndromes .... 163 *Walter B. Essman and Edward Sodaro*	
7. Localization of Substance P and Enkephalin in the Spinal Cord: Relationship to Pain Pathways............................. 187 *N. Eric Naftchi, Susan Abrahams, Henry St. Paul, and Linda Vacca*	
8. Gilles de la Tourette's Syndrome: An Overview .... 207 *Luigi Valzelli*	
9. Psychopharmacology of Clonidine .... 221 *Gary T. Shearman and Harbans Lal*	
10. The Clinical Profile of Psychotropic Drugs .... 257 *Frans de Jonghe, Jacob A.C. Bleeker, and Eliza D. J. Lindenberg*	
11. Clinical and Psyuchopharmacological Evaluation of L-5HTP in Depression... 279 *Motohisa Kaneko and Hisashi Kumashiro*	
12. Long-term Efficacy in the Treatment of Schizophrenia .... 309 *Sven J. Dencker*	
13. Central Cholinergic Mechanisms, Neuroleptic Action and Schizophrenia .... 337 *Man Mohan Singh and Harbans Lal*	

Preface

Research applications of neuropharmacology to clinical problems has, in recent years, enjoyed a growing interest and has, as a result, been increasingly explored. This tact has taken on a bidirectional effort through which neuropharmacological methodologies have been applied to investigate clinical problems in psychiatry and neurology, or basic mechanisms underlying such clinical problems have been investigated through more basic neuropharmacological models and methods. The results have served to increase our knowledge about clinical neuropharmacology.

The present volume was conceived as an overview of topics of clinical interest and concern that have been related to basic neuropharmacological concepts or techniques. These topics span a variety of areas of current interest including social deprivation, drug abuse, smoking behavior, memory dysfunction, the affective disorders, psychosis, and motor disturbances. In each instance the approach taken has been novel in that the directions through each subject have led to better understanding of the clinical entity through the neuropharmacological studies of the responses in question.

The present volume is not a textbook of clinical neuropharmacology. It is rather a source for the clinician to clarify areas of clinical interest through an understanding of the related neuropharmacodynamics. We, the editors hope that this volume will provide the reader with something new—clinically useful and conceptually clarified.

Walter B. Essman
Luigi Valzelli

Contributors

Susan Abrahams, Ph.D.
Laboratory of Biochemical
 Pharmacology
Institute of Rehabilitation
 Medicine
New York University Medical
 Center
New York, New York

Jacob A.C. Bleeker, M.D.
Psychiatric Department
Academic Hospital
University of Amsterdam
Amsterdam, Holland

Sven J. Dencker, M.D.
Department of Psychiatry
Lillhagen Hospital
Hisings Backa, Sweden

Walter B. Essman, M.D., Ph.D.
Departments of Psychology and
 Biochemistry
Queens College of the City
 University of New York
Flushing, New York

Frans de Jonghe, M.D.
Psychiatric Department
Academic Hospital
University of Amsterdam
Amsterdam, Holland

Motohisa Kaneko, M.D.
Department of Neuropsychiatry
Fukushima Medical College
Fukushima-ken, Japan

Athan Karras, Ph.D.
Division of Research
 and Evaluation
Queens Hospital Center
Long Island Jewish-Hillside
 Medical Center
Jamaica, New York

R. Kuman, M.D.
Departments of Psychiatry and
 Pharmacology
Institute of Psychiatry
London, England

Hisashi Kumashiro, M.D.
Department of Neuropsychiatry
Fukushima Medical College
Fukushima-ken, Japan

Harbans Lal, Ph.D.
Department of Pharmacology
Texas College of Osteopathic
 Medicine
Fort Worth, Texas

Eliza D.J. Lindenbergh, M.D.
Psychiatric Department
Academic Hospital
University of Amsterdam
Amsterdam, Holland

N. Eric Naftchi, Ph.D.
Laboratory of Biochemical
 Pharmacology
Institute of Rehabilitation
 Medicine
New York University Medical
 Center
New York, New York

Leonid Pevzner, M.D., Ph.D.
National Institute of Child Health
 and Human Development
Bethesda, Maryland

James W. Prescott, Ph.D.
Institute of Humanistic Science
West Bethesda, Maryland

Gary T. Shearman, Ph.D
Max Planck Institute for Psychiatry
Munich, Germany

*Man Mohan Singh, M.D., M.R.C.P.,
 M.R.C. Psych., D.P.M.*
Schizophrenia Program, V.A.
 Medical Center
Department of Psychiatry
University of Tennessee College
 of Medicine
Memphis, Tennessee

Edward Sodaro, M.A.
Department of Psychology
Queens College of the City
 University of New York
Flushing, New York

Henry St. Paul, Ph.D.
Laboratory of Biochemical
 Pharmacology
Institute of Rehabilitation
 Medicine
New York University Medical
 Center
New York, New York

Linda Vacca, M.D.
Department of Pathology
Medical College of Georgia
Augusta, Georgia

Luigi Valzelli, M.D.
Sections of Psychopharmacology
 and Biological Psychiatry
Mario Negri Institute for
 Pharmacological Research
Milan, Italy

NEUROPHARMACOLOGY
Clinical Applications

1

Neuronal-Glial Metabolic Interactions In Stress

Leonid Pevzner

INTRODUCTION

Classically Hans Selye's concept of stress (Selye, 1952, 1957) has emphasized, first of all, nonspecific reactions common to all stress factors, or kinds of stress. This idea has turned out to be quite promising, and it was subsequently confirmed under many different stress conditions. As will be demonstrated below, metabolic responses of neurons and glia in some cases are rather similar notwithstanding differences in the stress conditions used.

At the same time, however, in *in vivo* experiments, nervous and hormonal influences, both direct and indirect, upon various structures of nerve tissue form a too complicated pattern to result in identical metabolic changes in all these structures. Therefore the nonspecific components of stress can be added by individual specificity not only of particular kinds of stress under various experimental conditions but also of particular types of cells within the nervous system.

It should be mentioned that there hardly is a method of separate analysis of neurons and glial cells which can at present be claimed free from sufficient pitfalls (*vide infra*). All these considerations should be kept in mind when comparing the data of different authors which in some cases are rather contradictory.

Nevertheless, neuron-glia metabolic interactions are worth considering even at the present-day, perhaps somewhat unconvincing, state of this essential neurobiological problem. Historically, it was the neuron which initially became an object of functional biochemical studies of the nervous system at the cellular level (Hydén, 1943, 1947, 1955). Later on, however, evidence has been obtained by various authors which has indicated that the whole biochemical basis for nervous activity cannot be accounted for only by the metabolic properties of the neuron alone (for literature, see monographs by Hydén, 1972; Jakoubek, 1974; Pevzner, 1979a; Varon and Somjen, 1979).

A fruitful idea of the neuron-neuroglia metabolic unit put forward by Holger Hydén (1959, 1960, 1964) has stimulated a number of authors to deal with several aspects of neuronal-glial interactions including their interactions in stress.

MORPHOLOGICAL AND METHODOLOGICAL OUTLINES

In terms of histogenesis, both neurons and neuroglial cells originate from the same matrix cell, the medulloblast. Its initial differentiation leads to the formation of a neuroblast and a glioblast (as well as an ependymoblast). Final differentiation results in all types of neurons and glial cells, the latter consisting of two main classes, astrocytes and oligodendrogliocytes (Wechsler and Kleihues, 1968; Kuhlenbeck, 1970; Roots, 1978). It is worth indicating that evolutionarily the higher is the complexity of the whole organization of the animal, the greater is the number of glial cells relative to neurons, this ratio in mammalian brain becoming more than 10:1 (Hydén, 1972, Roots, 1978).

Whereas neurons are concentrated in some loci of the brain (cerebral and cerebellar cortex, basal ganglia, other nuclei of the brain or cerebellum), but absent in white matter or peripheral nerves, there are no loci in the central and peripheral nervous system free of glial cells. Their concentration may fluctuate there markedly depending upon localization but the total volume in the human cerebral cortex, for instance, which is occupied by astroglial and oligodendroglial cells may be roughly evaluated as about one third of the cortex tissue volume (Pope, 1978).

Both astrocytes and particularly oligodendrogliocytes have smaller sizes than neuronal bodies. The bodies and processes of glia form a network which surrounds every neuron and separates its body from brain capillaries (Peters et al., 1976). Such morphological interrelations make it extremely difficult for biochemists to separately analyze neuronal bodies and neuroglial cells.

At present, three chief approaches have been used for this purpose. The most recent and, perhaps, the most promising approach consists in obtaining large bulk of fractions enriched in neurons or, correspondingly, in glial cells. After initial disruption of brain tissue mechanically and/or enzymatically, a gradient ultracentrifugation is used which is based on different specific densities of neuronal bodies and glial cell bodies. There are many rather different schemes of this technique which result in enriched fractions with quite dissimilar degrees of purity, yield, morphological preservation of the cells, ratio of neurons and particular classes of glial cells as well as their viability and metabolic properties. Detailed description and critical evaluation of this approach can be found in reviews by Rose (1969), Johnston and Roots (1972), Sellinger and Azcurra (1975), Poduslo and Norton (1975), and Varon and Somjen (1979). Along with a number of advantages, this approach possesses some shortcomings, among which two are the most important: contamination of each kind of cells and lack of regional, topochemical analysis of individual types of neurons. To the same approach, although with some reservations, a method of *in vitro* culture of individual cell lines may be added, comprehensive analysis of this method recently being done by Fedoroff and Hertz (1977).

The second approach consists in microdissection of individual, as a rule sufficiently large neuronal bodies and surrounding clumps of glial cells. The samples obtained are so minute that their biochemical analysis requires application of microchemical or even ultramicrochemical methods. This requirement itself can be considered as a disadvantage of the approach which requires unique equipment and poses a number of methodical difficulties. Besides, the sample of perineuronal neuroglia contains all non-neuronal elements of the nerve tissue such as axons, dendrites, microglial cells, brain capillaries, etc. Due to necessity of microsurgical manipulations, only the largest neurons are most often studied: spinal ganglia neurons, spinal cord motoneurons, Deiters' neurons of medulla vestibular nuclei, etc. At the same time, the possibility of comparing several classes of individual neurons as well as their perineuronal glia represents an undoubted advantage of this approach. Its principles, description of procedure and criticism are exposed in papers by Lowry (1955, 1962), Hydén (1955, 1960, 1964), Giacobini (1956, 1964), Rose (1968, 1969).

The third approach is quantitative cytochemistry, *i.e.*, analysis of individual neurons and glial cells, under visual control, within histological sections of the nerve tissue. Combination of microscopy with spectroscopy (Caspersson, 1950, 1955, 1979) or interferometry (Barer, 1956; Davies, 1958; Wied, 1966) as well as some other procedures (autoradiography, fluorescence, immune and enzymatic reactions, etc.) allows determinations of chemical composition and metabolic responses of various kinds of neurons and neuroglia. This approach is particularly suitable to deal with a unique heterogeneity of the nerve tissue. Besides, it preserves morphological interrelations among individual cell structures of the nervous system, without any mechanical disruption of the tissue. This advantage of the cytochemical approach is counterbalanced by a comparatively low specificity of cytochemical procedures for individual chemical substances as well as by possible error sources which may decrease markedly the preciseness of cytochemical analysis (Wied, 1966). Critical comparison of all three approaches, their principles and literature can be found in monograph by Pevzner (1979a).

Whereas the majority of data concerning chemical composition of neurons and glia have been obtained by means of the first approach (enriched fractions), metabolic changes in neurons and glial cells at various kinds of stress have been revealed as a rule with the aid of microchemical or cytochemical methods.

EFFECTS OF HYPOXIA

When animals are subjected to *in vivo* hypoxia, its effect by no means can be restricted by merely an oxygen deficiency. The stress-like nature of general hypoxia results in participation of a number of adaptational mechanisms such as blood circulation, lung ventilation, tissue metabolism, etc. Among these mechanisms a hypothermic mechanism is worth mentioning. Data obtained by Chetverikov's group not too well known to western neurochemists have shown that the hypobaric hypoxia in rats (as a result of exposition of the animals in a low pressure chamber) induces rather rapidly a sufficiently pronounced hypothermia. It is this hypothermia rather than the hypoxia alone which evokes a decrease in brain phospholipid turnover. The same hypoxia but with an artificial warming of the rats which prevents the hypothermia gives rise, on the one hand, to quite normal phospholipid turnover but, on the other hand, to a marked mortality of these animals (Gasteva et al., 1966).

The most systematic studies on effects of *in vitro* hypoxia upon neuronal and glial metabolism have been carried out by Yanagihara (1973, 1974, 1976, 1979). He has provided for careful analysis of rates of RNA and protein synthesis taking into account essential methodical factors such as disruption of cells in the course of enriched fraction preparation, uptake of precursors of macromolecular syntheses, activity of corresponding enzymes, effects of ions and specific inhibitors. Basing on these data Yanagihara demonstrated that *in vitro* hypoxia produced similar effects on neuronal and glial macromolecular synthesis. In other words, sensitivity to hypoxia did not differ markedly between the two cellular elements of the nervous system.

As expected from all the considerations discussed above, an *in vivo* hypoxia evoked metabolic responses rather different in neurons and in glial cells. Hydén's group compared cytochrome oxidase activity in the bodies of Deiters' neurons and in perineuronal tissue containing glial cells after their microdissection. Micromanometric determinations have shown that if the animals had been exposed 12 h in an atmosphere containing as little as 8 percent oxygen, the cytochrome oxidase activity increased in the neurons but did not change in the glial cells (Hydén and Lange, 1961; Hamberger and Hydén, 1963; Hydén, 1964). Thus, microdissectional approach has provided for evidence in favor of a higher resistance of glial metabolism to *in vivo* hypoxia than of neuronal one.

Similar conclusion has been made with the aid of enriched fraction approach. According to Albrecht and Smialek (1975), 30-minute exposition of rats to an atmosphere of 4 percent O_2 or 1.5-h exposition in a hypercapnic atmosphere inhibited *in vivo* incorporation of ^{75}Se-methionine into proteins both of neuronal and of glial enriched fractions of the brain hemispheres. This inhibition was much more persistent in neurons than in glia.

More complicated pattern of changes in precursor incorporation into neuronal and glial proteins has been revealed at *in vivo* hypoxia by Blomstrand

(1970). In his experiments rabbits were kept in an atmosphere of 8 percent O_2 for 3 or 12 h, then their cerebral cortex slides were incubated with ^{3}H-leucine. Its incorporation into protein of the slides was decreased after 3 but increased after 12 h of hypoxia. If from the slides enriched fractions were isolated, the effect of 3-h hypoxia turned out to be localized in glial fraction only, while that of 12-h was much more pronounced in neuronal bodies. If the same precursor was administered to the animals intravenously, its incorporation into neuronal and glial proteins was changed after 12-h hypoxia in the same way as after the incubation of slides with ^{3}H-leucine. In this case, after 3-h hypoxia, incorporation of the precursor in glial enriched fraction was also decreased but in the neurons was somewhat augmented (Blomstrand, 1970).

Several contradictions of the data mentioned above are perhaps due to the fact that the authors studied either a single kind of neuron (Deiters' neurons) or all the cells of the whole brain (enriched fractions of cerebral hemispheres). Meanwhile similar conditions of hypoxia can evoke different effects in various kinds of neurons whose sensitivity to the cessation of oxygen and glucose supply has been shown to markedly differ (Van Liere and Stickney, 1963).

Indeed, cytospectrophotometric determinations have revealed individual differences in RNA changes in various central neurons and their perineuronal glia under several conditions of *in vivo* hypoxia (Pevzner, 1971, 1972, 1979b; Brumberg and Pevzner, 1976). In sodium barbital-anaesthetized cats, hypoxic hypercapnic hypoxia was induced by means of connection of an exposed tracheal cannula with a closed 3.5-*l* air jar. Duration of such hypoxia was 1 h. It resulted in a marked decrease in RNA content in the cytoplasm of visual and motor cortex neurons as well as in their glial satellite cells. In auditory cortex, such RNA decrease was observed only in the perineuronal neuroglia while in cerebellum neither in Purkinje cells nor in the surrounding glia. Rather similar pattern of RNA changes, with the only difference of glial RNA decrease being absent in visual cortex but present in cerebellum, was evoked by ischemic hypoxia due to bilateral ligation of vertebrae arteries in anaesthetized cats for 1 h together with an interrupted occlusion of both common carotid arteries every 5 min with 5-min pauses. In rats, acute or long-term hypoxia in a low pressure chamber (240 mm Hg, simulated altitude 8700 m, for the acute experiments while 290 mm Hg, simulated altitude 7000 m, for chronic experiments) gave rise in cerebellum to RNA accumulation both in Purkinje cells and in their perineuronal glia while in spinal cord ventral horns, only in neurons. In mice, acute histotoxic hypoxia due to intraperitoneal KCN injection (10 mg/kg) brought about in 15 min an activation of M-form of lactate dehydrogenase in spinal cord motor neurons and spinal ganglia neurons without statistically significant changes in their perineuronal glia. In cerebellar and cerebral cortex neurons, there was an augmentation of H-form activity whereas in the glial cells adjacent to cerebellum Purkinje cells both H-form and M-form of lactate dehydrogenase were activated (Brumberg and Pevzner, 1976).

EFFECTS OF COOLING

Cooling is one of the most often used forms of stress. A great number of physiological data summarized by Mrosovsky (1971) and Hensel (1973) have presented an evidence in favor of direct involvement of various hypothalamus nuclei in an adaptation reaction to this kind of stress.

If laboratory albino rats raised in thermostatically controlled animal house were placed in a cold room at 2-4° C, the nuclear histone content per cell was increased in 24 h both in medial preoptic area and in supraoptic nucleus neurons (Krichevskaya et al., 1976). In glial cells there was a simultaneous decrease in the histone content in supraoptic nucleus while no changes in medial preoptic area. In the latter, a decrease in the histone content was observed in the whole neuron-neuroglia unit after 3-day exposure of the animals to the cold whereas in supraoptic nucleus the initial reciprocal changes were replaced by the inverse ones: a decrease of the neuronal and accumulation of the glial histones. After 15-day constant cooling, the content of neuronal and glial histones returned completely to the norm in the hypothalamus area studied (Krichevskaya et. al., 1976).

In the experiments described above, the stress seemed to be rather mild. Although laboratory rats are accustomed to live at a room temperature, living under conditions of as moderate cooling as 2-4° C hardly represents too severe stress for the given species. Therefore the metabolic response in hypothalamic structures was not too pronounced and disappeared as result of cold adaptation by a fortnight. Another pattern of metabolic response to a cooling was revealed in the case of much more severe cooling suggested by LeBlanc (1967). A modification of LeBlanc's scheme of cold adaptation consisted in that rats in individual cages were placed for 2 min in a cold room a -20° C, then kept for 5 min at 25° C, and then again cooled at -20° C for 2 min, this cycle being repeated 15 times (Filipchenko et al., 1978). As a result, the whole experiment lasted about 1.5 h, *i.e.*, twice as short as that in LeBlanc's work, and included a total of 30 min cooling. On the end of the cooling, the animals were returned to standard vivarium where they were kept up to 30 days. One hour on the cessation of the cooling, the RNA content per cell was shown cytospectrophotometrically to increase both in neurons and in perineuronal glia of medial preoptic area. This increase was observed also 2 days after the end of the cooling, with a return to the control value in another 3 days. More persistent increase in the RNA content was revealed in the neurons and perineuronal glia of mamillary bodies: it was found out as late as 5 and 15 days after the rats were returned to the animal house. It was only 30 days after the cessation of the cooling that the RNA content returned to the norm in the neurons and decreased somewhat lower than the norm in their glial satellite cells (Filipchenko et al., 1978).

EFFECT OF CONVULSIONS

Convulsions due to administration of various analeptics represent rather a convenient model of stress. Biochemical studies on this point at cellular level have dealt as a rule with neurons only. Parallel analysis of neurons and glial cells carried out by a few authors has shown a marked decrease in RNA and protein content both in motor neurons and perineuronal glial cells at the acute convulsions evoked by injections of picrotoxin (Rubinskaya, 1971) or Metrazol (pentamethylenetetrazol) (Pevzner, 1971; Pevzner and Saudargene, 1971). The degree of these changes and their stability depended much on whether the neurons investigated had been motor or sensory (Pevzner and Saudargene, 1971), secretory or nonsecretory (Schmidt and Zimmermann, 1978), cortical or spinal ones (Rubinskaya, 1971). But the whole pattern of RNA and protein reduction was rather similar in all cases. The same decrease in RNA content in neurons and perineuronal glia as result of a convulsive state was observed by Pevzner (1979c) even when the seizures were induced by hyperbaric hyperoxy rather than by any analeptics. Perhaps this similarity is a consequence of general changes in blood circulation, carbohydrate and energy metabolism shown during experimental status epilepticus by Plum's group (Plum et al., 1968; Duffy et al., 1975).

Much more individual was a dynamics of postconvulsive reparation. Thus, after cessation of Metrazol convulsions, the restoration of initial content of RNA and proteins occurred much quicker in perineuronal glial cells than in spinal motor neurons (Pevzner and Saudargene, 1971). In hyperoxia-induced convulsions which were more severe than Metrazol convulsions, the postconvulsive reparation was characterized by more pronounced and stable changes which in many cases proceeded parallely in neurons and in neuroglia (Pevzner, 1979c).

Metrazol-evoked convulsions resulted in quantitative changes in protein content only, as far as cytospectrophotometric evaluation can be relied on. In the course of postconvulsive restoration, however, there were also some qualitative changes in protein molecules. They were found out by parallel determinations of the total protein content and of the protein SH-group content (Pevzner and Saudargene, 1971). On cessation of convulsions, the relative SH-group content (per mass unit of total protein) increased, this augmentation being absent in spinal motor neurons and their glia but present in spinal ganglia neurons and to a greater degree in their glial satellite cells.

EFFECT OF FOOT-SHOCK

This stress factor is also used quite often in studies on changes of metabolism in the nervous system under effects of stress. These changes at the level of the whole brain are exposed and critically discussed in a comprehensive monograph by Jakoubek (1974). As to comparison of stress-induced metabolic responses in neurons and in neuroglia, the foot-shock has been applied only in single works.

Short-term foot-shock in rats has been shown to bring about reciprocal changes in RNA content: increase in spinal cord motor neurons but decrease in their perineuronal neuroglia, these changes being detected as soon as 5 min after beginning of the foot-shock (Pevzner, 1971). More prolonged foot-shock (20 min) resulted in a return of the neuronal and glial RNA content to the control level. At last, 60-min foot-shock gave rise to a pronounced reduction of RNA content both in the motor neurons and in adjacent glial cells. On cessation of the foot-shock, restoration of the control value of RNA content, like in the case of postconvulsive reparation (see above), was completed considerably sooner in the glial cells than in the motor neurons.

Since the foot-shock represents a kind of a most intensive sensory stimulation, it seemed that the most pronounced metabolic response should be revealed in sensory neurons. Meanwhile, in the whole course of 60-min foot-shock in rats there were no changes in the cytoplasmic RNA content in the spinal ganglia neurons (Pevzner, 1979a). In the period of a rest after the end of the foot-shock, the RNA content increased 4 h on cessation of the stress but completely returned to norm afterwards. It is not unreasonable to suggest that the macromolecular changes in the neuronal body take place mainly as a metabolic response to a synaptic multi-step stimulation rather than to a direct excitation of a sensory neuron through its peripheral receptors (Pevzner, 1979a).

An interesting kind of the foot-shock stress, anticipation stress, has been analyzed by Jakoubek (1974). Rats were placed in a cage with an electrical grid floor and a foot-shock was given to the animals after a waiting period of 45 min. This trial was repeated daily for 7 days, the animals were killed after 7 trials.

Biochemical analysis of the rats after 7 daily anticipation stress trials has shown that such an anticipation of a painful stimulation can alter essentially active transport of precursors into the brain tissue and biosynthesis of macromolecules from these precursors (Jakoubek, 1974).

Comparison of a metabolic response of neurons and of glial cells to the anticipation stress has revealed a number of intercellular differences (Jakoubek et al., 1979). At once after the 7th trial of the anticipation stress there was an augmentation of the cytoplasmic RNA content in spinal cord motor neurons while no changes were found out in the adjacent glial cells. A part of the animals were administered with a tranquilizer diazepam (10 mg/kg), on the 8th day of the experiment. Forty minutes later, the rats were placed into the same grid floor cage and killed after the 45-min waiting. Diazepam turned out to prevent any change in the neuronal RNA content. At the same time, an increase in glial RNA content was observed in the animals injected with diazepam (Jakoubek et al., 1979).

EFFECT OF RESTRAINT

Restraint, fixation of the animal to prevent any free movement is rather severe form of stress, so-called immobilization stress. However, neuron-glia interrelations have been studied only in experiments by Brumberg and her co-authors who applied a milder condition of restraint. Experimental animals, mice (Brumberg, 1969; Brumberg and Pevzner, 1972) and rats (Brumberg et al., 1972) were placed in individual cages which restrained movements of the animals but did not produce actual immobilization. As a result, such experiment could last two and even three weeks; it is only in the latter case that a discoordination, light paresis of hind legs and a loss of body weight were revealed. Cytospectrophotometric determinations have demonstrated no changes in the cytoplasmic RNA content in spinal cord motor neurons and spinal ganglia neurons as well as in the bodies of perineuronal glial cells of spinal cord ventral horns by the end of 3-week restraint. In neuroglia of spinal ganglia there was a marked reduction of the RNA content. After such prolonged hypokinesia, free motor activity of these mice outside the cages gave rise rapidly to a total decrease in RNA content both in the neurons and in the adjacent glial cells of the spinal cord and spinal ganglia (Brumberg and Pevzner, 1972). Subsequent return of the glial RNA to the control level, like in the cases of foot-shock or several kinds of convulsions (*vide supra*), was achieved more rapidly than that of the neuronal RNA. At the same time, as late as 3 days after the end of the hypokinesia, when all the symptoms of it completely disappeared, a normalization of the neuronal RNA content was accompanied by a secondary, delayed decrease in the content of glial RNA.

Still milder and shorter (for 2 weeks) hypokinesia in rats which had not resulted in any visible motor disturbances brought about different metabolic responses in spinal cord cells depending on their localization. In the lumbar enlargement of which motor neurons are responsible for hind leg muscular activity a marked increase was observed in the RNA content of the motor neurons while a decrease in that of perineuronal glia. In the cervical enlargement of the spinal cord no statistically significant changes were detected in the same animals. It is interesting that if this hypokinesia was combined with a moderate hypoxic hypoxia (the individual cages with animals were kept for two weeks in a low pressure chamber), the content of neuronal RNA remained normal or augmented in the cervical or lumbar intumescence resp. while the content of glial RNA markedly increased in both intumescences (Brumberg et al., 1972).

EFFECT OF A FORCED MUSCULAR ACTIVITY

In a series of works by Brumberg, adult male mice were put into a swimming pool for 3-4 h (Brumberg, 1968, 1969; Brumberg and Pevzner, 1972). According to her cytospectrophotometric data, such a forced muscular activity induced an accumulation of cytoplasmic RNA in spinal cord motor neurons and a temporary decrease of cytoplasmic RNA in spinal ganglia. These changes in neurons were accompanied by no statistically significant alterations in glial RNA content. Subsequent rest of the animals after the cessation of the swimming was characterized by a return of the augmented RNA content in motor neurons to the norm while by a parallel decrease in the glial RNA.

Much more severe stress was achieved through swimming in experiments by Geinisman (1971, 1972). He was dealing with rats made to swim with an attached load which amounted to 1/11 of their body weight. This resulted in the animals beginning usually to submerge as soon as after 50 min of the swimming. Therefore the whole experiment lasted only 40 min. In the large motor neurons of the lumbal spinal cord intumescence, the content of cytoplasmic RNA somewhat increased while in the small motor neurons decreased by the end of the 40-min swimming. The content of glial RNA decreased, the change being localized only in perineuronal neuroglia rather than in the glial cells characterized by no visible contact with spinal motor neurons (Geinisman, 1971, 1972).

Another kind of a forced muscular activity was chosen by Tiplady et al. (1974): rats were running for one hour in the wheel. This gave rise to an accumulation of RNA both in nuclei and in the cytoplasm of pyramidal neurons of the motor area of cerebral cortex while no statistically significant changes in the RNA content were detected in perineuronal glial cells. It is interesting that the content of nuclear or cytoplasmic RNA in the motor neurons of the lumbar intumescence of the spinal cord, as well as in their glial satellite cells, remained unchanged in the same animals (Tiplady et al., 1974).

EFFECT OF ADRENALECTOMY

In the course of analysis of stress mechanisms, adrenalectomy is often used as one of the most efficient experimental approaches. Strangely enough, this approach was applied for studies on neuron-neuroglia metabolic interrelations only in a single paper.

Male rats were adrenalectomized under ether anaesthesia. They subsequently received normal food *ad libitum* while drinking water contained 1 percent NaCl. In cerebellum Purkinje cells as well as in spinal cord motor neurons, at the fourth day after the operation, the cytoplasmic RNA content was decreased. This decrease hardly could be considered specific because it persisted in a group of adrenalectomized rats administered daily with hydrocortisone. In perineuronal neuroglial cells the content of RNA remained constant in all cases. Quite opposite pattern appeared in hypothalamus, a brain area more specifically involved in a whole response to stress (hypothalamo-pituitary-adrenal system). Whereas no RNA alterations were revealed in hypothalamus supraoptic neurons in all groups of animals, a marked RNA reduction occurred in perineuronal glia of the supraoptic nucleus. This metabolic glial response, unlike the neuronal one mentioned above, was, in all probability, rather specific because it disappeared completely under effect of the injections of hydrocortisone to adrenalectomized rats (Pevzner, 1979a).

These data are interesting to compare with earlier results which have demonstrated an accumulation of RNA and protein in perineuronal glial cells after injections of adrenaline to rats and cats (Pevzner, 1965, 1968). Daily administration of 30 μg to rats and of 60 μg to cats for 2 weeks gave rise to a pronounced augmentation of RNA and protein content in neuroglial cells adjacent to neurons of cervical sympathetic ganglion, of spinal cord lateral horns and of spinal cord ventral horns. Such augmentation was not found out in the corresponding neurons; on the contrary, in some cases (particularly in spinal motor neurons) there was a decrease in the RNA and protein content.

It is reasonable to suggest that neuroglial cells are more sensitive to hormonal, or more broadly, to any trophic influences upon the whole nervous system (Pevzner, 1968). This suggestion seems to have found a support in studies on glial cell cultures: metabolism of cultivated cells of glial types was substantially altered due to alimentary deficiency (Clos, 1978) and effects of corticosteroids (de Vellis and Kukes, 1973; de Vellis et al., 1977; Vernadakis et al., 1979), thyroid hormones (Clos, 1978), estradiol and progesterone (Vernadakis et al., 1979). Even pharmacological drugs such as neuroleptics (Henn et al., 1978) or morphine (Oguri et al., 1976) of which primary targets should have been neuronal receptors actually affected phosphorylation in isolated glial enriched fractions.

CONCLUSION. "DIVISION OF LABOR" WITHIN THE NEURON-NEUROGLIA UNIT

Data reviewed above demonstrate that stress evokes a number of metabolic changes in neurons and glial cells, these changes being rather universal in various kinds of the stress. When the stress effect upon the nervous system is sufficiently pronounced the content of macromolecules in neurons and glia is reduced. Thereby an initial, control equilibrium between anabolic and catabolic processes is shifted to the latter. This metabolic response involves both chief classes of the nerve tissue cells.

On cessation of stress, a restoration of cell metabolism occurs in the nervous system. In spite of individual character of various types of the stress, there is a common feature of that post-stress restoration: it proceeds as a rule more rapidly in perineuronal glial cells than in corresponding neurons. This seems to contradict to numerous data about a more intensive macromolecular biosynthesis in neurons than in glia (for literature, see reviews by Jakoubek, 1974;

Hertz, 1977; Lange, 1978; Varon, 1978; Varon and Somjen, 1979; Pevzner, 1979a). However, this higher intensity (which was demonstrated only in rest conditions by the enriched fraction method) does not necessarily indicate actual effectiveness of the reparation process. The latter could have been not less, or even greater, in glial cells as compared with neurons. Indeed, when the content of macromolecules in the neurons is markedly reduced, its increase up to the normal level is hindered by several factors. One of them is axonal flow, it is a powerful source of constant macromolecular losses from the neuronal body which trigger an intensive work of neuronal biosynthetic machinery (see, for instance, Droz, 1973; Kerkut, 1975; Heslop, 1975). Another factor is a topographical relationship between neurons and glia, the latter being located in direct contacts with brain capillary network. Therefore all precursors for macromolecular synthesis from blood circulation reach initially glia and only subsequently neurons. Besides, glial cells have been shown to possess much more intensive than neurons uptake of amino acids from the surrounding medium (Rose, 1973; Hamberger et al., 1975; Minchin and Beart, 1975; Schon and Kelly, 1975). This active amino acid transport seems to be provided for by Na^+, K^+-activated ATPase of which the activity is markedly higher in glial cells than in neurons, although the content of APT is much lower in glia as compared with neurons (for literature, see review by Hertz, 1978).

At the same time, several individual kinds of stress can induce some changes peculiar to a particular stress. Thus, rather mild, not too severe stress conditions can give rise only to intraneuronal metabolic response. Perhaps, this failure to involve neuroglial metabolism depends on a degree of hormonal disbalance in the whole pattern of a given stress. The more pronounced is participation of adrenal cortex in the total adaptation syndrome, the more evident seems to be metabolic response in glial cells, too. It can, therefore, be suggested that the neuronal metabolism is controlled to a greater degree by synaptic events, by effects of transmitters and/or ions, whereas glial metabolism is preferably regulated by hormones or other physiologically active substances entering glial cell body from blood circulation or extracellular space.

This "division of labor," on the one hand, unites neuron and neuroglia into a single functional-metabolic unit. In spite of an autonomy, metabolic and functional independence which both neurons and glial cells manifest, for instance, *in vitro* when cultivated in nutritionally enriched media, neither neuron nor glia can be considered, under actual *in vivo* conditions, an independent morphological, functional or biochemical elementary unit of the nervous system. It is only the whole neuron-neuroglia unit which possess a maximally effective set of properties peculiar to the highly specific tissue such as the nerve tissue.

On the other hand, within the single neuron-neuroglia unit, the metabolic "division of labor" between two main cellular compartments provides for a greater effectiveness of functioning of the whole unit. The latter operates, in fact, as a self-controlling system with a stable self-regulation through intercellular negative feed-back. Biochemical indicators of this feed-back in the neuron-neuroglia activity and metabolism are exposed and discussed in a monograph by Pevzner (1979a). The most important signals which code information about intracellular metabolism of each partner of the unit and transfer this information to the other party are, beyond any doubts, ions, neurotransmitters, physiologically active amino acids and in some cases, perhaps, even some macromolecules (Herz, 1977; Schoffeniels et al., 1978; Pevzner, 1978, 1979a; Varon and Somjen, 1979).

Both initial stages of the stress and the subsequent multi-step time course of adaptation syndrome involve, to a various degree, metabolic response of the single functional neuron-neuroglia unit.

REFERENCES

Albrecht, J. and Smialek, M. (1975): Effect of hypoxia, ischemia and carbon monoxide intoxication on in vivo protein synthesis in neuron and glia cell enriched fractions from rat brain. *Acta Neuropathol. 31:* 257-262.
Barer, R. (1956): Phase-contrast and interference microscopy in cytology. *Physical Techniques in Biol. Res. 3:* 29-90.
Blomstrand, C. (1970): Effects of hypoxia on protein metabolism in neuron and neuroglia enriched fractions from rabbit brain. *Exp. Neurol. 29:* 175-188.
Brumberg, V.A. (1968): The influence of different lengths of time of swimming on the RNA content in the neurons and neuroglia of the motor and sensory parts of the spinal cord. *Doklady Akad. Nauk SSSR, Biol. Sci. Section* (Engl. Transl.) *184:* 158-160.
Brumberg, V.A. (1969): Changes in the volumes of the cell bodies of motor and sensory spinal-cord neurons and surrounding glial cells at different motor-activity levels. *Doklady Akad. Nauk SSSR, Biol. Sci. Section* (Engl. Transl.) *184:* 158-160.
Brumberg, V.A., Gazenko, O.G., Demin, N.N., Malkin, V.B., and Pevzner, L.Z. (1972): Topochemical differences in the content of RNA in the motor neurons of the spinal cord during hypoxia and hypokinesia. *Doklady Akad. Nauk SSSR, Biol. Sci. Section* (Engl. Transl.) *205:* 500-503.
Brumberg, V.A. and Pevzner, L.Z. (1972): Ribonucleic acid content in neuron-neuroglia unit of the spinal cord. *Neuropathol. Polska 10:* 343-357.
Brumberg, V.A. and Pevzner, L.Z. (1976): Cytospectrometric studies on the lactate dehydrogenase isoenzymes in functionally different neuron-neuroglia units. II. Species and strain differences and effects of histotoxic hypoxia and audiogenic convulsions. *Acta Histochem. 55:* 1-7.
Caspersson, T. (1950): *Cell Growth and Cell Function.* Norton, New York.
Caspersson, T. (1955): Quantitative cytochemical methods for the study of cell metabolism. *Experientia 11:* 45-60.
Caspersson, T. (1979): On the development of quantitative cytochemical techniques for studies of cell nuclei. *Acta Histochem Suppl. XX:* 15-28.
Cos, J. (1978): Hormonal and nutritional effects on the development of glia. In: E. Schoffeniels et al., (Eds.) *Dynamic Properties of Glia Cells.* Pergamon Press, Oxford et al., 247-256.
Davies, H.G. (1958): The determination of mass and concentration by microscope interferometry. *Gen. Cytochem. Methods 1:* 55-161.

de Vellis, J. and Kukes, G. (1973): Regulation of glial cell functions by hormones and ions. *Tex. Repts. Biol. Med. 31:* 271-293.
de Vellis, J., McGinnis, J.F., Breen, G.A.M., Leveille, P., Bennett, K., and McCarthy, K. (1977): Hormonal effects on differentiation in neural culture. In: S. Fedoroff and L. Hertz (Eds.) *Cell, Tissue and Organ Cultures in Neurobiology* Academic Press, New York et al., 485-511.
Droz, B. (1973): Renewal of synaptic proteins. *Brain Res. 62:* 383-394.
Duffy, T.E., Howse, D.C., and Plum, F. (1975): Cerebral energy metabolism during experimental status epilepticus. *J. Neurochem. 24:* 925-934.
Federoff, S. and Hertz, L. (Eds.). (1977): *Cell, Tissue, and Organ Cultures in Neurobiology.* Academic Press, New York et al.
Filipchenko, R.E., Pevzner, L.Z., and Slonim, A.D. (1978): Delayed RNA changes in various neuron-neuroglia units of rat hypothalamus after short-term intermittent deep cooling, with special reference to a concept of vegetative memory. *Acta Histochem. 61:* 23-39.
Gasteva, S.V., Dvorkin, V. Ya., and Chetverikov, D.A. (1966): On the cause of the decrease in metabolic rate of individual fractions of the rat brain phospholipids during oxygen starvation of the organism. *Doklady Akad. Nauk SSSR, Biol. Sci. Section* (Engl. Transl.) *169:* 570-572.
Geinisman, Yu. Ya. (1971): Nucleic acid content of spinal motoneurons and their satellites under orthodromic and antidromic stimulation. A cytospectrophotometric study. *Brain Res. 28:* 251-262.
Geinisman, Yu. Ya. (1972): Effects of excitatory and inhibitory synaptic actions on RNA content of spinal motoneurones. *Brain Res. 44:* 221-229.
Giacobini, E. (1962): A cytochemical study of the localization of carbonic anhydrase in the nervous system. *J. Neurochem 9:* 169-177.
Giacobini, E. (1964): Metabolic relations between glia and neurons studied in single cells. In: M.M. Cohen and R.S. Snider (Eds.) *Morphological and Biochemical Correlates of Neural Activity.* Harper & Row, New York, 15-38.
Hamberger, A., Babich, J.A., Blomstrand, C., Hansson, H.-A., and Sellström, Å. (1975): Evidence for differential function of neuronal and glial cells in protein metabolism and amino acid transport. *J. Neurosci. Res. 1:* 37-56.
Hamberger, A. and Hydén, H. (1963): Inverse enzymatic changes in neurons and glia during increased function and hypoxia. *J. Cell Biol. 16:* 521-525.
Henn, F.A., Anderson, D.J., and Sellström, Å. (1978): The role of neuroleptic drug receptors on astroglial cells. In: E. Schoffeniels et al. (Eds.) *Dynamic Properties of Glia Cells.* Pergamon Press, Oxford et al., 435-441.
Hensel, H. (1973): Neural processes in thermoregulation. *Physiol. Rev. 53:* 948-1017.
Hertz, L. (1977): Biochemistry of glial cells. In: S. Fedoroff and L. Hertz (Eds.) *Cell, Tissue, and Organ Cultures in Neurobiology.* Academic Press, New York et al., 39-71.
Hertz, L. (1978): Energy metabolism of glial cells. In: E. Schoffeniels et al. (Eds.) *Dynamic Properties of Glia Cells.* Pergamon Press, Oxford et al., 121-132.
Heslop, J.P. (1975): Axonal flow and fast transport in nerves. *Adv. Comp. Physiol. Biochem. 6:* 75-163.
Hydén, H. (1943): Protein metabolism in the nerve cell during growth and function. *Acta Physiol. Scand. 6:* Suppl. 17.
Hydén, H. (1947): Protein and nucleotide metabolism in the nerve cell under different functional conditions. *Symp. Soc. Exp. Biol. 1:* 152-162.
Hydén, H. (1955): The chemistry of single neurons: a study with new methods. In: H. Waelsch et al., (Eds.) *Biochemistry of Developing Nervous System.* Academic Press, New York et al., 358-370.

Hydén, H. (1959): Quantatitive assay of compounds in isolated, fresh nerve cells and glial cells from control and stimulated animals. *Nature 184:* 433-435.
Hydén, H. (1960): The neuron. In: J. Brachet and A.E. Mirsky (Eds.) *The Cell,* vol. 4. Academic Press, New York et al., 215-323.
Hydén, H. (1964): Biochemical and functional interplay between neurons and glia. In: J. Wortis (Ed.) *Recent Advances in Biological Psychiatry,* vol. 6. Plenum Press, New York, 31-54.
Hydén, H. (1972): *Macromolecules and Behaviour. Arthur Thomson Lectures,* G.B. Ansell and P.B. Bradley (Eds.). MacMillan Press, Birmingham.
Hydén, H. and Lange, P. (1961): Differences in the metabolism of oligodendroglia and nerve cells in the vestibular area. In: S.S. Kety and J. Elkes (Eds.) *Regional Neurochemistry.* Pergamon Press, Oxford et al., 190-199.
Jakoubek, B. (1974): *Brain Function and Macromolecular Synthesis.* Pion Ltd., London.
Jakoubek, B., Pevzner, L.Z., and Pavlik, A. (1979): Changes of the protein metabolism in rat spinal motoneurons and perineuronal glial cells induced by anticipation stress and the administration of diazepam. A cytospectrophotometric study. *Neuroscience 4:* 1179-1186.
Johnston, P.V. and Roots, B.I. (1972): *Nerve Membranes. A Study of the Biological and Chemical Aspects of Neuron-Glia Relationships.* Pergamon Press, Oxford et al.
Kerkut, G.A. (1975): Axoplasmic transport. *Comp. Biochem. Physiol. 51A:* 701-704.
Krichevskaya, A.A., Mogilnitskaya, L.V., and Pevzner, L.Z. (1976): Nuclear histone level in neurons and neuroglia in certain parts of the hypothalmus during prolonged cooling of animals. Doklady Akad, Nauk SSSR, Biol. Sci. Section (Engl. Transl.) 226: 85-87.
Kuhlenbeck, H. (1970): *The Central Nervous System of Vertebrates.* Vol. 3, Part I. Structural Elements: Biology of Nervous Tissue. S. Karger, Basel.
Lange, P.W. (1978): Nucleic acids and proteins. In: E. Schoffeniels et al. (Eds.) *Dynamic Properties of Glia Cells.* Pergamon Press, Oxford et al., 231-245.
LeBlanc, J. (1967): Adaptation to cold in three hours. *Amer. J. Physiol. 212:* 530-532.
Minchin, M.C.W. and Beart, P.M. (1975): Compartmentation of amino acid metabolism in the rat dorsal root ganglion; a metabolic and autoradiographic study. *Brain Res. 83:* 437-449.
Mrosovsky, N. (1971): *Hibernation and Hypothalamus.* Appleton-Century-Crofts, New York.
Oguri, K., Lee, N.M., and Loh, H.H. (1976): Apparent protein kinase activity in oligodendroglia chromatin after chronic morphine treatment. *Biochem. Pharmacol. 25:* 2371-2376.
Peters, A., Palay, S.L., and Webster, H. deF. (1976): *The Fine Structure of the Nervous System. The Neurons and Supporting Cells.* W.B. Saunders, Philadelphia et al.
Pevzner, L.Z. (1965): Topochemical aspects of nucleic acid and protein metabolism within the neuron-neuroglia unit of the superior cervical ganglion. *J. Neurochem. 12:* 993-1002.
Pevzner, L.Z. (1968): Nucleic acids in the neuron-neuroglia unit in various functional states of the nervous system. In: Z. Lodin and S.P.S. Rose (Eds.) *Macromolecules and Function of the Neuron.* Excerpta Medica Foundation, Amsterdam, 335-358.
Pevzner, L.Z. (1971): Topochemical aspects of nucleic acid and protein metabolism within the neuron-neuroglia unit of the spinal cord anterior horn. *J. Neurochem. 18:* 895-907.
Pevzner, L.Z. (1972): Topochemical aspects of nucleic acid metabolism within the neuronal-neuroglial unit of cerebellar Purkinje cells. *Brain Res. 46:* 329-339.
Pevzner, L.Z. (1978): Phasic interrelations between neuronal and neuroglial metabolism. In: E. Schoffeniels et al. (Eds.) *Dynamic Properties of Glia Cells.* Pergamon Press, Oxford et al., 223-229.

Pevzner, L.Z. (1979a): *Functional Biochemistry of the Neuroglia*. Plenum Press, New York.
Pevzner, L.Z. (1979b): Cytochemical comparison of two kinds of experimental hypoxia: changes of RNA content per cell in cerebellar and cerebral cortex neurons and perineuronal glia. *Exper. Neurol. 65:* 237-241.
Pevzner, L.Z. (1979c): RNA and protein changes in spinal motoneurons and perineuronal glia under effects of two kinds of experimental convulsions. *Acta Histochem. 64:* 237-242.
Pevzner, L.Z. and Saudargene, E.-D. (1971): Two-wave length visible cytospectrophotometry of nucleic acids and proteins in the motor and sensory neurons and their glial cell-satellites of rat spinal cord during Corazol seizures. *Acta Histochem. 39:* 101-117.
Plum, F., Posner, J.B., and Troy, B. (1968): Cerebral metabolic and circulatory responses to induced convulsions in animals. *Arch. Neurol. 18:* 1-13.
Poduslo, S.E. and Norton, W.T. (1975): Isolation of specific brain cells. In: J.M. Lowenstein (Ed.) *Methods in Enzymology*, Vol. 35. Lipids. Academic Press, New York et al., 561-579.
Pope, A. (1978): Neuroglia: quantitative aspects. In: E. Schoffeniels et al. (Eds.) *Dynamic Properties of Glia Cells*. Pergamon Press, Oxford et al., 13-20.
Roots, B.I. (1978): A phylogenetic approach to the anatomy of glia. In: E. Schoffeniels et al. (Eds.) *Dynamic Properties of Glia Cells*. Pergamon Press, Oxford et al., 45-54.
Rose, S.P.R. (1968): The biochemistry of neurons and glia. In: *Applied Neurochemistry*. Oxford-Edinburgh, 332-355.
Rose, S.P.R. (1969): Neurons and glia: separation techniques and biochemical interrelationships. In: A. Lajtha (Ed.) *Handbook of Neurochemistry*, Vol. II. Plenum Press, New York, 183-193.
Rose, S.P.R. (1973): Cellular compartmentation of metabolism in the brain. In: R. Balázs and J.E. Cremer (Eds.) *Metabolic Compartmentation in the Brain*. MacMillan Press, London, 287-304.
Rubinskaya, N.L. (1971): RNA content in spinal motorneurons, cerebellar Purkinje cells and their glial cell-satellites during picrotoxin convulsions. *Vopr. Med. Khim. 17:* 306-311 (in Russian).
Schmidt, M. and Zimmermann, P. (1978): Reactivity patterns of nerve cell-glia-complexes in mice during pentylenetetrazole-induced seizures. Cytometric-cytophotometric studies. *Acta Neuropathol. 43:* 243-250.
Schoffeniels, E., Franck, G., Hertz, L., and Tower, D.B. (Eds.) (1978): *Dynamic Properties of Glia Cells. An Interdisciplinary Approach to Their Study in the Central and Peripheral Nervous System*. Pergamon Press, Oxford et al.
Schon, F. and Kelly, J.S. (1975): Selective uptake of [^{3}H] β-alanine by glia: association with glial uptake system for GABA. *Brain Res. 86:* 243-257.
Sellinger, O.Z. and Azcurra, J.M. (1974): Bulk separation of neuronal cell bodies and glial cells in the absence of added digestive enzymes. In: N. Marks and M. Rodnight (Eds.) *Research Methods in Neurochemistry*, vol. 2. Plenum Press, New York, 3-38.
Selye, H. (1952): *The Story of the Adaptation Syndrome* (told in the form of informal, illustrated lectures). Med. Publ., Montreal.
Selye, H. (1957): *The Stress of Life*. Longmans Green, London et al.
Tiplady, B., Glushchenko, T.S., and Pevzner, L.Z. (1974): Effect of forced motor activity on the RNA content of neurons and neuroglial cells of the brain and spinal cord. *Doklady Akad. Nauk SSSR, Biol. Sci. Section* (Engl. Transl.) *214:* 78-80.
Van Liere, E.J. and Stickney, J.C. (1963): *Hypoxia*. Chicago.
Varon, S. (1978): Macromolecular glial markers. In: E. Schoffeniels et al. (Eds.) *Dynamic Properties of Glia Cells*. Pergamon Press, Oxford et al., 93-103.

Varon, S. and Somjen, G.G. (1979): Neuron-Glia Interactions. *Neurosci. Res. Progr. Bull.* *17:*1-239.

Vernadakis, A., Nidess, R., Culver, B., and Arnold, E.B. (1979): Glial cells: modulators of neuronal environment. *Mech. Aging and Devel. 9:* 553-566.

Wechsler, W. and Klienhues, P. (1968): Protein metabolism and cytodifferentiation in the nervous system. An autoradiographic and electron microscopic study. In: Z. Lodin and S.P.R. Rose (Eds.) *Macromolecules and Function of the Neuron.* Excerpta Med. Foundation, Amsterdam, 73-90.

Wied, G.L. (Ed.) (1966): *Introduction to Quantitative Cytochemistry.* Academic Press, New York-London.

Yanagihara, T. (1973): Cerebral anoxia: an improved *in vitro* model for biochemical study. *Stroke 4:* 409-411.

Yanagihara, T. (1974): Cerebral anoxia: effect on transcription and translation. *J. Neurochem. 22:* 113-117.

Yanagihara, T. (1976): Cerebral anoxia: effect on neuron-glia fractions and polysomal protein synthesis. *J. Neurochem. 27:* 539-543.

Yanagihara, T. (1979): Protein and RNA synthesis and precursor uptake with isolated nerve and glial cells. *J. Neurochem. 32:* 169-177.

2

Somatosensory Affectional Deprivation (SAD) Theory of Drug and Alcoholic Behaviors

James W. Prescott

Part I

The *Somatosensory Affectional Deprivation* (SAD) theory of drug and alcoholic behaviors is a developmental psychobiological theory that is proposed to account for the common ground of the many and diverse theories of substance abuse. The basic proposition of this theory is that the neurobiology of our behavior is not only inseparable from culture but is, in fact, largely shaped by culture. The shaping process of culture upon the developing brain (the organ of behavior) is accomplished through our various sensory modalities and through the sensory processes of deprivation and stimulation.

With few exceptions the developing mammalian brain, particularly the primate brain, is highly immature at birth and is dependent upon sensory stimulation for its normal growth, development, and functional and structural organization. The richness or paucity of dendritic structures of the neurone (brain cell), for example, are largely influenced by the sensory processes of stimulation and deprivation during the formative periods of brain development. The *complexities* and *possibilities* of neuronal communication (and thus behavior) are dependent upon the richness or paucity, *i.e.*, complexity of dendritic structures of brain cells. The dendritic structures are analogous to cables that interconnect with other cables of other dendritic structures (brain cells) which form a structural basis of interneuronal communication. Another major element in the story of interneuronal communication are neurochemical transmitter substances which are present at synaptic junctions between dendrites and which make possible the transfer of "energy-information" from one brain cell to another. These events are accompanied by electrophysiological activity which is another manifestation of interneuronal communication. The point of this synaptic overview of interneuronal communication is to emphasize that the morphology (structural), neurochemical, and electrophysiological (functional) processes of interneuronal communication are all strongly influenced by the sensory processes of stimulation and deprivation. Thus, the effects of the social, physical, and cultural environment are ultimately transformed into perceptual experiences through the encoding and decoding of sensory processes. Further, whether certain perceptual experiences *can ever be realized* will be dependent upon the quality and quantity of our sensory experiences, as structured by our social, physical and cultural environment, during the formative periods of brain development (Prescott, 1967, 1971a, 1971b, 1972a, 1972b, 1973, 1975, 1976a, 1976b, 1977, 1978).

The second basic proposition of the *Somatosensory Affectional Deprivation* (SAD) theory of substance abuse is that certain sensory modalities and processes are more important than others in accounting for substance abuse. Specifically, it is the emotional senses of somesthesis (touch); vestibulation (movement); and olfaction (smell) in contrast to the cognitive senses of vision and hearing that are central and indispensable to understanding our emotional/affective behaviors where substance abuse is one manifestation of our emotional/affective state. It is the deprivation of our emotional senses and not our cognitive senses during the formative periods of brain development that can account for and predict our emotional/affective-social behaviors which include not only substance abuse but abusive behaviors in general. Thus, the question of destructive and exploitive behaviors toward ourselves and others (in contrast to nurturant and altruistic behaviors) becomes a question of whether affectional bonds are formed or not formed during the formative periods of brain development. Within an evolutionary context it should be noted that olfaction assumes a greater role in lower mammals and vestibular functions assumes a greater role in higher mammalian forms, specifically the primate, in the formation of affectional bonds (Prescott, 1975, 1976a).

In previous studies the *Somatosensory Affectional Deprivation* (SAD) theory has been successful in predicting physical violence (high and low) in 100 percent of 49 primitive cultures distributed throughout the world. This was made possible by evaluating the degree of physical affection (touching, holding, carrying) of the infant by its mother or caretakers and by the degree of physical affection that was permitted to be expressed through the acceptance or rejection of premarital sexuality. The issue of violence, *i.e.,* the failure of nurturance and the failure to form affectional bonds is highly related to the issue of substance abuse in several respects. First, in a very general sense, the body needs and "searches" for a state of harmony, contentment and in higher life forms (homo sapiens) an altered and transcendent state of conscious "Being." A necessary condition for the attainment of the "State-of-Being" is the experiencing of physical (somatosensory) pleasure that is essential for the formation of affectional bonds. When this somatosensory pleasure and affectional bonds are denied then compensatory behaviors to reduce tension, discomfort and "anomie" became imperative. The common compensatory behaviors are physical violence (toward others and oneself); alcoholism and drug abuse and preseverative stimulus-seeking behaviors that attempt to provide the sensory stimulation that was deprived early in life. The stereotypical rocking behaviors of the isolation-reared Harlow monkeys and of institutionalized children is a case in point. Similarly, the chronic toe and penis sucking of the Harlow isolation-reared monkeys; the self-mutilation of isolate reated monkeys and dogs; the paradoxical "supersensitivity" to touch and impaired pain perception in isolate reared monkeys and dogs; and the chronic stimulus-seeking behaviors, particularly of a sexual and violent nature, in the American culture (massage parlors, pornography; violent films; and rape) are all illustrative of this basic principle of stimulus-seeking behaviors consequent to early somatosensory deprivation (Prescott, 1972, 1973, 1975, 1976a, 1976b; Ainsworth, 1972; Cairns, 1972; Bowlby, 1969; Harlow, 1971; Harlow et al., 1963; Dokecki, 1973; Lichstein and Sackett, 1971; Lynch, 1970; Mason, 1968. 1971; Mason and Kenney, 1974; Mason and Berkson, 1975; Cairns, 1966; Fuller, 1967; Freedman, 1968; Friedman et al., 1968; Melzack and Burns, 1965; Malzack and Thompson, 1956; Melzack and Scott, 1957; Mitchell, 1968, 1970, 1975; Mitchell and Clark 1968; Sackett, 1970; Rienson, 1960, 1961a, 1961b, 1964; Schaffer, 1964a, 1964b; Spitz, 1945, 1965; Suomi and Harlow, 1972; Zubek, 1969). The findings of Behling (1979) highlight the relationship between alcohol abuse, violence of child abuse and failure of nurturance where 69 percent of 51 instances of child abuse had a history of alcohol abuse in at least one parent.

In the context of the *Somatosensory Affectional Deprivation* (SAD) theory it is not surprising to find the compensatory behaviors of violence in the primitive culture study cited above and the finding of Barry (1976) that the single greatest predictor of drunkenness in 13 primitive cultures was the high amount of crying during infancy ($r=.77$). Drunkenness was also significantly correlated with low general indulgence during infancy ($r=.40$; $n=26$) and low duration of bodily contact with caretaker during later stages of infancy ($r=.42$; $n=23$). Significant relationships between deprivation of parental physical affection and use of drugs and alcohol have been reported for college students (Prescott, 1975); for prisoners (Prescott and Wallace, 1978); and for institutionalized alcoholics and participants in a drug treatment program (Prescott and Wallace, 1976). Significant relationships between drug and alcohol usage with rejection of premarital and extramarital sex have also been reported for college students (Prescott, 1975).

An interpretive statement of the above relationships with respect to somatosensory pleasure-seeking; isolation rearing (somatosensory deprivation); altered neuronal communication; and altered states of "consciousness" appears necessary. Briefly, the SAD theory postulates that somatosensory deprivation of isolation-rearing leads to impaired neuronal systems that mediate pleasure which now lack the neuronal structural bases to influence higher brain centers (neocortex) and thus prevents an *integration* of somatosensory pleasure with higher brain centers and, thus, altered states of consciousness or states of "Transcendent-Being." (See Teilhard de Chardin's essay "Evolution of Chastity" on this point.) Consequently, most of the somatosensory pleasure stimulus-seeking behaviors of contemporary western civilization (not just America) appear to be "non-integrative" in nature, *i.e.,* it is primarily "reflexive." This means the "pleasure experience" is a momentary and transitory phenomena that produces a temporary reduction of tension and discomfort but does not represent a true positive state of "integrative-pleasure." Thus, *anomie* remains: a high need for another "pleasure-fix" remains; and the complex of *perseverative* behaviors remains. Drugs and alcohol "by-pass" the somatosensory process and provide a direct route to higher brain centers and altered states of consciousness or states of "Transcendent-Being." It should be noted that SAD of social isolation results in an aversion to touch and thus constitutes a barrier to "touch-therapy" that is essential for rehabilitation.

Within the context of SAD theory three basic groups of substance abusers exist and need to be evaluated and treated differently. These are (a) the pleasure users (marijuana, heroin, etc.); (b) pleasure avoider users (alcohol, depressants, tranquilizers); and (c) altered "states-of-consciousness" users (hallucinogens).

A factory analytic study involving items of drug and alcoholic usage produced orthogonal factors for alcohol and marijuana usage (Prescott and Wallace, 1976). Unfortunately, time and space do not permit review of this data or an elaboration of SAD theory of drug typologies and their implications for research and therapy. It is suggested, however, that sensory process orientation would be highly heuristic, *i.e.,* special attention should be given to evaluating vestibular-cerebellar processes in alcoholics; somesthetic-cerebellar processes in pleasure drug users; and visual/auditory-neocortical processes in hallucinogenic users. It should be recognized that these suggestions are highly speculative and have many limitations but, nevertheless, may have some heuristic merit in attempting to specify specific neurobiological brain processes with specific choices of substance use and abuse.

Evidence that social isolation rearing alters neurochemistry of brain function has been partially reviewed elsewhere (Prescott, 1971, 1976a; Laletal, 1972; Essman, 1971; Welch and Welch, 1969; Valzelli, 1975; DeFeudis and Marks, 1973; Rosenberg et al., 1968). Certain studies, however, deserve special commentary and recent developments with respect to the endorphins are especially relevant to somatosensory affectional deprivation theory and data, as is the basic alteration of the CNSs response to drugs that are induced by SAD of isolation rearing.

In this specific social-neurobiological context, Lal et al. (1972) have demonstrated that social isolation rearing of mice (somatosensory deprivation) significantly altered the pharmacological effects of Hexobarbital, Phenobarbital, Cloral Hydrate, Barbital and Chlorpromazine. Specifically, social isolation enhances stimulant drug effects and reduces CNS depressant effects.

Bonnet et al. (1976), reported that mice reared in social isolation (somatosensory affectional deprivation) for twenty weeks showed a significant reduction in narcotic agonist and antagonist binding. No differences could be found in stereospecific binding between the rearing groups with 15 weeks of differential rearing but were found at 17 and 21 weeks of rearing. These authors also reported a significant reduction of the number of opiate binding sites in the brains of isolation-reared mice compared to aggregation-reared mice. This loss of opiate receptor sites in isolation-reared mice is analogous to the loss of dendrites consequent to social isolation rearing.

Panksepp et al. (1978), reported a significant decrease in distress vocalizations of puppies who were *briefly* separated from their mothers (15 min) with an injection of .125 mg/rg of oxymorphone; and that naloxone increased group vocalization of 2-5-day-old white Leghorn chicks that were briefly separated from their mother. These authors discuss the parallels between the biological nature of narcotic addiction and the formation of social bonds and their theoretical position is consistent with SAD theory and this writer's conviction that the brain endorphin systems may be one of the most important neurobiological systems that mediate the development of affectional bonds that includes sexual affectional bonding as well.

The role of endorphins in sexual behavior has been studied by Gesa et al. (1979), where they have reported the following findings from their rat study:

(a) DALA (D-Ala^2-MeI- enkephalinamide) given intracerebroventricularly at a dose of 6 mg completely inhibited copulatory behavior and the ability to ejaculate in sexually active rats. Naloxone (4 mg/kg) given intraperitoneally completely reversed this effect;

(b) Naloxone does not enhance sexual behavior in sexually active rats;

(c) Naloxone (4 mg/kg) given intramuscularly significantly enhances mounting, intromission and ejaculation in sexually *inactive* rats.

These authors suggest that endorphins may underlie sexual disorders and that opioid antagonists "might become potentially useful therapeutic agents for sexual disturbances in man" (p. 204). A similar statement might be said for the treatment of alcoholics whose somatosensory pleasure system is dysfunctional and often inoperable. Pleasure inducing drugs such as marijuana and the opioids may prove to be a useful first step in a program of somatosensory rehabilitation for alcoholics. Different therapeutic stratagems appear indicated, however, for other classes of substance abusers.

The above studies are cited because of the increasing evidence that has linked early social isolation (somatosensory affectional deprivation) to: (a) violence, drug/alcohol abuse, and sexual dysfunctioning; (b) altered neurochemistry, electrophysiology, and dendritic structures (neuronal communication) in somatosensory and motor cortex and cerebellar cortex; (c) altered narcotic agonist and antagonist binding; and (d) altered CNS response to stimulant and depressant drugs. The role of sexual functioning and sexual pleasure as part of the developmental continuum of affectional bonding and its relationship to endorphins, drug/alcohol usage, and violence, particularly alcohol-induced violence, bring a convergence of theories and experimental evidence that, heretofore, were considered disparate entities and phenomena.

The findings of Gesa et al. (1979), and of Panksepp (1978), however, appear contradictory and inconsistent with this proposed convergence. In the former study stimulation of opiate receptors induced pleasure-deficit behaviors (failure to copulate and ejaculate); whereas in the latter study stimulation of opiate receptors induced pleasure-enhancement behaviors (decrease in distress vocalizations). Similarly, in the former study, naloxone enhanced pleasure behaviors (increased copulation and ejaculation); whereas naloxone in the latter study decreased pleasure behaviors (enhanced distress vocalization). These apparent fundamental contradictions are proposed to be resolvable within SAD theory and Cannon's Law of Denervation Supersensitivity which is an integral and essential neurophysiological mechanism of SAD theory (Prescott, 1971, 1972).

Briefly, fundamental distinctions must be made between CNS that are characterized or not characterized by *Denervation Supersensitivity* which is induced by Deafferetation, *i.e.*, a loss of afferent input. Sexual inactivity, like social isolation rearing, involves somatosensory deprivation which constitutes a special case of functional deafferentation. As reported by Struble and Riesen (1978), primate isolation rearing results in loss of dendrites in somatosensory cortex. The loss of opiate receptor sites; reduced narcotic agonist and antagonist binding; enhancement of stimulant drug effects and inhibition of depressant drug effect are all consequent to social isolation and thus share, in this writer's view, a common explanatory mechanism, namely Cannon's Law of Denervation Supersensitivity (Cannon, 1939; Cannon and Rosenbleuth, 1949; Collier, 1968; Sharpless, 1969). It is within this context that it is relevant to emphasize that the effect of opioid substances upon their receptors is to depress the activity of cells bearing these receptors and consequently are classed as inhibitory neurotransmitters (Goldstein, 1981). The enhancement of these inhibitory neurotransmitters through the mechanism of denervation supersensitivity might account for the inhibition of copulatory and ejaculatory behavior as reported by Gesa et al. (1979). Similarly, the *absence* of denervation supersensitivity in Panksepp's experimental subjects could account for his endorphin stress reducing (pleasure enhancement?) effects.

The findings of Gispen et al. (1976), that low doses of B-endorphin (.01-.30 ug) induced excessive grooming behavior in rats, and of Meyerson and Terenius (1977) that higher doses of B-endorphin (1 and 3 ug) significantly reduced mounting copulatory behavior in wistar rats exposed to estrous females confirm the "bidirectionality" of endorphin mechanisms. Naltrexone given subculaneously 30 minutes before the peptide blocked the effect of 1 ug B-endorphin thus confirming that impaired sexual functioning was mediated via opiate receptors. It should be noted that 1 ug B-endorphin did not interfere with sexual exploratory behavior that included active pursuit and investigation of the anogenital area of the female.

The above reports of "bidirectionality" of endorphin activity as a function of dosage level; the *endorphin antagonistic* effects; and the *naloxone agonistic* effects concerning sexual behaviors are not unrelated to the naloxone agonistic effects concerning pain perception.

Levine et al. (1979), in a study of human clinical pain (tooth extraction) found that naloxone produced analagesia at low doses (0.4 and 2 mg) and hyperalgesia at high doses (7.5-10 mg) for a placebo-respondent group. Interestingly, naloxone had little effect on placebo non-responders. Questions must be raised whether placebo responders and those experimental preparations that manifest naloxone agonistic effects (bi-directionality) could be characterized by SAD or other forms of induced denervation supersensitivity. These questions are relevant to the findings of Buchsbaum et al. (1977), where they divided their subjects into "pain-sensitive" and "pain-insensitive" groups as determined by their ratings of an electric shock. They found that only the pain-sensitive subjects reported a naloxone (2 mg) analgesia effect, and that "pain-insensitive" subjects showed a naloxone hyperalgesia.

Although the studies of Levine et al. (1979), and Buchsbaum et al. (1977), are not directly comparable since Levine employed multiple dosages of naloxone and Buchsbaum employed a single naloxone dosage it is of interest to contrast the two naloxone hyperalgesia groups with respect to the issue of placebo responding. Levine reported a naloxone bi-directional effect for placebo responders whereas Buchsbaum's "pain-insensitive" bi-directional responders were characterized as placebo "non-responders" since their placebo response was less than half of the "pain-sensitive" group. These "inconsistencies" require further experimental study.

These observations only complicate an already very complicated set of issues and phenomena of endorphin related behaviors. However, the "bir-directionality" phenomena of naloxone (low dosage producing analgesia and high dosages producing hyperalgesia) first reported by Lasagna (1965) and reported elsewhere Buchsbaum et al. (1977); Levine et al. (1979); and the *naloxone agonist* effects and *endorphin antagonist* effects involving not only pain phenomena but sexual-social and motor behaviors (Gesa et al., 1979; Meyerson and Terenius, 1977;

Gispen et al., 1976; Bloom et al., 1976; Jacquet and Marks, 1976) suggest an extremely complex role of modulation, regulation, and integration of sensory, social, emotional, and motor behaviors by the endorphin system.

It is perhaps heuristic to mention the findings of Reis et al. (1973), that low levels of electrical stimulation in the cerebellar rostral fastigial nucleus of the cat elicited grooming behavior but with increasing levels of electrical stimulation the grooming behavior changed to consumatory behaviors and ultimately to predatory attack behaviors with high levels of electrical stimulation. This study is cited because of its remarkable analagous results to B-endorphin reported above where "low" dosage of B-endorphin results in positive pleasurable behaviors (grooming, mounting, and ejaculation) and "high" dosage of B-endorphin results in decreased pleasurable behaviors (impaired pursuit of estrous female, mounting, copulation, and ejaculation).

This writer has previously elaborated a theory of cerebellar regulation and integration of sensory, social, emotional and motor behaviors within the context of SAD theory (Prescott, 1971, 1976, 1978). Heath and his co-workers have established a wealth of data describing cerebellar-limbic relationships which were postulated by SAD theory and have further dramatized how cerebellar stimulation can modulate extreme states of emotional expression (positive and negative) in human subjects (Heath, 1972, 1975a, 1975b, 1976, 1977, 1978, 1979; Heath et al., 1979). According to SAD theory the cerebellum is not itself the site of these behaviors but exerts a regulatory influence on limbic, reticular, and frontal cortical structures to modulate these behaviors. Cerebellar modulation of limbic-endorphin activity would be a natural extension of SAD theory and could be tested in both animal and human studies. It would be expected, for example, that endorphin/naloxone behaviors would be altered with chronic cerebellar electrical stimulation that resulted in profound changes in emotional behavior, as described by Heath et al. (1979). In particular, since Heath (1972, 1975a, 1975b) has documented abnormal electrical spike discharges in the limbic and cerebellar structures of isolation-reared primates; and Saltzberg et al. (1971, 1976, 1980), have developed signal analysis methods to detect these deep brain spike discharges from scalp EEG recordings it makes possible a series of exciting studies that could link a known history of somatosensory affectional deprivation to abnormal deep brain spike activity; to specific patterns of endorphin/naloxone induced behaviors; to therapeutic regimens that, if effective, *e.g.,* chronic cerebellar stimulation; endorphin/naloxone therapy; and somatosensory stimulation therapies; than these effective therapies should be reflected in altered spike discharges; altered endorphin/naloxone behaviors; and altered social emotional behaviors, particularly in response to drugs and alcohol.

The role of the cerebellum in somatosensory affectional deprivation has been given support by Berman et al. (1974); and Floeter and Greenough (1979) who reported significant increases in spiny branchlets of Purkinje cells in the para flocculus and the nodulus of the cerebellum in monkeys reared in colony conditions compared to isolate reared and socially experienced animals (environmental variation of SAD). Although, denervation supersensitivity mechanisms inherent in somatosensory affectional deprivation are offered as a major explanatory process in accounting for the variety of diverse and often apparently inconsistent and contradictory findings from the endorphin/naloxone behavioral literature, it is recognized that other factors, *e.g.,* neonatal anoxia can induce denervation supersensitivity (Berman and Berman, 1975; Burch et al., 1975); and that the "family" of endorphins and their antagonists are additional factors that can contribute to the complexity of findings reported in the literature and their interpretation.

The major theoretical orientation of this paper is to emphasize that any study of endorphin/naloxone behaviors or drug/alcohol behaviors must take into acacount the developmental history of the organism to determine whether the CNS of that organism is characterized by denervation supersensitivity whether induced by somatosensory affectional deprivation or other etiological developmental factors.

The phenomena of "hyperendorphinism" of affective disorders (Buchsbaum et al., 1980) which may well be an expression of "neurotransmitter density" due to denervation supersensitivity is an example of a construct that perhaps can be benefited by a developmental perspective. Neurotransmitter Density in neurochemistry is analagous to Current Density (mA/cm^2) in electrophysiology and expresses the relationship of the amount of released neurotransmitter substance available to the number of available receptors (ANT/R_N).

Since isolation rearing results in a reduction of the number of opioid receptors, a state of "hyperendorphinism" may not reflect a change in absolute volume of released endorphin but rather a change in the number of opioid receptors (endorphin density). The converse could also occur (increased volume of endorphin with receptor number remaining constant) for different etiological reasons. This is mentioned for the prupose of suggesting that "hyper-endorphinism" may not be a unitary phenomena since different mechanisms and etiologies could mediate this effect.

It would be a serious omission not to mention the classic theoretical system developed by Petrie (1976, 1978) which has unusual relevance to the issues of substance abuse and to somatosensory affectional deprivation theory. Briefly, Petrie (1967, 1978) has proposed a theoretical system that postulates CNS processes of *Reduction* and *Augmentation* of the sensory environment which describes an individual's "reactance" to pain and sensory deprivation. The "CNS Augmenters" are characterized by an intolerance for pain and a tolerance for sensory deprivation. This pattern of "reactance" occurs because the CNS of these individuals acts to "augment" or "enhance" the impact of a sensory event upon the CNS. Conversely, the "CNS Reducers" are characterized by a tolerance for pain and an intolerance for sensory deprivation. This pattern of "reactance" occurs because the CNS of these individuals acts to "reduce" or "inhibit" the impact of a given sensory event upon the CNS. Thus, the "CNS Reducers" are characterized by a chronic state of insufficient afferent stimulation (stress of sensory insufficiency or sensory deprivation) and engage in behaviors that are designed to maximize afferent stimulation of the CNS. Consequently, these "CNS Reducers" are those who engage in a variety of stimulus-seeking behaviors, *e.g.,* delinquents who are CNS Reducers when punished with solitary confinement will frequently engage in self-mutilative behaviors that involve cutting their flesh with razors and burning their flesh with cigarette ends (note self-mutilation of isolation-reared animals).

Petrie (1978) described the response of Reducer, Moderates, and Augmenters to alcohol where she found that Augmenters were most affected by dramatically changing from an *Augmenting* "reactance" mode to a *Reducing* reactance mode. Similar but less strong "reducing" effects were obatined with "Reducers." Comparable results were obtained with other drugs, such as aspirin and chlorpromazine. Thus, "Augmenters" as a group were shifted more away from pain intolerance to pain tolerance. Buchsbaum (1978) has provided a review of a number of neurophysiological studies from his laboratory and others on "Reducers" and "Augmenters." Without reviewing all of his findings, suffice it to point out that he reported that reduction of the amplitude of sensory evoked potentials to increased stimulus intensity was associated with pain tolerance and analgesia and that "augmentation" was linked to substance abuse. The studies of Buchsbaum and Lugwig (in press), and Knorring and Oreland (1978), are also relevant to these issues.

This writer has previously suggested that somatosensory affectional deprivation of isolation rearing is a major contributing factor to the developmental neuropsychobiological substrate of Petrie's typology of "Reducers" and "Augmenters" (Prescott, 1967). Chronic or perservative stimulus-seeking behaviors and impaired pain perception, for example, are predominate characteristics of somatosensory affectional deprivation (denervation supersensitivity) and the "CNS Reducer." There are however, significant differences in the communality of the two theoretical asystems where SAD is characterized by "paradoxical" behaviors, *e.g.,* simultaneous supersensitivity to touch and impaired pain perception that is not accounted for by Petrie's typology. Zuckerman's (1979) theory of *Sensation seeking* is also intrinsically related to the theories of Petrie (1978) and Prescott (1967, 1971a, 1971b, 1972a, 1972b, 1973, 1975, 1976a, 1976b, 1977).

This writer has attempted to link these basic developmental neurobiological processes of SAD to cross-cultural characteristics of childrearing practices; social-religious mores and customs that regulate sexual behaviors; to personality characteristics of authoritarianism, exploitation, and narcissism in contrast to egalitarianism, nurturance, and altruism. Further, that these contrasts in personality characteristics, considered at the micro-social level, constitute the bases for the political structure of a culture, namely, egalitarian-democratic societies vs. authoritarian-fascist societies (Prescott, 1975, 1976, 1977). It is of some significance that Petrie (1978) in her second edition draws exactly the same parallels from her theory to the characteristics of both personality and culture with her typologies of "Compassions" vs. "Callousness," *i.e.,* the "Augmenter" vs. "Reducer" (pp. xii-xiv).

In concluding this theoretical essay, it hardly needs to be emphasized that the social-emotional dysfunctioning of the individual in society, whatever form that it may be expressed, is not only an intrinsic aspect of neurobiological functioning of the individual but also of the social-psychological forces of culture that shape the individuality of neurobiological functioning through the formative developmental process of sensory stimulation and deprivation; and through a culture of chemical and physical environments that influence fetal, neonatal, and postnatal development. Maternal habits of chemical ingestion, *e.g.,* alcohol, drugs, food/spice preferences or exposure to certain chemical environments during gestation may well "imprint" upon the developing fetus certain "sensitivities" and "predispositions" for use or avoidance of these chemical agents during postnatal life with all the implications that this has for behavior.

It necessarily follows that preventive and therapeutic programs cannot be restricted to molecular biological stratagems that are directed at the individual organism. The reconstruction of the individual requires also the reconstruction of society and culture.

The elements of societal and cultural reconstruction involve not only shaping a safe, beneficient physical environment but also a nurturant, caring, and affectionate environment of human relationships. The latter touches deeply upon philosophical and religious idealogies that regulate the morality of pain and pleasure in human relationships and the role of women in society. These issues have been cogently framed by two writers in the early 1930s who could not have been more separated by developmental life experiences, profession, and geography, yet arrived at the same insights upon the human condition.

The first of these is Wilheim Reich, a psychoanalyst, who in the Germany of 1933 wrote the following about sexuality, authoritarianism, and women in society:

> More than the economic dependency of the wife and children on the husband and father is needed to preserve the institution of the authoritarian family. For the suppressed classes, this dependency is endurable only on condition that the consciousness of being a sexual being is suspended as

completely as possible in women and children. *The wife must not figure as a sexual being, but solely as a child-bearer. Sexually awakened women, affirmed and recognized as such, would mean the complete collapse of the authoritarian ideology.* (p. 105)

The second person is Teilhard de Chardin, a Jesuit paleontologist, who in the Peking of 1934 wrote the following about sexuality, women in society and knowledge in his essay on *The Evolution of Chastity:*

Woman is, for man, the symbol and personification of all the fulfillments we look for from the universe. The theoretical and practical problem of the attainment of knowledge has found its natural 'climate' in the problem of the sublimation of love. At the term of the spiritual power of matter, lies the spiritual power of the flesh and of the feminine.

It is here, if I am not mistaken, that we reach the source of the divergence which seems to detach our modern sympathies from the traditional cult of chastity. The Christian code of virtue seems to be based on the presupposition that woman is for man essentially an instrument of generation. Either woman exists for the propagation of the race—or woman has no place at all: such is the dilemma put forward by the moralists. All that is most dear to us in our experiences, and most certain, revolts against this simplification. However fundamental woman's maternity may be, it is almost nothing in comparison with her spiritual fertility. Woman brings fullness of being, sensibility, and self-revelation to the man who has loved her. (p. 70)

...The feminine is the most formidable of the forces of matter (p. 74)...
The truth is, indeed, that love is the threshold of another universe (p. 78)

...And so we cannot avoid this conclusion: it is biologically evident that to gain control of passion and so make it serve spirit must be a condition of progress. (p. 86)

The above philosophical and moral commentaries may appear remote from the specific issues of a theory of alcohol, drug abuse, and violence. From this writer's perspective they could not be more central. The chaos of human relationships in our culture: between parents and children; husband and wife; male and female are all intrinsically related to unbearable human conditions where alcohol and drugs provide not only an apparent escape but insidiously maintains and facilitates the "anomie" and destructiveness of interpersonal relationships.

A moral reconstruction of the role of pleasure in human relationships and of women in society are essential prerequisites if any meaningful and lasting solution to alcoholism, drug abuse and violence in our culture is to be realized; and where the realization of this reconstruction must necessarily involve the replacement of the authoritarian structure of patrilineal cultures with the nurturant/affectional structure of matrilineal cultures (Prescott, 1978, 1979).

PART II

INITIATION OF SUBSTANCE USAGE

Factors that are responsible for the initiation of drug and alcohol use are many and varied. From the perspective of Somatosensory Affectional Deprivation (SAD) theory there is first the establishment of a neuropsychobiological predisposition or need for drugs and alcohol. Any factor that contributes to a reduction of afferent activity in the somesthetic (touch) and vestibular (movement) sensory modalities (partial functional deafferentation) from the fetal period of development and throughout the formative periods of postnatal life can be considered as contributing factors to potential substance abuse. Fetal conditioning to maternal substance using during gestation may be a variable of some significance in this context (stimulus-seeking behavior at the neurophysiological level). Early separation of newborns from their mothers—a common hospital practice—and continuing "institutionalization" of infants and children (infant nurseries and child day care centers that are characterized by SAD) are considered to be contributing factors. Failure to breast-feed or short-term breast-feeding (less than two years) that reflects low nuturance or avoidance of intimacy; and breast-feeding that is "mechanical" (duty and responsibility) and not "joyous" are additional factors for consideration. Permitting infants and children to cry for prolonged periods without providing immediate nurturance and to permit them to cry themselves to sleep are additional contributing factors as is the intentional infliction of pain upon infants and children. The failure of *fathers* to be physically affectionate to their infants and children (sons and daughters) is considered to be a major variable of significance for future substance abuse. The failure to provide continuous vestibular stimulation by not carrying the infant throughout the day results in impaired neuro-integrative vestibular-somesthetic and other sensory processes that now require artificial psychochemical stimulation later in life or other forms of compensatory stimulus-seeking behaviors.

Finally, the failure of children to develop close friendships among their peers; and the failure of adolescents to develop not only close friendships but intimate caring and affectionate sexual relationships among their peers are considered to be significant factors that help establish a neuropsychobiological foundation for substance abuse.

CONTINUATION OF SUBSTANCE USAGE

The continuation of substance usage is dependent, in part, upon the continuation of somatosensory affectional deprivation and the need to maintain friendships and "social positions" where those friendships and "social positions" are contingent upon the use of drugs or alcohol. Support for the continuing use of drugs is facilitated by the practices of modern medicine and the advertisement industry of the pharmaceutical corporations. Social learning processes operate at all levels of development (childhood to adulthood) which capitalizes upon the need for the body to find relief from tension and pain that is created in large part by somatosensory affectional deprivation. Societal and moral values that are intrinsically opposed to somatosensory pleasure and sexual pleasure, in particular, provide support for the alternatives of drugs and alcohol. Societal opposition to massage parlors and prostitution but open acceptance and support of the alcohol industries is a case in point. Societal acceptance of addicting drugs that impair somatosensory pleasure, *e.g.*, alcohol and methadone; and opposition to drugs that facilitate pleasure, *e.g.*, marijuana and heroin is another case in point. Carstairs' (1966) classic study should be consulted in this context because it is a dramatic illustration of the reciprocal inhibitory relationship between drug usage and behaviors that are culturally determined. Carstairs reported on the use of Bhang (marijuana) and alcohol in the two highest caste groups, *Rajput* and *Brahmin,* in a village in northern India. The *Rajput* was the warrior class and indulged in alcohol, which facilitated the expression of sexuaity and violence, and they avoided Bhang; the *Brahmin* was the religious class and they indulged in Bhang which facilitated religious experiences and enhanced their spiritual life. The holy men avoided alcohol which they considered destructive to salvation and would not permit a Hindu who had consumed alcohol to "enter one of his temples (not even a goddess temple) without first having a purgatory bath and change of clothes" (p. 105).

The continuation and *choice of drug* for use and abuse are culturally influenced. A culture will support the use of certain drugs that are consistent with and support its own mores and values and opposes the use of those drugs that interfere with those mores and values. Thus, the American culture which is predominantly an extroverted, violent, and exploitive culture (sexually and economically) supports the use of alcohol which facilitates these behaviors; and, conversely, opposes the "pleasure" drugs (marijuana and heroin) which inhibit violence and exploitation and facilitates introspective and contemplative behaviors. The issue is not whether a drug is addicting or non-addicting since alcohol is addicting (culturally supported) and marijuana is non-addicting (culturally opposed); heroin is addicting (culturally opposed); and methadone is addicting (culturally supported). It is both the fabric and loom of culture which must be understood if the continuation and choice of specific drugs for use and abuse are to be understood.

TRANSITION – USE TO ABUSE

Given the theory statement in Part I and a synopetic review of many but not all factors contributing to the *Initiation* and *Continuation* of substance abuse in Part II, the transition from use to abuse of psychochemical substances according to somatosensory affectional deprivation (SAD) theory is dependent upon the following factors:

a) time of onset of SAD
b) duration of SAD
c) severity of SAD
d) nature, quality, duration, and time period during formative periods of development of intervien, restorative, and rehabilitative experiences of somatosensory affectional relationships. Absence of such experiences are considered to be particularly pathogenic for abusive behaviors.
e) nature, quality, duration, and time period during formative periods of development of other experiences or factors that result in impaired somesthetic and vestibular functioning which interferes with the rehabilitation of somatosensory affectional processes. In general, it is the chronic failure, for whatever reasons, to experience the enrichment of somatosensory affectionate experiences in the context of meaningful relationships that sets the condition for the transition from use to abuse. Individuals who do not or cannot make the transition from states of "reflexive" pleasure to states of "integrative" pleasure are also "at risk" for making the transition from substance use to substance abuse (10).

CESSATION OF USE

Cessation of use is dependent to a very large degree upon an individual's ability to change the social, physical, and cultural environment that would make possible the restoration of somatosensory affectionate experiences within the context of meaningful human relationships. Without this change, cessation of use becomes extremely difficult and short-lived. Purely cognitive strategies to induce change are highly unlikely to be successful. The basic psychophysiology of attachment processes must be treated so that affectional bonds can be restored in order that cessation of use can be effectively realized. Psychopharmacological therapies that directly stimulate somatosensory and somatopleasure processes of the CNS/ANS may be a necessary first step in the process of somatosensory affectional rehabilitation in particularly difficult cases. The transition from psychopharmacological therapies to somatosensory affectional therapies is a necessary and essential transition for the realization of cessation of substance abuse. Altered vestibular functioning; hydro-flotation and hydro-suspension therapies; massage and somesthetic therapies to reintegrate the vestibular-somesthetic and other sensory processes appear necessary for the reconstruction and rehabilitation of the psychophysiological mechanisms of attachment behaviors. The extent to which those psychophysiological mechanisms can be rehabilitated for the purpose of establishing affectional bonds will determine to a large extent the nature and extent of cessation of substance abuse.

RELAPSE OF USE

Relapse of substance abuse will occur when only cognitive behavioral restructuring is achieved without the concomitant changes in the neuropsychobiological mechanisms of somatosensory affectional processes. The disassociation of cognitive behaviors from psychophysiological behaviors in the processes of rehabilitation provide a basis for relapse of substance abuse. The establishment or reestablishment of neuro-integration of somatosensory affectional processes with "higher brain centers" (altered status of consciousness) would constitute an effective barrier to relapse of substance abuse. If early deprivations are sufficiently severe such that there is a permanent neuronal alteration of the brain then the neuronal dendritic networks necessary for the integration of somatosensory affectional processes with "higher brain centers" would be absent and, thus, preclude a permanent rehabilitation. Under such circumstances, continued enriched somatosensory affectional experiences would be required to prevent relapse. An instructive analogy is the diabetic who requires constant injections of insulin to maintain normative functioning.

REFERENCES

Ainsworth, M.D.S. (1972): Attachment and dependency: A comparison. In: J.L. Gewirtz (Ed.) *Attachment and Dependency.* V.H. Winston and Sons, Washington, D.C. 97-138.
Barry, H., III(1976): Cross cultural evidence that dependency conflict motivates drunkenness In: M.W. Everett, J.O. Waddell and D.B. Health (Eds.) *Cross-Cultural Approaches to the Study of Alcohol.* Mouton Publishers, Paris; Aldine, Chicago.
Behling, D.W. (1979): Alcohol Abuse as Encountered in 51 Instances of Reported Child Abuse. *Clinical Pediatrics 18* (2): 87-91.
Berman, A.J., Berman, D., and Prescott, J.W. (1974): The Effect of Cerebellar Lesions on Emotional Behavior in the Rhesus Monkey. In: I.S. Cooper, M. Riklan, and R. Snider (Eds.) *The Cerebellum, Epilepsy, and Behavior.* Plenum Press, New York. pp. 277-284.
Bloom F., Segal, D., Ling, N., Guillemin, R. (1974): Endorphins: Profound behavioral effects in rats suggest new etiological factors in mental illness. *Science 194:* 630.
Bonnet, K.A., Miller, J.M., and Simon, E.J. (1976): The Effects of Chronic Opiate Treatment and Social Isolation on Opiate Receptors in the Rodent Brain. In: H.W. Kosterlitz (Ed.) *Opiates and Endogenous Opioid Peptides.* Elsevier, Amsterdam.
Bowlby, J. (1969): *Attachment and Loss. Vol. I. Attachment.* Basic Books, New York.
Buchsbaum, M.S. (1978): Neurophysiological Studies of Reduction and Augmentation. In: A. Petrie *Individuality In Pain and Suffering* (2nd Ed.). University of Chicago Press, Chicago.

Buchsbaum, M.S., Davis, G.C., Bunney, W.E., Jr. (1977): Naloxone alters pain perception and somatosensory evoked potentials in normal subjects. *Nature 270 (5638).* December 15, 620-622.

Buchsbaum, M.S. and Ludwig, A.M. (In press): Effects of sensory input and alcohol administration on visual evoked potentials in normal subjects and alcoholics. In: H. Begleiter (Ed.), *Biological Effects of Alcohol.* Plenum Press, New York.

Buchsbaum, M.S., Davis, G.C., and Kahmen, Van D.P. (In press): Diagnostic classification and the endorphin hypothesis of schizophrenia: Individual differences and psychopharmacological strategies. In: C.F. Baxter (Ed.), *VA Advisory Conference on Chronic Schizophrenia.* Raven Press, New York.

Burch, N.R., Dossett, R.G., Berman, A.J., and Berman, D. (1975): Period Analysis of the Electroencephalogram: Maturation and Anoxia. In: J.W. Prescott, M.S. Read, and D.B. Coursin (Eds.), *Brain Function and Malnutrition: Neuropsychological Methods of Assessment.* John Wiley & Sons, New York.

Cairns, R.B. (1966): Attachment behavior of mammals. *Psychol. Rev. 73:* 409-426.

Cairns, R.B. (1972): Attachment and dependency: A psychobiological and social-learning synthesis. In: J.L. Gewirtz (Ed.), *Attachment and Dependency.* V.H. Winston and Sons, Washington, D.C.

Cannon, W.B. (1939): A law of denervation. *Am. J. Medical Science 198:* 737-749.

Cannon, W.B. and Rosenbleuth, A. (1949): *The Supersensitivity of Denervated Structures.* MacMillan, New York.

Carstairs, G.M. (1966): Bhang and Alcohol: Culutral Factors in the Choice of Intoxicants. In: D. Solomon (Ed.) *The Marijuana Papers.* Mentor Paperback. New American Library, Bobbs Merrill, Indianapolis.

Collier, H.O.J. (1968): Supersensitivity and dependence. *Nature,* Lond. *220:* 228-231.

DeFeudis, F.V. and Marks, J.H. (1973): Brain to serum distribution of radioactivity of injected (^{3}H)-d-amphetamine in differentially housed mice. *Biol. Psychiat. 6:* 85-88.

Dokecki, P.R. (1973): When the bough breaks...what will happen to baby. Review of: *Rock-a-bye baby.* In: Lothar Wolff (Exec. Prod.), Time-Life Films, Inc., New York. *Contemp. Psychol. 18:* 64.

Essman, W.B. (1971): Neurochemical changes associated with isolation and environmental stimulation. *Biol. Psychiat. 3:* 141.

Floeter, M.K. and Greenough, W.T. (1979): Cerebellar Plasticity: Modification of Purkinje Cell Structure by differential rearing in Monkeys. *Science 206 (4415):* October 12, 227-229.

Freedman, D.A. (1968): The influence of congenital and perinatal sensory deprivation on later development. *Psychosomatics 9 (5):* 272-277.

Friedman, C.J., Sibinga, M.S., Steisel, I.M., and Sinnamon, H.M. (1968): Sensory restriction and isolation experiences in children with phenylehetonuria. *J. Abnorm. Psychol. 73 (4):* 294-303.

Fuller, J.L. (1967): Experimental deprivation and later behavior. *Science 158:* 1645-1652.

Gesa, G.L., Paglietti, E., and Quarantotti, B.P. (1979): Induction of Copulatory Behavior in Sexually Inactive Rats by Naloxone. *Science 204:* April 13, 203-205.

Gispen, W.H., Wiegant, V.M., Bradbury, A.F., Hulme, E.C., Smyth, D.G., Snell, C.R., and DeWied, D. (1976): Induction of excessive grooming in the rat fragments of lipotropin. *Nature 164:* 794.

Goldstein, H., *Endorphins.*

Harlow, H.F. (1971): *Learning to Love.* Albion, San Francisco.

Harlow, H.F., Harlow, M.K., and Hansen, E.W. (1963): The maternal affectional system of rhesus monkeys. In: H.L. Rheingold (Ed.), *Maternal Behaviors in Mammals.* Wiley, New York.

Heath, R.G. (1975): Maternal-Social Deprivation and Abnormal Brain Development: Disorders of Emotional and Social Behavior. In: J.W. Prescott, M.S. Read, and D.B. Coursin (Eds.), *Brain Function and Malnutrition: Neuropsychological Methods and Assessment.* John Wiley, New York.

Heath, R.G. (1972): Pleasure and brain activity in man: Deep and surface electroencephalograms during orgasm. *J. Nerv. Ment. Dis. 154:* 3-18.

Heath, R.G. (1975): Brain function and behavior: I. Emotion and sensory phenomena in psychotic patients and in experimental animals. *J. Nerv. Ment. Dis. 160:* 159-175.

Heath, R.G. (1976): Brain function in epilepsy: Midbrain, medullary, and cerebellar interaction with the rostral forebrain. *J. Neurol. Neurosurg. Psychiat. 39:* 1037-1051.

Heath, R.G. (1977): Modulation of emotion with a brain pacemaker: Treatment for intractable psychiatric illness. *J. Nerv. Ment. Dis. 165:* 300-317.

Heath, R.G., Cox, A.W., and Lustick, L.S. (1974): Brain activity during emotional states. *Amer. J. Psychiat. 131:* 858-862.

Heath, R.G., Dempsey, C.W., Fontana, C.J., and Myers, W.A. (1978): Cerebellar stimulation: Effects on septal region, hippocampus, and amygdala of cats and rats. *Biolog. Psychiat. 13:* 501-529.

Heath, R.G., Dempesy, C.W., Fontana, C.J., and Fitzjarrell, A.T. (1979): *Biolog. Psychiat.,* in press.

Heath, R.G., Llewellyn, R.C., and Rouchell, A.M. (1979): Brain mechanisms in psychiatric illness: Rationale for and results of treatment with cerebellar stimulation. In: E.R. Hitchcock, H.T. Ballantine, Jr., and B.A. Meyerson (Eds.), *Modern Concepts in Psychiatric Surgery,* Elsevier/North-Holland Biomedical Press, pp. 77-84.

Jacquet, Y.F., and Marks, N. (1976): The C-fragment of B-lipotropin: An endogenous neuroleptic of anti-psychotogen. *Science 194:* 632.

Knorring, Von L. and Oreland, L. (1978): Visual evoked responses and platlet MAO as an aid to identify a risk group for alcoholic abuse. In: *Progress in Neuropsychopharm. 2:* 385-392.

Lal, H., DeFeo, J.J., Pitterman, A., Patel, G., and Baumel, I. (1972): Effects of prolonged social deprivation or enrichment on neuronal sensitivity for CNS depressants and stimulants. In: *Drug Addiction: Experimental Pharmacology, Vol. I.,* Futura Publishing, New York. pp. 255-266.

Lasagna, L. (1965): *Proc. R. Soc. Med. 58:* 978-983.

Levine, J. (1978): The narcotic antagonist naloxone enhances clinical pain. *Nature 272:* 826-827.

Lichstein, L. and Sackett, G.P. (1971): Reactions by differentially raised rhesus monkeys to noxious stimulation. *Developmental Psychobiology 4:* 339-352.

Lynch, J.J. (1970): Psychophysiology and development of social attachment. *Psychophysiology, 151:* 231-244.

Mason, W.A. (1968): Early social deprivation in the non-human primates: implications for human behavior. In: D.E. Glass (Ed.), *Environmental Influences.* The Rockefeller University Press and Russell Sage Foundation, New York.

Mason, W.A. (1971): Motivational factors in psychosocial development. In: W.J. Arnold and M.M. Page (Eds.), *Nebraska Symposium on Motivation.* University of Nebraska Press.

Mason, W.A. and Kenney, M.D. (1974): Redirection of filial attachments in rhesus monkeys: dogs as mother surrogates. *Science 183:* 1209-1211.

Mason, W.A. and Berkson, G. (1975): Effects of maternal mobility on the development of rocking and other behaviors in rhesus monkeys: a study with artificial mothers. *Developmental Psychobiology 8:* 197-211.

Melzack, R. and Burns, S.K. (1965): Neurophysiological effects of early sensory restriction. *Exp. Neurology 13:* 163-175.

Melzack, R. and Thompson, W.R. (1956): Effects of early experience on social behavior. *Canad. J. Psychol. 10:* 82-90.

Melzack, R. and Scott, T.H. (1957): The effects of early experience on the response to pain. *Journal of Comparative Physiology and Psychology 50:* 155-161.

Meyerson, B.J. and Terenius, L. (1977): Endorphin and male sexual behavior. *European Journal of Pharmacology 42:* 191-192.

Mitchell, G.D. (1968): Persistent behavior pathology in rhesus monkeys following early social isolation. *Folia Primatology 8:* 132-147.

Mitchell, G.D., and Clark, D.L. (1968): Long-term effects of social isolation in nonsocially adapted rehsus monkeys. *The Journal of Genetic Psychology 113:* 117-128.

Mitchell, C.D. (1970): Abnormal behavior in primates. In: L.A. Rosenblum (Ed.), *Primate Behavior: Developments in Field and Laboratory Studies.* Academic Press, New York. 195-249.

Mitchell, G. (1975): What monkeys can tell us about human violence. *The Futurist.* April: 75-80.

Panksepp, J., Herman, B., Conner, R., Bishop, P., and Scott, J.P. (1978): The biology of social attachments: Opiates alleviate separation distress. *Biological Psychiatry 13:* 607-618.

Petrie, A.S. (1978): *Individuality In Pain and Suffering.* University of Chicago Press, Chicago, 1976; Revised and Ed.

Prescott, J.W. (1967): Invited commentary: Central nervous system functioning in altered sensory environments (Cohen, S.I.). In: M.H. Appley, and R. Trumbull (Eds.), *Psychological Stress.* Appleton-Century-Crofts, New York.

Prescott, J.W. (1971): Early somatosensory deprivation as an ontogenetic process in the abnormal development of the brain and behavior. In: I.E. Goldsmith and Moor-Jankowski (Eds.), *Medical Primatology 1970.* Karger, Basel.

Prescott, J.W. (1972): Before ethics and morality. *The Humanist.* Nov/Dec., 19-21.

Prescott, J.W. (1973): Commentary: sexual behavior in the blind. In: A.E. Gillman and A.R. Gordon (Eds.), *Medical Aspects of Human Sexuality.* June: 59-60.

Prescott, J.W. (1975): Body pleasure and the origins of violence. *The Futurist.* April: 64-74.

Prescott, J.W. (1976a): Somatosensory deprivation and its relationship to the blind. In: Z.S. Jasirzembska (Ed.), *The Effects of Blindness and Other Impairments on Early Development.* American Foundation for the Blind, New York.

Prescott, J.W. (1976b): Violence, pleasure and religion. In: *The Bulletin of the Atomic Scientists.* March.

Prescott, J.W. (1977): Phylogenetic and Ontogenetic Aspects of Human Affectional Development. In: R. Gemme and C.C. Wheeler (Eds.), *Selected Proceedings of the 1976 International Congress of Sexology.* Human Sexuality Series (R. Green, Ed.), Plenum Press, New York.

Prescott, J.W. (1979): Deprivation of physical affection as a primary process in the development of physical violence: A comparative and cross-cultural perspective. In: D.G. Gil (Ed.), *Child Abuse and Violence.* American Orthopsychiatric Association, AMS Press, New York. pp. 66-137.

Prescott, J.W. (1971): Sensory deprivation vs. sensory stimulation during early development: A comment on Berkowitz's study. *The Journal of Psychology 77:* 189-191.

Prescott, J.W. (1972): Cannon's Law of Denervation Supersensitivity: Implications for Psychophysiological Assessment. *Psychophysiology 9:* 279 (Abstract).

Prescott, J.W. (1978): Why men dehumanize women: Patriarchy, dualism and monotheism revisited. *Invited Address.* Western Psychological Association Annual Meeting. San Francisco, CA. April 21.

Prescott, J.W. (1979): Alienation of affection. *Psychology Today.* December.

Prescott, J.W. and Wallace, D. (1978): Role of pain and pleasure in the development of destructive behaviors: a psychometric study of parenting, sexuality, substance abuse and criminality. In: Marvin E. Wolfgang, Chair., Laura Otten (Ed.), *Proceedings of Colloquium on the Correlates of Crime and the Determinants of Criminal Behavior.* Center for the Study of the Correlates of Crime and the Determinants of Criminal Behavior. National Institute of Law Enforcement and Criminal Justic. LEAA, Washington, D.C., March.

Prescott, J.W. and Wallace, D. (1976): Developmental sociobiology and the origins of aggressive behavior. *XXIst International Congress of Psychology.* (Read by Dr. Dalmas Taylor.) July, 1976, Paris.

Reich, W. (1973): *The Mass Psychology of Fascism.* Farrar, Straus and Giroux, New York. (New Trans. 1969, 5th Printing.)

Reis, D.J., Doba, N., and Nathan, M.A. (1973): Predatory attack, grooming, and consummatory behaviors evoked by electrical stimulation of cat cerebellar nuclei. *Science 182:* 845-847.

Riesen, A.H. (1961): Excessive arousal effects of stimulation after early sensory deprivation. In: P. Solomon et al., (Eds.), *Sensory Deprivation.* Harvard University Press, Cambridge, Mass. 34-40.

Riesen. A.H. (1960): Effects of stimulus deprivation on the development and atrophy of the visual sensory system. *Amer. J. Orthopsychiat. 30:* 23-36.

Riesen, A.H. (1961): Stimulation as a requirement for growth and function. In: Fiske and Maddi (Eds.), *Functions of Varied Experience.* Dorsey Press, Homewood.

Riesen, A.H. (1964): Effects of visual deprivation of perceptual function and the neural substrate. In: d'ajuriaguerre (Ed.), *Deafferentation Experimentale et Clinique.* Symposium, Bel Air. 47-66.

Rosenzweig, M.R., Drech, D., Bennett, E.L., and Diamond, M.C. (1968): Modifying brain chemistry and anatomy by enrichment or impoverishment of experience. In: G. Newton and S. Levine (Eds.), *Early Experience and Behavior.* Charles C. Thomas, Springfield. 258-298.

Sackett, G.P. (1970): Unlearned responses, differential rearing experiences, and the development of social attachments by rhesus monkeys. In: L.A. Rosenblum (Ed.), *Primate Behavior: Developments in Field and Laboratory Research,* Vol. 1. Academic Press, New York. 111-140.

Saltzberg, B. (1976): A model to relating ripples in the EEG power spectral density to transient patterns of brain electrical activity induced by sucortical spiking. In: *IEEE Transactions of Biomedical Engineering 23:* 355-356.

Saltzberg, B. Lustick, L.S., and Heath, R.G. (1971): Detection of focal depth spiking in the scalp EEG of monkeys. *Electroencephal. Clin. Neurophysiol. 31:* 327-833.

Saltzberg, B. and Lustick, L.S. (1975): Signal analysis: An overview of EEG applications. In: J.W. Prescott, M.S. Read, and D.B. Coursin (Eds.), *Brain Function and Malnutrition: Neuropsychological Methods of Assessment.* John Wiley & Sons, New York.

Schaffer, H.R. and Emerson, P.E. (1964): Patterns of response to physical contact in early human development. *J. Child Psychol. and Psychiat. 5:* 1-13.

Schaffer, H.R. and Emerson, P.E. (1964): The development of social attachment in infancy. *Monogr. Soc. Res. Child Develop. 3:* 1-77.

Sharpless, S.K. (1975): Disuse supersensitivity. In: A.H. Riesen (Ed.), *The Developmental Neuropsychology of Sensory Deprivation*. Academic Press, New York.

Spitz, R.A. (1945): Hospitalism: An inquiry into the genesis of psychiatric conditions in early childhood. *Psychoanalytic Study of the Child 1:* 53-74.

Spitz, R.A. (1965): *The First Year of Life*. International University Press, New York.

Struble, R.G. and Riesen. A.H. (1978): Changes in cortical dendritic branching subsequent to partial social isolation in stumptailed monkeys. *Developmental Psychobiology 11:* 479-486.

Suomi. S.J. and Harlow, H.F. (1972): Social rehabilitation of isolate-reared monkeys. *Developmental Psychology 6:* 487-496.

Teilhand de Chardin, P. (1975): The evolution of chastity (1933). In: *Toward the Future*. Harcourt-Brace Jovanovich, New York.

Valzelli, L. (1967): Drugs and aggressiveness. In: *Advances in Pharmacology, V. 5,* 79-108.

Welch, B.L. and Welch, A.S. (1969): Aggression and the biogenic amine neurohumors. In: Garattini and Sigs (Eds.), *The Biology of Aggressive Behavior*. Excerpta Medica Foundation, Amsterdam.

Zubek, J.P. (Ed.) (1969): *Sensory Deprivation: Fifteen Years of Research*. Appleton-Century-Crofts, New York.

Zuckerman, M. (1979): *Sensation Seeking: Beyond the Optimal Level of Arousal*. Lawrence Erlbaum Assoc., Hillsdale, New Jersey.

3

Neurotransmitter and Neuropeptide Correlates of Cigarette Smoking

Athan Karras

Cigarette smoking is a well-recognized pernicious habit that is difficult to break. Nicotine, the alkaloid in cigarette smoke, is considered the primary reinforcer in smoking (Jarvik, 1970; Russell, 1976; Schachter, 1977). Thus smoking is the means by which the habitual user (addict) receives his nicotine fix. As with other addictions, its maintenance is considered to be the resultant of pharmacological, social, and psychological factors. In fact, smokers themselves attribute many reasons for their smoking, ranging from tension release and satisfaction from sensori-motor manipulation of a cigarette and feeling comfortable in social situations, to preventing withdrawal symptoms (McKennell, 1970).

A powerful drug, nicotine affects many biological systems. A review of its pervasive biological effects may be found in *Smoking and Health: A Report of the Surgeon General* (1979). We will concentrate on its neuro-humoral actions. In addition to reviewing the literature on its addicting potential, we shall survey its effects on the cholinergic and adrenergic receptor systems, and its effects on the adrenopituitary axis (ACTH and corticosteroids). Implications regarding the release of Beta endorphin and its role in smoking maintenance will be reviewed, with reference to pilot work in our laboratory that supports the hypothesis that the endorphins, and especially Beta endorphin, are involved in smoking maintenance.

NICOTINE AS THE SUBSTANCE OF INTEREST

It is possible that chronic smoking may be solely or primarily psychologically maintained. A pack-a-day smoker takes more than 50,000 puffs yearly, and reasons given by the smoker often seem to reflect psychological factors, such as the reduction of stress from daily life events by indulging in a familiar habit that offers oral satisfaction (Jacobs et al., 1970). Thus engaging in smoking behaviors (overt and covert) are positively reinforcing (Hunt, 1970; Mausner and Platt, 1971).

An alternative explanation attributes the maintenance of smoking through the positive reinforcing properties of pharmacological agents and the negative reinforcing properties of the smoking abstinence syndrome. That is, smoking is the manifestation of physical dependence on one or more substances taken in by the smoker. Of all the constituents that have been extracted from cigarettes, nicotine is the primary contender, with tar being considered a weak but possible runner up. Tar is defined as all particulate phase constituents minus nicotine and water vapor (*Smoking and Health*, 1979).

The essential criterion for establishing the addicting properties of a substance is the development of dependence upon it, preceded by tolerance, that is less reactivity (behaviorally and physiologically) to it. It is obvious that those who continue to smoke develop tolerance to many of its effects: nausea disappears, as does choking on the smoke inhaled; tachycardia in the novice subsides into a moderately accelerated heart rate in the chronic smoker. Tolerance can begin immediately; Stolerman et al. (1973) found that tolerance developed in rats regarding locomotor behavior after only a single pretreatment of nicotine.

It is less obvious that there is physical dependence upon any of the constituents of cigarette smoke, including nicotine. Criteria for physical dependence, in addition to tolerance, include the primary reinforcing qualities of a substance, the precipitation of an abstinence syndrome in its absence, and the avoidance of the abstinence syndrome. We find that the overwhelming body of the research on the dependence potential of tobacco substances investigates dose-effect relationships between nicotine and various physiological and behavioral responses. The methods used are titration effects, the appearance of an abstinence syndrome and its avoidance. In fact reports on titration effects can be considered investigations of the abstinence syndrome.

An excellent and comprehensive review of the titration studies that suggest that nicotine produces dependence may be found in Russell (1976). Briefly, a number of investigators have shown that when cigarettes with greater amounts of nicotine are substituted for the smoker's usual brand, the number of cigarettes consumed drops; there is an opposite effect when lower than usual nicotine cigarettes are smoked (*e.g.*, Finnegan et al., 1945; Russell et al., 1975). However, these studies were not conducted blind. Further, it appears that subjects easily adjust downward but do not appear to compensate upward adequately when they smoke low nicotine cigarettes. Some of the reasons for the latter effect are that the subject may have had to increase smoking to such an extent, because nicotine content was extremely low, that puffing became too hard and too much effort was required.

In a study conducted double-blind, Schachter (1977) found that subjects who were chronic, heavy smokers smoked significantly fewer high nicotine than low nicotine cigarettes in a natural setting. When they smoked low nicotine cigarettes the heavy smokers reported that they were dissatisfied with the cigarettes and experienced withdrawal. For the light smokers (15 or fewer cigarettes per day and with erratic smoking habits) there was no significant difference in the number smoked for the two types of cigarettes.

It appears however that the means by which nicotine is delivered may be important. For example, nicotine administered intravenously must be administered in large doses for smoking to be reduced (Lucchesi et al., 1967); if it is not, no effect is apparent (Kumar et al., 1977). Kumar et al. (1977) found that tobacco smoke with varying amounts of nicotine that were inhaled through a special apparatus did cut down on cigarette consumption, but that nicotine received intravenously did not. This study presents a problem however; the baseline values on days when nicotine was administered intravenously were very similar to the final values of the inhaled tobacco condition, suggesting that for the intravenous condition subjects were at their minimum level at the start of the session. The use of other kinds of substitutes for cigarette smoking, such as nicotine or lobeline-impregnated gum have led to mixed results, with the best results, when obtained under double-blind conditions, indicating only small decreases in cigarette consumption with nicotine-dosed gum (Gritz and Jarvik, 1977).

Thus the consistent findings with the use of titration methods are obtained when cigarettes with varying nicotine doses are used. But, as nicotine content is correlated with the amount of tar, it is possible that the smoker is titrating tar intake. This possibility seems a weak one. Finnegan et al. (1945) and Schachter et al. (1977) had wide variations in the nicotine levels of their cigarettes while tar was held constant or virtually so. Goldfarb et al. (1976) manipulated both variables. All three studies, the latter two conducted blind, found that subjects regulated the number of cigarettes according to the nicotine content of the cigarette.

Virtually all studies using the titration model report the number of cigarettes smoked or puffs taken but do not give actual nicotine levels of the body fluids of the subjects. Exceptions are the studies by Goldfarb et al. (1976) and Russell et al. (1975), with the former measuring urinary nicotine levels and the latter the amount of nicotine in blood plasma. When low nicotine brands were smoked both urinary and blood plasma levels were noticeably below levels found when the subject smoked his own brand. With the high nicotine cigarettes urine and blood plasma nicotine levels were very similar to those found with the subject's usual brand. The latter finding for urinary levels was found with the second substudy in Goldfarb et al. (1976), which was the one in which the subject was blind as to the nicotine content of the experimental cigarettes.

As nicotine probably stimulates the release of peripheral adrenergic transmitters, Beta adrenergic antagonists have been used to determine the addiction potential of nicotine. Carruthers (1976), in a randomized cross-over double-blind study, had smokers smoke three high and three low nicotine cigarettes, while receiving placebo or oxprenolol, a Beta adrenergic blocker. Each batch of cigarettes was smoked within a half hour. Many of the physiological effects usually associated with rapid smoking were inhibited, such as rapid heart beat and elevated blood pressure, but not the rise in catecholamines, especially in this instance noradrenaline (NA). Smoking satisfaction was unimpaired, suggesting that autonomic arousal was not a factor in the satisfaction derived from smoking.

Stolerman et al. (1973) tested the effects of two nicotine antagonists on *ad lib* smoking; one pentolinium, acts peripherally, while the other, mecamylamine, has central as well as peripheral effects. The theory was that the blockade of peripheral and/or central nicotine receptors of the cholinergic system would enhance the amount of smoking and decrease smoking satisfaction, since the antagonist(s) would displace nicotine at the receptor sites. Drugs or placebo were administered double-blind to all subjects. Mecamylamine produced these effects and more, as subjects also reported feeling dysphoric in general. As hand steadiness improved, which has been noticed by others when smokers have no nicotine or low levels of it (Frankenhaeuser et al., 1968; Myrsten et al., 1972), the beginnings of an abstinence syndrome may have been induced, which would also account for feelings of dysphoria. However, as the subjective effects of the drug on nonsmokers were not reported, the possibility of an abstinence syndrome should be only tentatively considered. In contrast, various pentolinium dosages primarily had no effects.

A partial animal analogue of the titration paradigm is the self-administration of nicotine in animals. Hanson et al. (1979) have shown that rats self-administered nicotine at rates significantly higher than control levels and that there appeared to be a positive relationship between nicotine dose level and rate of responding. The animals also appeared to exhibit tolerance, as their response rate dropped over time when nicotine dose was kept constant. Further, the rats showed the usual extinction pattern associated with cessation of positive reinforcers following the cessation of nicotine during their responding: there was an upsurge in response level before extinction. Finally, an acute dose of mecamylamine but not of pentolinium increased response rate, indicating the central action of nicotine through nicotine-sensitive cholinergic receptors. Goldberg et al. (1981), using a different species and method, have also demonstrated that nicotine can function as an effective reinforcer under a second-order schedule of administration (*i.e.*, the development of conditioned reinforcing properties through nicotine intake).

Very recently Abood and his colleagues appear to have located noncholinergic sites for the action of nicotine in the brain (Abood et al., 1978, 1979).

The usual anticholinergic drugs, such as d-tubocurarine, were not effective antagonists in reversing prostration effects in rats administered nicotine intraventricularly. However derivatives of nicotine or piperdine, such as N-benzyl, acted as antagonists. Pursuing these leads, Romano and Goldstein (1980) strongly suggest that these findings do not necessarily imply that nicotine effects are produced through another, as yet unchartered, receptor system. Their findings still implicate the cholinergic system; however the anomalous effects of nicotine in *in vitro* studies need investigating.

When a drug that supposedly produces physical dependence is withdrawn an abstinence syndrome is expected to appear. Using the term "syndrome" implies a typical symptom picture associated with the condition, with the appearance of symptoms dependent on the length of dependence and drug dosage. The abstinence syndromes in opiate and ethanol withdrawal are the most thoroughly documented and serve as models.

Although the large majority of chronic smokers report discomfort upon cessation, there appears to be a variety of cessation symptoms rather than a syndrome. Other than craving and irritability some smokers report attacks of anxiety, weepiness, diarrhea, and profuse sweating, whereas others describe a very different set of symptoms. Shiffman and Jarvik (1976) found that smoking symptoms could be grouped into four factors through factor analysis, namely stimulation, craving, physical and psychological symptoms, each with its own time course in appearing and subsiding. However, in addition to a small sample size, there is no information on the factor loadings of the items within each grouping, which would determine the consistency of their appearance as a cluster.

Another expected characteristic of an abstinence syndrome is that the strength of the addiction determines the appearance of symptoms and their severity. The evidence is inconsistent in smoking withdrawal. *Smoking and Health* (1979) summarizes the different findings on this issue and offers an excellent and pithy exposition of the problems that cloud the answer, one of which will be elaborated upon.

It is clear that abstinence symptoms can also appear with deprivation of stimuli upon which a person is only psychologically dependent. Homesickness is one such example. Certain kinds of physiological signs, such as body temperature, are considered to be more likely the result of abstinence from a physically dependent substance. Fägerström (1978) found such a statistically significant relationship with a questionnaire that measured strength of smoking dependence. The body temperature of the more dependent smoker decreased more upon smoking cessation. Other examples of changes in physiological reactivity with extended abstinence are reduced adrenalin but not noradrenalin excretion (Myrsten et al., 1977). The comparatively heightened NA values may explain the irritability often found in abstemious smokers, as excessive

NA has often been associated with aggression (Buck, 1976). Changes in EEG patterns may also help to define an abstinence syndrome. Rhythmical activity decreased and tended to resemble sleep-like patterns during a period of smoking deprivation (Itel et al., 1971; Ulett and Itel, 1969). The effects were reversed when smoking was resumed.

This review of the possibly physically addicting potential of nicotine strongly supports such a claim. The evidence from each of the various viewpoints is never sufficient however for clear confirmation, but Schachter and his colleagues (1977) note that the apparently large number of striking exceptions to the rule that smokers smoke to titrate their nicotine levels can readily be matched by the ease with which the evaluation of such incidents, whether anecdotal or research, demonstrates that they were poorly documented or investigated. As with other addictions, smoking maintenance most probably includes psychological and sociological factors, which we have not reviewed, our point being that nicotine is the necessary condition.

If nicotine is addicting, what systems does it affect that may be responsible for its effects? We shall review two that are often cited, namely the cholinergic and adrenergic receptor systems and two others that our pilot work appears to implicate, the adreno-corticotropic-Beta endorphin systems.

THE CHOLINERGIC SYSTEM

Nicotine has complex effects on the nervous system that are a result of its action on a variety of neurotransmitters. It has two phases of action, mimicking cholinergic activity in small doses, but with larger doses first stimulating cholinergic neurons and then blocking their firing (Volle and Koelle, 1975). Its effects are so pervasive that about the only receptors that are seldom affected are muscarinic-type cholinergic receptors; otherwise it readily alters synaptic transmission in the central nervous system, autonomic ganglia and at postjunctional autonomic sites (Russell, 1976). As we have seen earlier, its effects on ganglionic cholinergic receptors, however, do not seem to be as important as those on the brain for regulating the smoker's requirements for nicotine.

Nicotine appears to have a variety of effects on the cholinergic receptor system in the brain. Mecamylamine, a nicotine antagonist that acts centrally as well as peripherally, lowered systolic blood pressure in smokers and non-smokers alike, and increased the number of cigarettes smoked by chronic smokers (Stolerman et al., 1973). This finding suggests that nicotine has stimulus-cueing properties that act through the cholinergic system. The question arises as to whether neurotransmitters other than acetylcholine (Ach) share in such nicotine stimulus properties. Hirshhorn and Rosecrans (1974) found that nicotine could be used to cue rats when food was available. Its stimulus property could be antagonised only by mecamylamine; muscarinic, adrenergic (A), and NA antagonists were ineffective.

The effects of nicotine on electrical cortical activity appear to be mediated however by both muscarinic (Guha and Pradhan, 1976) and nicotinic receptors (Domino, 1967; Hall, 1970). Guha and Pradhan (1976) showed that initial nicotine effects on the EEG and auditory-evoked potentials were suppressed by scopolamine, a muscarine antagonist; no nicotine antagonists were applied to determine if muscarine activity was mediated through nicotine receptors. Domino (1967) and Hall (1970) showed that EEG changes from nicotine and their behavioral consequences could be eliminated with mecamylamine. A comprehensive review of the neuropharmacology of nicotine can be found in Domino (1973).

The above studies imply that nicotine has a direct effect on Ach release in the brain (such effects have been found in other areas of the central nervous system, namely for Renshaw cells; see Domino, 1973). Essman (1973) has recently shown that nicotine uptake in the rat cerebral cortex affects concentrations of total bound and vesicular Ach; these decrease, whereas the concentration of the Ach pool is unaffected.

Segal et al. (1978) have actually demonstrated that there are cholinergic muscarinic and nicotinic receptors in rat brain through biochemical and autoradiographic techniques. Most of the limbic forebrain structures contain nicotinic receptors, with the hippocampus and hypothalamus displaying especially high concentrations. The neocortex has an abundance of both receptors; in fact in contrast to the above sites there was no clear anatomical dissociation of the two receptors in this area, which may explain why Guha and Pradhan (1976) found that scopolamine suppressed nicotinic effects (see above).

This review of the effects of nicotine on the cholinergic receptor system, in conjunction with our earlier summary of its role in self-administration, strongly suggests that the cholinergic influence on perception and behavior is profound when nicotine is administered.

THE CATECHOLAMINE SYSTEM

Several investigators have suggested that nicotine, mimicking Ach, releases NA peripherally and perhaps centrally, and that its release is primarily responsible for self-stimulation in animals receiving nicotine (Pradhan and Bose, 1978; Schechter and Rosecrans, 1972), and in smoking maintenance (Carruthers, 1976; Jarvik, 1970). Several lines of research suggest a brain reward system that implicates amine pathways, especially NA, although the dopamine and serotonin systems may be involved (Olds, 1977). Thus, through elevated NA secretion, smokers can supposedly modulate their level of arousal, leading to optimal performance and subjective comfort (Frankenhaeuser et al., 1971). Schildkraut et al. (1975) observed that heroin addicts who had stronger rushes from intravenous injections of opiates and were more aggressive in demanding their drugs had NA levels during the addiction phase that were above those at the preaddiction phase; those who had less pronounced positive effects and less aggressive drug seeking behavior had no differences in NA values for the two phases.

The idea that nicotine releases NA derives from the formulation of Burn and Rand (1959) that Ach is the means by which a post-ganglionic sympathetic nerve impulse releases NA. Their hypothesis is analgous to the mechanism for the release of A from the adrenal medulla and would account for such physiological effects of smoking as elevations in blood pressure, heart rate and free fatty acids. With few exceptions, investigators report increased A levels in chronic smokers (*e.g.*, Kershbaum et al., 1968; Watts and Bragg, 1956; Winternitz and Quillen, 1977), with higher levels being associated with higher nicotine levels (Frankenhaeuser et al., 1970; Watts and Bragg, 1956). The exceptions include Cryer et al. (1974) and Tucci and Sode (1972), who found no differences between smokers and nonsmokers on a variety of biochemical measures.

The release of NA with smoking is less clearly established, even in those studies that report the release of A. In a series of controlled studies by Frankenhaeuser and her colleagues, urinary NA values under various smoking conditions were either the same as under a nonsmoking condition (Frankenhaeuser et al., 1970; Myrsten et al., 1972) or less than it (Frankenhaeuser et al., 1968). The latter finding was calculated by the present author from the data in the graphs and by statistically comparing the combined smoking conditions against the nonsmoking one. In fact a similar trend was found in the Frankenhaeuser et al. (1970) study. Yet all of these studies found higher A levels for the smoking conditions.

Similarly Watts and Bragg (1956) and Winternitz and Quillen (1977) found no difference in NA levels between smoking and nonsmoking conditions. Nicotine content of the cigarettes used and frequency of smoking appeared to meet the conditions of having the smokers absorb adequate amounts of the drug. In fact in some of the studies relatively high doses of nicotine were absorbed in short periods of time.

Similar negative results have been reported for urinary NA when smokers have been compared to nonsmokers over an eight hour (Watts and Bragg, 1956) or 24 hour period (Tucci and Sode, 1972). Thus under smoking conditions urinary NA levels do not appear unusually high when examined under conditions in which the smoker (a) is his own control, (b) is compared to nonsmokers, (c) performs in a laboratory setting, or (d) performs under (brief) natural conditions.

However, when plasma NA levels are measured, then greater amounts are found when chronic smokers smoke than when they do not (Carruthers, 1976; Cryer et al. 1974). A careful examination of the procedures in both of these studies indicates that (a) subjects were chronic smokers; (b) the smoking regimen approximated natural smoking conditions; (c) the heightened excretion could not be accounted for by exertion from smoking, as Cryer et al. (1974) had a sham smoking condition; and (d) the NA release appeared to be dose-related, with more excretion occurring from cigarettes with relatively high nicotine content (1.9 mg) (Carruthers, 1976).

Another important question is the source of plasma NA, whether it is peripheral or central in origin. Both Carruthers (1976) and Cryer et al. (1974) introduced NA antagonists with primarily peripheral blocking action, oxprenolol and propranolol (Beta blockers), and phenotolamine (alpha blocker). Both studies reported that the blockers suppressed many physiological responses that can be peripherally augmented by NA, such as blood pressure, heart beat and fatty acids. But NA levels were unaffected by the blockers and Carruthers (1976), who determined smoking satisfaction during the blockade, found it unaffected. Cryer et al. (1974) found that measurements of central biochemical effects of NA were intact or almost so, even under blockade. For example plasma levels of cortisol were unaffected by the blockade and growth hormone levels were only mildly so. However, as we shall see below, he may have been misled as to which transmitter activates cortisol.

It would be important to know of any direct evidence of central NA release. We know of no studies that measure 3 methoxy-4-hydroxy-phenylglycol (MHPG) levels in the cerebral-spinal fluid in relation to cigarette smoking. Anywhere from 30 to 70 percent of urinary MHPG reflects brain release of NA (Maas et al., 1976). Schildkraut et al. (1975) found that their addicts who had a more profound heroin effect had elevated NA levels, as indicated by urinary MHPG values, but not through other measures of NA that presumably are more likely to reflect peripheral levels.

Thus it appears that NA is released in a dose-dependent manner by the nicotine that accumulates under normal smoking conditions. In addition, blood plasma levels may be the more appropriate measure for measuring peripheral effects, and urinary MHPG values for roughly estimating central effects.

EFFECTS ON THE ADRENOPITUITARY SYSTEM

We have already noted some of the stimulant effects of smoking on cardiovascular responses. Other cardiovascular consequences are an increase in cardiac output and stroke volume (Irving and Yamamoto, 1963; Kerrigan et al., 1968). Its long-term effects on the heart are considered to be profoundly unhealthful and coronary heart disease appears to be the most important single cause of mortality among cigarette smokers (*The Smoking Digest,* 1977). Most research has concentrated on the effects on sympathetic stimulation of the catecholamines on cardiovascular performance, but more recently interest has turned to examining the possibility of increased adrenal cortical activity. This condition may result in chronically high corticosteroid levels and a consequent step-up of cholesterol synthesis which may have atherogenic implications (Barrett, 1966).

Several investigators have reported that corticosteroid levels were higher in smokers during a smoking condition as compared to an abstinence condition (Kershbaum et al., 1968; Winternitz and Quillen, 1977), or when compared to nonsmokers (Cheraskin et al., 1975; Cryer et al., 1974; Kershbaum et al., 1968). Differences were found whether plasma levels of cortisol or 24 hour urinary levels of hydroxycorticoids were measured. Cheraskin et al. (1975) also reported that heavier smokers had higher urinary steroid levels than a mixed group of nonsmokers and light smokers.

On the other hand Hökfelt (1961) and Tucci and Sode (1972) did not find differences in blood or urine between nonsmoking and smoking conditions for smokers or between smokers and nonsmokers. Hökfelt (1961) found however that nonsmokers who smoked and inhaled did have higher plasma cortisol levels, and concluded that the release of corticosteroids may be the consequence of an acute stress condition to which the chronic smoker has adapted.

A review of the methods of the studies that yield both kinds of findings reveals nothing startlingly different between them. Winternitz and Quillen (1977) heavily saturated their subjects with nicotine, but then Cryer et al. (1974) did not. One possible difference with regard to cortisol plasma levels is that positive findings were obtained by having frequent blood samples drawn (Cryer et al., 1974; Kershbaum et al., 1968) or by having an indwelling catheter (Winternitz and Quillen, 1977). Hökfelt (1961) and Tucci and Sode (1972) did not use such procedures. Sauerbier and Mayersbach (1977) have demonstrated that 24 hour mean values and the circadian pattern of NA plasma levels are affected by the mode of sampling. Frequent venipuncture in the course of 24 hours results in more stable and lower NA levels throughout the sampling period than venipuncture samples from subjects used only once. These findings may also be relevant to the activation of cortisol, which is released under conditions of stress. Infrequent sampling may lead to a stress reaction in smokers and nonsmokers that may mask the effects of nicotine.

If corticosteroids are released, is the mechanism peripheral through increased sympathetic activity, or central, through ACTH? No one has measured ACTH release during smoking. There is indirect evidence from animal and human studies that ACTH should be released during smoking. Kershbaum et al. (1968) reviewed earlier studies using animal work which indicated that nicotine did not appear to act directly on adrenal cortical tissue. However from the findings from the animal preparations in their study they proposed that ACTH release was the result of a nicotine-induced increase in sympathetic and adrenergic activity. Rubin and Warner (1975) have gone even further and have shown that nicotine can stimulate directly isolated adrenocortical cells of the cat; these results were from *in vitro* studies so that the effect of inducing a significant release of corticosteroids through this means under *in vivo* conditions has not been established.

Cam et al. (1979) have recently reported that acute administration of nicotine *in vivo* increases plasma steroid levels in rats, which is completely abolished by hypophysectomy. These findings indicate that the adrenal response to nicotine is most probably mediated through pituitary ACTH. Of importance to the present review is that the plasma nicotine concentrations and the elevated plasma steroid levels in their animals were extremely similar to those typically found in chronic smokers (Isaac and Rand, 1972; Russell and Feyerabend, 1975).

There is also a problem in evaluating the degree of involvement of ACTH through measuring cortisol. ACTH is secreted periodically spontaneously in quantities that do not release corticosteroids (Krieger, 1977). It is possible that chronic smoking may enhance such slippage in order to control corticosteroid levels.

A review of the role of the adrenopituitary axis in smoking indicates that the conditions under which it is activated (if at all) in chronic smoking is unclear and the means for measuring its activation may not be valid. It is important to resolve these problems not only for their health implications, but as we shall see, for their role in maintaining the smoking habit.

EFFECTS ON THE ENDORPHINS AND BETA LIPOTROPIN HORMONE (BLPH)

If corticosteroids are released in chronic smoking and if the release is through ACTH, then BLPH and Beta endorphin (BE) should also be released. Guillemin et al. (1977) first reported that every acute stress that they applied that released ACTH into rat blood also released simultaneously BE in equimolar amounts. Mains et al. (1977) have shown that ACTH and BLPH have a common precursor and that ACTH, BLPH and BE are stored and released together. Loh (1979) has recently reported that these peptides may derive from two common peptides. At this time BLPH appears to be the prohormone for BE, which corresponds to the C fragment of BLPH (residues 61-91) which Li and Chung (1976) obtained from camel pituitaries. Li et al. (1978) reported that the human pituitary synthesizes BE. This work has been confirmed by Chrétien et al. (1979) who have also reported that human BE is synthesized de novo from BLPH. It appears that all three peptides also coexist in brain cells (Akil et al., 1978). However, depending on the brain region, BLPH levels are at least 70 to 700 times less than those found in the pituitary (Akil et al., 1978). Coexistence of the three in the brain should have been expected once brain ACTH was reported in animals (Krieger et al., 1977) and humans (Pelletier and Desy, 1978). It also appears that ACTH and BE levels closely parallel each other under resting or stress conditions in humans; this association may not be detected if cortisol is used to infer ACTH activity (Carr et al., 1981; Wiedemann et al., 1979).

BE is one of the peptides of one of two subsystems of the endogenous opiate system; the other group is called the enkephalins. The generic term for the opioid peptides of the two systems is endorphin and all appear to derive from BLPH (Loh and Li, 1977), with the enkephalins being smaller fractions (pentapeptides). These substances appear to be the endogenous ligands of the receptors of their respective subsystems. Their distribution, which is being mapped by several research teams, includes the neural pain system (peripheral and central), pituitary, the brain, such as the hypothalamus, amygdala, periaqueductal gray matter, and other organs, such as the gut and adrenal medulla. Each subsystem has its own pathways (*e.g.,* Jacquet, 1978; Schultzberg et al., 1978; Snyder et al., 1975; Wiegant et al., 1977). At this time enkephalin pathways have been mapped in all these areas but not in regions of the pituitary which contain ACTH, BLPH and BE (Cox et al., 1978; Rossier et al., 1979a). Because the two more frequently studied enkephalins—leu and met—are degraded very rapidly their role is postulated to be analogous to transmitters, whereas the much longer lasting BE is considered to have hormone-like activity and to exhibit greater opiate-like activity than the enkephalins with regard to producing analgesia, inducing physical dependence and in displacing nalaxone (NAL), an opiate antagonist (see Kosterlitz and Hughes, 1978, for a summary). However its greater potency may be the result of its longer lasting action.

One of the major riddles is to determine the physiological role of the endorphins. The first predicted effect was their mediation of pain, which has been firmly established through animal and human studies. The most consistent effects found were that NAL blocked acupuncture analgesia in mice (Pomeranz and Chiu, 1976) and in man (Mayer et al., 1977), reduced the latency in mice and rats for escape from a noxious stimulus (Jacob et al., 1974) and lowered pain threshold in human placebo responders (Levine et al., 1978, 1979). All of these findings support the notion that endorphins may be involved in pain but they do not prove it.

More recent studies have shown directly that human BE has analgesic activity in people suffering from chronic, clinical pain but not from acute pain experimentally inflicted (Hosobuchi and Li, 1978). Pomeranz (1978) has reported a series of studies in which endorphins have been implicated more directly through the use of acupuncture. Hypophysectomy, which abolished acupuncture analgesia by removing the primary source of BE, and genetic studies which showed that mice deficient in opiate receptors did not show acupuncture analgesia (whereas their parent strains, which have no such deficiency, do) seem to be convincing. Most recently stimulation of human periaqueductal gray matter has brought relief for chronic pain sufferers and increases in BE in their ventricular fluid (Hosobuchi et al., 1979).

The effects of the endorphins appear to extend to other behaviors and physiological systems not previously considered opiate-related. NAL relieves endotoxin hypotension (Holaday and Faden, 1978), suppresses behavioral effects of d-amphetamine (Dettmar et al., 1978), may reverse acute alcohol intoxication (Markley and Mezery, 1978) and nitrous oxide analgesia (Berkowitz et al., 1977), and enhances copulatory behavior in sexually inactive animals (Gessa et al., 1979). This list is far from being complete. We shall summarize in more detail its possible relationship to food and water consumption, and smoking, all of which appear to implicate BE and the adrenopituitary axis to a greater degree than other endorphins. The putative interactions of all of these behaviors with the endorphins is made via NAL, a drug with remarkably high specificity for some classes of opiate receptors. It is possible however, that because of the diversity of the behaviors and systems it affects, it is less specific in its action than is currently recognized.

Margules et al. (1978) have found that excessive BE (but not leu-enkephalin) appears to be associated with overeating in genetically obese mice and rats. These mice also have markedly elevated ACTH levels as compared to their normal litter mates. NAL produced a dose-related suppression of food intake in both the obese and normal animals, but the effect was profound for the obese groups. The authors point out that BE acts on the pancreas to stimulate insulin release and appetite increase, and that the implication is that the blockade of BE by NAL reduces insulin release and a decrease of appetite. Rossier et al. (1979b) have shown that the enkephalins may very well play a role in the early stages of the animal's becoming obese and dispute the primacy of BE as the endorphin contributing to the evolution of the condition. However, it may help maintain it once it is established.

The effects of the endorphins appear to apply to the food and water consumption of normal animals. Holtzman (1979) obtained similar results in a different strain of rats with normal weight. He measured water consumption as well as food consumption and found that water consumption in thirsty animals provided the more reliable findings. In order to determine if the effect was due to possible suppression of behavior in general, he tested the effect on animals that had been morphine-dependent but had undergone opiate abstinence for several days prior to being tested. There were no differences between this group and a nonaddicted group in appetite suppression, even though the previously addicted subjects still exhibited greater analgesic tolerance to morphine than the nonaddicted ones. Similar findings have been obtained for food intake in animals under normal conditions (Brands et al., 1979) and under diazepam-enhanced intake (Stapleton et al., 1979).

It appears that only one study has attempted to associate the endorphins with smoking. Malizia et al. (1978) treated 15 abstinent chronic smokers with electropuncture to reduce their withdrawal symptoms. A subgroup of smokers (size unknown) that responded to the acupuncture by "experiencing the repulsion against tobacco" (p. 362) were given NAL or saline solution shortly before the end of the treatment for that day. NAL reversed the tobacco repulsion, and in fact, a strong urge to smoke returned. Saline solution had no effect on repulsion. The report appears to be a preliminary one, and no data are provided. Another problem in evaluating it is that NAL was always given first, so that at best the study is single-blind. In response to a letter by the author, Dr. Malizia stated that in many cases abstinent smokers needed additional treatment cycles, which were progressively less effective (personal communication, dated 4/23/79).

Even if BE, released through acupuncture, reduced craving and other abstinence symptoms of smoking, this fact would not necessarily involve it in smoking maintenance. It is possible that smoking abstinence enhances comparative NA levels (Myrsten et al., 1977). The release of BE during abstinence could then reduce the relative imbalance, relieving the abstinence symptoms. This model has been proposed by Gold et al. (1979) to account for the amelioration of the opiate abstinence syndrome with clonidine, an alpha-2-adrenergic agonist that blocks the action of NA in the locus coeruleus; empirical verification of the hypothesis has been reported by Aghajanian (1978) through recordings of individual neurons in the locus coeruleus which are affected either by NAL or clonidine but not by both.

However, there is other circumstantial evidence that implicates BE in smoking. Smokers smoke more during the afternoon (Meade and Wald, 1977) and those abstaining are most uncomfortable in the afternoon (Shiffman and Jarvik, 1976). These findings coincide with the larger amount of ACTH (and presumably BE) excreted during the morning than during the latter part of the day. Such diurnal variation has also been noticed for rats regarding pain sensitivity, except the hours are reversed because of their nocturnal habits (Frederickson et al., 1977), in normal humans in pain (Davis et al., 1978), and in intractable pain sufferers (Folkard et al., 1976). Further, these same studies showed that NAL lowered the thresholds for the rats in the evening and for normals in the morning, but had little or no effect on pain thresholds in morning for rats (when BE would be at its lowest) and in the afternoon for normals (when BE would be at its lowest). Again, the findings are circumstantial but they strongly support the hypothesis that BE is probably involved in smoking.

If the endorphins, and especially BE, are involved in smoking maintenance, should NAL cause an abstinence syndrome in smokers? Before answering the question, we believe that from the data presented above a two-factor theory of addiction is needed to predict narcotic antagonist effects. If the endorphin sytem is the primary system involved, as in opiate addiction, then NAL should enhance craving and precipitate an abstinence syndrome. If it is an intermediary, then NAL should moderate the action of endorphins on the primary system, without necessarily precipitating an abstinence syndrome. For example, no abstinence symptoms were found as part of the effects of NAL on the systems reported above which previously had not been thought of as primarily involving opiate receptor sites (*e.g.,* food and water consumption). In order to avoid circular reasoning, a means must be found to determine the nature of involvement of the endorphins that is not based solely on NAL effects.

Perhaps applying one or more of the following three criteria can avoid circularity: (a) nonopiate receptors for which the drug (substance) is a ligand have been identified (*e.g.,* nicotine receptors); (b) a naturally occurring physiological or biochemical imbalance is controlled to some extent by another system (*e.g.,* appetite or thirst); and (c) chronic administration of standard doses of the drug (substance) do not produce intoxication (*e.g.,* food or water), even if addicting (*e.g.,* nicotine). Using criteria (a) and (c) for nicotine, we would expect NAL to suppress smoking without inducing an abstinence syndrome. Our pilot data, reported below, confirm this prediction.

THE CHOLINERGIC ACTIVATION OF THE ADRENOPITUITARY AXIS

In addition to probably activating NA during smoking, nicotine may also be responsible for releasing ACTH and BE and for regulating corticosteroid levels through cholinergic pathways. The model we use relies partly on the one developed by Lewis and Shute (1978). Ach releases ACTH-releasing hormones in the hypothalamus and Segal et al. (1978) have demonstrated that this area of the brain has a great number of nicotine-sensitive cholinergic sites. As we have noted above, ACTH and BE appear to be released together.

Further, nicotine may affect plasma corticosteroid levels. Krieger (1977) summarized her studies and those of others that implicate the major neural areas in the regulation of corticosteroid periodicity. These include the suprachiasmatic nucleus, the retinal-hypothalamic tract and the midbrain raphe. All of these are rich in cholinergic-nicotine receptors in animals (Segal et al., 1978).

However, there is the strong possibility that nicotine in the brain also releases NA in the hypothalamus, as there are numerous adrenergic receptor sites in this region. NA release in this region may suppress ACTH release by acting on ACTH-releasing hormones (Axelrod, 1977). The interaction of Ach and NA on ACTH and BE release is unknown, although from the literature review we would expect Ach effects to predominate.

SMOKING EFFECTS ON COGNITIVE PERFORMANCE[1]

The effects of smoking on cognitive functioning have generally been examined in two areas: the differences between smokers and nonsmokers, and the effects of abrupt withdrawal on habitual smokers. In both cases the dependent measures have generally been performance on simple learning tasks, and the literature on the effects has been inconclusive.

Jarvik (1970), surveying the then-existing literature on smoking and cognitive functioning, concluded that, due to the great variability in results among the different studies, the effects on cognitive performance had to be weak, at best. Research conducted since then has done little to change this conclusion. Kleinman et al. (1973), in a study primarily investigating the effects of smoking deprivation, found that non-deprived smokers and nonsmokers did not differ on the number of trials to learn paired-associates of either low or high meaningfulness; but opposite results were found by Stevens (1976). Using standardized learning measures of increasing complexity, Stevens (1976) found that nonsmokers did significantly better than smokers on three of the four tests used. Carter (1974) also reported differences between smokers and nonsmokers on a cognitive task, letter-digit substitution, but because he did not report whether the difference favored smokers or nonsmokers, his results are uninterpretable.

Research on the effects of smoking cessation on habitual smokers, like research on smoker-nonsmoker differences, has also been characterized by variability of results. Myrsten et al. (1977) investigated the effects of abstinence on physiological and psychological arousal and on cognitive functioning. Although there were some slight differences between groups on cognitive tasks, in general, physiological arousal and subjective variables (*i.e.*, irritation, depression, anxiety, etc.) were relatively more affected than mental performance. There was no support for the common belief among smokers that to abstain from smoking would impair their mental ability and efficiency.

However, an earlier report from the same laboratory arrived at a different conclusion (Elgerot, 1976). Performance on three complex cognitive tests (Raven's Progressive Matrices, a letter series test, and a mental arithmetic test) were facilitated by abstinence, while two simpler tests (a perceptual speed test, and a proof-reading test) were unaffected. One difference between the two studies that might account for the discrepant results is the length of the abstinence period: five days in the Myrsten et al. (1977) study and 15 hours in Elgerot's (1976). However, it is not clear when during the abstinence period Myrsten et al. (1977) administered their tests.

Whereas Elgerot (1976) found that smoking facilitated complex tasks, Kleinman et al. (1973) found the opposite for their 24 hour deprived subjects. The deprivation periods in both studies were relatively similar to each other. In direct contrast to the conclusions of Myrsten et al. (1977) Kleinman et al. (1973) concluded: "If it is assumed that the majority of learning tasks smokers engage in outside the laboratory may be classified as difficult, then...the immediate effects of withdrawal from cigarettes would result in a learning deficit" (p. 966). In agreement with these results, Heimstra et al. (1967) found that smoking produced consistently inferior performance on a simulated driving task.

In general, the literature on the effects of deprivation on cognitive tasks, like the literature on smoker-nonsmoker differences, appears to be characterized by inconclusive results. Jarvik (1970) concluded that this was the result of a weak or nonexistent relationship, although it is also possible that this is due to the variablility of methods used. The problem of comparing different abstinence lengths has already been discussed. Two additional methodological problems are differing smoker criteria and characteristics, and the use of different cognitive tasks. For example, the differences between the results of Kleinman et al. (1973) and Stevens (1976) may be due to the different smoker characteristics in the two studies (a minimum of 20 cigarettes per day for Kleinman et al., and a mean daily consumption of 12.8 cigarettes for Stevens). Elgerot's (1976) conclusion that complex tasks were facilitated by smoking and Kleinman et al.'s (1973) and Heimstra et al.'s (1967) conclusion that these tasks were hindered cannot be meaningfully compared until it is known how their complex cognitive tasks compare. Until researchers use more comparable smoking populations and cognitive tasks that can be meaningfully compared, it may not be known how smoking affects cognitive processes.

PRELIMINARY WORK BY THE AUTHOR[2]

Based on the findings that cortisol is probably released during smoking and that acupuncture may relieve the craving for smoking, my colleague, Dr. Kane, and I speculated that perhaps BE is involved in smoking maintenance. We therefore decided to test the effects of NAL on smoking. The two-factor theory of addiction had not yet been formulated. We assumed that NAL would have an effect, without its direction being specified.

A relatively large dose of NAL (10 mg) was decided upon because BE competes more successfully with NAL at receptor sites and because we wished to test its effects over several hours. We also decided to use a double-blind procedure because comparably large doses injected intravenously into normal human subjects seemed very safe (*e.g.*, Levine et al., 1978, 1979; Yanagida, 1978).

Seven employees of the medical center, 3 men and 4 women, aged 29 to 54 ($\bar{X} = 37.63$) volunteered as subjects. They smoked from 20 to 50 cigarettes per day ($\bar{X} = 30.00$), and had been smoking at their present rate for from 9 to 25 years ($\bar{X} = 14.75$). All were in good health and none was on any medication. All signed informed voluntary consent forms.

Subjects were instructed to smoke no more than two cigarettes on both mornings of testing, and none after 8:00 A.M. They were also asked not to drink coffee for at least one hour prior to testing. On the two testing occasions they smoked their usual brand of cigarettes, which ranged in nicotine content from .5 mg per cigarette to 1.3 mg ($\bar{X} = .86$ mg).

A session began between 9:15 A.M. and 10:15 A.M. After having filled out forms on their desire for a cigarette and mood, and having had their blood pressure and pulse recorded, 10 mg/ml of NAL or 1 ml of placebo (inert NAL vehicle) was administered subcutaneously. Beginning 30 min after the injection, and every 30 min for the next 3 hr six trials were introduced in which subjects first rated their desire for a cigarette, smoked one for 2 min, if they wished, and then rated their satisfaction (if a cigarette were smoked) and mood. These subjective reports were made by marking vertical visual analog scales, 100 mm long, with appropriate end point statements, a procedure similar to that used by Levine et al. (1978). The interval between the two sessions varied between 2-3 days.

During a trial, the experimenter recorded the number of puffs taken and then saved the unsmoked portion, the butt, for later weighing (in mg), after discarding the filter. On the first and fourth trials subjects reported the number and severity of side effects from a list of 31 possible adverse reactions; the experimenter recorded blood pressure and pulse rate.

Only the behavioral measures showed that NAL affected smoking. Table 1 reports trial means and standard errors of the placebo condition regarding the number of puffs and trials smoked and the weight of the butts; change scores for each variable during the NAL condition are reported as percentages of the placebo condition. Subjects took 32 percent fewer puffs, smoked 30 percent less often, and had butts that were 13 percent heavier. The effects of the treatment are sturdy and highly consistent, as the eta^2 for each variable indicates (see Table 1). Intercorrelations (product-moment) between the three variables are all statistically significant ($p < .05$), and consistent in direction, ranging between .79 and .86 (disregarding sign).

Although none of the subjective reports (including side effects), blood pressure, and pulse rate, differentiated between the conditions, their mean change scores were consistent with behavioral outcomes. Change in desire was in fact significantly correlated ($p < .05$) with the change scores of puffs (.86) and butt weight (-.82), and approached significance for change scores of trials smoked (.70; $p = .07$). The latter finding is surprisingly large when we realize that the range of percent change scores for this variable was restricted.

The total amount of nicotine available on a daily basis (daily number of cigarettes multiplied by nicotine content per cigarette) was significantly ($p < .05$) correlated with improvement in mood (.82) and the number of side effects (-.87) for the NAL condition. Correlations of the behavioral measures with amount of available nicotine, mood and side effects were small as well as nonsignificant.

The greater improvement in mood and reduction in side effects associated with greater daily nicotine intake may be another instance of nicotine being the principal agent in maintaining smoking behavior. As an organism grows tolerant to a substance, it becomes more susceptible to its antagonist. Usually, as with opiates, heightened susceptibility is associated with severer withdrawal symptoms, rather than their reduction. Regardless of the direction of the susceptibility, endogenous opiates seem to be involved in smoking.

These findings suggest that the endorphins, and possibly BE, are activated in cigarette smoking and may be partially responsible for its maintenance. Failure of NAL to enhance desire or to induce withdrawal symptoms suggests that the endorphin system(s) acts as an intermediary in nicotine maintenance. Of the three criteria we proposed to apply to determine the role of the endorphins in addictive or repetitive behavior, two of them (nonopiate ligands, and lack of intoxication) apply to smoking. We would therefore expect NAL to suppress smoking without inducing an abstinence syndrome. Our data confirm this prediction.

TABLE 1. Trial Means and Standard Errors (S.E.) of Placebo Condition and of Percentage Change Scores for the Naloxone Condition

	Variable		
	Number of Puffs	Butt Weight (mg)	Number of Trials Smoked
Placebo Mean	5.34	761.14	4.57
S.E.	.87	48.40	.43
% Change			
Mean	32.28%	-13.00%	30.00%
S.E.	10.83	4.52	10.91
p value	.05	.05	.05
Eta^2	.53	.51	.48

Change scores for puffs, butt weight (minus filter) and number of trials smoked are reported as mean percentage change from placebo, corrected for baseline (placebo) differences by calculating percentages for each subject in the following manner:

$$\frac{\text{Puffs (e.g.) on Placebo day} - \text{Puffs on NAL day}}{\text{Puffs on Placebo Day}} \quad (100).$$

Mean raw scores were considered an unsatisfactory metric across subjects because of differences among brands in weight, length, nicotine load and ease of inhaling. Two-tail p values were determined by t tests for paired observations. As subjects had to return to their work sites following the injections, the first trial was considered a practice one, leaving 5 scores per session for measuring treatment effects. Subjects were tested individually in private either in their own office or in one nearby to their worksite.

CONCLUSION

Smoking maintenance appears to be regulated centrally and to a significant degree by nicotinic receptor sites and the endorphin system. There are methods to investigate the probable effects of nicotine as it is mediated through the cholinergic receptor system and the endorphin system.

With regard to the endorphin system, the effects on BE and on the adrenopituitary system of which it is a part, should first be studied. Investigating the role of BE is also necessary to confirm our preliminary findings regarding the effects of NAL on smoking and to support the two-factor theory of addiction.

Briefly, if the endorphin system is the primary system involved, as in opiate addiction, then NAL should enhance craving and precipitate an abstinence syndrome. If it is an intermediary, then NAL should suppress the action of endorphins on the primary system, without necessarily precipitating an abstinence syndrome. We believe that BE is involved as an intermediary system, based on two of the three criteria.

We also need to determine whether activation of nicotinic receptors is a primary and necessary step to other central effects. Some of the basic questions are: (1) Are BE, BLPH, and ACTH peptides released during smoking? (2) Is central NA, which can have a modulating effect on these peptides and may be in part responsible for abstinence effects, also released? (3) How would the blockade of nicotine at cholinergic sites affect the release of these substances, affect smoking behavior and satisfaction, mood, and cognitive performance? (4) Are these effects dose-related, and what are normal values against which to compare dose-related changes?

Most studies have used too few variables, constrained the subject's smoking behavior, and have had the smoker (or nonsmoker) observed for short periods of time so that diurnal effects of the biochemical substrate and consequently on smoking and performance have not been well-characterized. When these limitations are coupled with the fact that the key variables may have been overlooked, it is probable that our current store of information provides little insight into the biochemical mechanisms of smoking maintenance.

FOOTNOTES

1. This section was researched and written by James Stone, research assistant at the Hillside Division.
2. The study was carried out by Betty Chandler Caldwell and James Stone at the Hillside Division.

REFERENCES

Abood, L.G., Lowy, K., Tometsko, A., and Booth, H. (1978): Electro-physiological, behavioral and chemical evidence for a noncholinergic, stereospecific site for nicotine in rat brain. *J. Neurosci Res. 3:* 327-333.
Abood, L.G. Lowy, K., Tometsko, A., and MacNeil, M. (1979): Evidence for a noncholinergic site for nicotine's action in brain: psychopharmacological, electrophysiological and receptor binding studies. *Arch. Intl. Pharmacodyn. 237:* 213-229.
Aghajanian, G.K. (1978): Tolerance of locus coeruleus neurones to morphine and suppression of withdrawal response by clonidine. *Nature 276:* 186-188.
Akil, H., Watson, S.J., Berger, P.A., and Barchas, J.D. (1978): Endorphins, B-LPH, and ACTH. In: E. Costa and M. Trabucchi (Eds.), *Advances in Biochemical Psychopharmacology.* Raven Press, New York, pp. 125-139.
Axelrod, J. (1977): Catecholamines: effects of ACTH and adrenal corticoids. In: D. Krieger and W. Ganong (Eds.), *ACTH and Related Peptides: Structure, Regulation, and Action.* The New York Academy of Sciences, New York, pp. 275-283.
Barrett, A.M. (1966): The role of plasma free fatty acids in the elevation of plasma cholesterol and phospholipids produced by adrenaline. *J. Endocrin. 36:* 301-316.
Berkowitz, B.A., Finck, A.D., and Ngai, S.H. (1977): Nitrous oxide analgesia: reversal by naloxone and development of tolerance. *J. Pharmacol. Exp. Ther. 203:* 539-547.
Brands, B. Thornhill, J.A., Hirst, M., and Gowdey, C.W. (1979): Suppression of food intake and body weight gain by naloxone in rats. *Life Sci. 24:* 1773-1779.
Buck, R. (1976): *Human Motivation and Emotion.* J. Wiley, New York.
Burn, J.H., and Rand, M.J. (1959): Sympathetic postganglionic mechanism. *Nature 184:* 163-165.
Cam, G.R., Bassett, J.R., and Cairncross, K.D. (1979): The action of nicotine on the pituitary-adrenal cortical axis. *Arch. Intl. Pharmacodyn. 237:* 49-66.
Carr, D.B., Bullen, B.A., Skrinar, G.S., Arnold, M.A., Rosenblatt, M., Beitins, I.Z., Martin, J.B., and McArthur, J.W. (1981): Physical conditioning facilitates the exercise-induced secretion of Beta-endorphin and Beta-Lipotropin in women. *New Eng. J. Med. 305:* 560-563.
Carruthers, M., (1976): Modification of the noradrenaline related effects of smoking by beta-blockade. *Psychol. Med. 6:* 251-256.
Carter, G.L. (1974): Effects of cigarette smoking on learning. *Percept. Mot. Skills 39:* 1334-1346.
Cheraskin, E., Ringsdorf, W.M., and Medford, F.H. (1975): Tobacco consumption and adrenocortical activity. *J. Orthomolec. Psychiat. 4:* 261-263.
Chrétien, M. Crine, P., Lis, M., Benjannet, S., and Seidah, N.G. (1979): Beta-lipotropin = pro-endorphin. In: R. Collu, A. Barbeau, J. Ducharme and J. Rochefort (Eds.), *Central Nervous System Effects of Hypothalamic Hormones and Other Peptides.* Raven Press, New York, pp. 237-251.
Cox, B.M., Baizman, E.R., Su, T., Osman, O.H., and Goldstein, A. (1978): Further studies on the nature and functions of pituitary endorphins. In: E. Costa and M. Trabucchi (Eds.), *Advances in Biochemical Psychopharmacology.* Raven Press, New York, pp. 183-189.
Cryer, P.E., Santiago, J.O., and Shah, S. (1974): Measurement of norepinephrine in small volumes of human plasma by a single isotope derivative method: response to the upright posture. *J. Clin. Endocrin. Metab. 39:* 1025-1029.
Davis, G.C., Buchsbaum, M.S., and Bunney, W.E., Jr. (1978): Naloxone decreases diurnal variation in pain sensitivity and somatosensory evoked potentials. *Life Sci. 23:* 1449-1459.

Dettmar, P.W., Cowan, A., and Walter, D.S. (1978): Naloxone antagonizes behavioral effects of d-amphetamine in mice and rats. *Neuropharmacology 17:* 1041-1044.

Domino, E.F. (1967): Electroencephalographic and behavioral arousal effects of small doses of nicotine: A neuropsychopharmacological study. *Ann. N.Y. Acad. Sci. 142:* 216-244.

Domino E.F. (1973): Neuropsychopharmacology of nicotine and tobacco smoking. In: W.L. Dunn (Ed.), *Smoking Behavior: Motives and Incentives.* Winston, Washington, D.C., pp. 5-31.

Elgerot, A. (1976): Note on selective effects of short-term tobacco-abstinence on complex versus simple mental tasks. *Percept. Mot. Skills. 42:* 413-414.

Essman, W.B. (1973): Nicotine-related neurochemical changes: some implications for motivational mechanisms and differences. In: W.L. Dunn (Ed.) *Smoking Behavior: Motives and Incentives.* Winston, Washington, D.C., pp. 51-65.

Fägerström, K.O. (1978): Measuring degree of physical dependence to tobacco smoking with reference to individualization of treatment. *Addict. Beh. 3:* 235-241.

Finnegan, J.K., Larson, P.S., and Haag, H.B. (1945): The role of nicotine in the cigarette habit. *Science 102:* 94-86.

Folkard, S., Glynn, C.J., and Lloyd, J.W. (1976): Diurnal variation and individual differences in the perception of intractable pain. *J. Psychosomat. Res. 20:* 289-301.

Frankenhaeuser, M., Myrsten, A., and Post, B. (1970): Psychophysiological reactions to cigarette smoking. *Scand. J. Psychol. 11:* 237-245.

Frankenhaeuser, M., Myrsten, A.L., Post, B., and Johansson, G. (1971): Behavioral and physiological effects of cigarette smoking in a monotonous situation. *Psychopharmacologia 22:* 1-7.

Frankenhaeuser, M., Myrsten, A., Waszak, M., Neri, A., and Post, B. (1968): Dosage and time effects of cigarette smoking. *Psychopharmacologia* (Berl.) *13:* 311-319.

Frederickson, R.C.A., Burgis, V., and Edwards, J.D. (1977): Hyperanalgesia induced by naloxone follows diurnal rhythm in responsivity to painful stimuli. *Science 198:* 756-758.

Gessa. G.L., Paglietti, E., and Quarantotti, B.P. (1979): Induction of copulatory behavior in sexually inactive rats by naloxone. *Science 204:* 203-205.

Gold, M.S., Redmond, O.E., and Kleber, H.B. (1979): Noradrenergic hyperactivity in opiate withdrawal supported by clonidine reversal of opiate withdrawal. *Am. J. Psychiat. 136:* 100-103.

Goldberg, S.R., Spealman, R.D., and Goldberg, D.M. (1981): Persistent behavior at high rates maintained by intravenous self-administration of nicotine. *Science 214:* 573-575.

Goldfarb, T., Gritz, E.R., Jarvik, M.E., and Stolerman, I.P. (1976): Reactions to cigarettes as a function of nicotine and "tar." *Clin. Pharmacol. Therap. 19:* 767-772.

Gritz, E.R., and Jarvik, M.E. (1977): Pharmacological aids for the cessation of smoking. In: J. Steinfeld, W. Griffith, K. Ball and R.M. Taylor (Eds.), *Proceedings of the Third World Conference on Smoking and Health.* U.S.D.H.E.W. Publication No. 77-1413, pp. 575-591.

Guha, D., and Pradhan, S.N. (1976): Effects of nicotine on EEG and evoked potentials and their interactions with autonomic drugs. *Neuropharmacology 15:* 225-232.

Guillemin, R., Vargo, T., Rossier, J., Minick, S., Ling, N., Rivier, C., Vale, W., and Bloom, F. (1977): B-endorphin and adrenocorticotropin are secreted concomitantly by the pituitary gland. *Science 197:* 1367-1369.

Hall, G.H. (1970): Effects of nicotine and tobacco smoke on the electrical activity of the cerebral cortex and olfactory bulb. *Br. J. Pharmacol. 38:* 271-286.

Hanson, H.M., Ivester, C.A., and Morton, B.R. (1979): Nicotine self-administration in rats. In: N.A. Krasnegor (Ed.), *Cigarette Smoking as a Dependence Process.* U.S.D.H.E.W. Publication No. 79-800, pp. 70-90.

Heimstra, N.W., Bancroft, N.R., and DeKock, A.R. (1967): Effects of smoking upon sustained performance in a simulated driving task. *Ann. N.Y. Acad. Sci. 142:* 295-307.
Hirschhorn, I.D., and Rosecrans, J.A. (1974): Studies on the time course and the effect of cholinergic and adrenergic receptor blockers on the stimulus effect of nicotine. *Psychopharmacologia* (Berl.) *40:* 109-120.
Hökfelt, B. (1961): The effect of smoking on the production of adrenocortical secretion. *Acta Med. Scand.* (Supplement 369): 123-124.
Holaday, J.W., and Faden, A.I. (1978): Naloxone reversal of endotoxin hypotension suggests role of endorphins in shock. *Nature 275:* 450-451.
Holtzman, S.G. (1979): Suppression of appetitive behavior in the rat by naloxone: lack of effect of prior morphine dependence. *Life Sci. 24:* 219-226.
Hosobuchi, Y., and Li, C.H. (1978): The analgesic activity of human Beta-endorphin in man (1, 2, 3). *Commun. Psychopharm. 2:* 33-37.
Hosobuchi, Y., Rossier, J., Bloom, F.E., and Guillemin, R. (1979): Stimulation of human periaqueductal gray for pain relief increases immunoreactive Beta-endorphin in ventricular fluid. *Science 203:* 279-281.
Hunt, W.A. (Ed.) (1970): *Learning Mechanisms in Smoking.* Aldine, Chicago.
Irving, D.W., and Yamamoto, T. (1963): Cigarette smoking and cardiac output. *Br. Heart J. 25:* 126-132.
Isaac, P.F., and Rand, M.J. (1972): Cigarette smoking and plasma levels of nicotine. *Nature 236:* 308-310.
Itil, T.M., Ulett, G.A., Asu, W., Klingenberg, H., Ulett, J.A. (1971): The effects of smoking withdrawal on quantitatively analyzed EEG. *Clin. Electroencephal. 2:* 44-51.
Jacob, J.J., Tremblay, E.C., and Colombel, M. (1974): Facilitation de réactions nociceptives par la naloxone chez la souris et chez le rat. *Psychopharmacologia* (Berl.) *37:* 217-223.
Jacobs, M.A., Spiken, A.Z., Norman, M.N., and Anderson, L.S. (1970): Life stress and respiratory illness. *Psychosomat. Med. 32:* 233-242.
Jacquet, Y.F. (1978): Opiate effects after adrenocorticotropin or Beta-endorphin injection in the periaqueductal gray matter of rats. *Science 201:* 1032-1034.
Jarvik, M. (1970): The role of nicotine in the smoking habit. In: W.A. Hunt (Ed.), *Learning Mechanisms in Smoking.* Aldine, Chigago, pp. 155-190.
Kerrigan, R., Jain, A.C., and Doyle, J.T. (1968): The cirulatory response to cigarette smoking at rest and after exercise. *Amer. J. Med. Sci. 255:* 113-119.
Kershbaum, A., Pappajohn, D.J., Bellet, S., Hirabayashi, M., and Shafiiha, H. (1968): Effect of smoking and nicotine on adrenocortical secretion. *J. Amer. Med. Assoc. 203:* 275-278.
Kleinman, K.M., Vaughn, R.L., and Christ, V.T., (1973): Effects of cigarette smoking and smoking deprivation on paired-associate learning of high and low meaningful nonsense syllables. *Psychol. Rep. 32:* 963-966.
Kosterlitz, H.W., and Hughes, J. (1978): Development of the concepts of opiate receptors and their ligands. In. E. Costa and M. Trabucchi (Eds.), *Advances in Biochemical Psychopharmacology,* vol. 18. Raven Press, New York, pp. 31-44.
Krieger, D.T. (1977): Regulation of circadian periodicity of plasma ACTH levels. In: D.T. Krieger and W.F. Ganong (Eds.), *ACTH and Related Peptides: Structure, Regulation, and Action.* N.Y. Acad. Sci., New York, pp. 561-567.
Krieger, D.T. Liotta, A., and Brownstein, M.J. (1977): Presence of corticotropin in brain of normal and hypophysectomized rats. *Proc. Natl. Acad. Sci.* USA *74:* 648-652.
Kumar, R., Cooke, E.C., Lader, M.H., and Russell, M.A.H. (1977): Is nicotine important in tobacco smoking? *Clin. Pharmacol. Therap. 21:* 520-529.
Levine, J.D., Gordons, N.C., and Fields, H.L. (1978): The mechanism of placebo analgesia. *Lancet ii:* 654-657.

Levine, J.E., Gordons, N.C., and Fields, H.L. (1979): Naloxone dose dependently produces analgesia and hyperalgesia in postoperative pain. *Nature 278:* 740-741.
Lewis, P.R., and Shute, C.C.D. (1978): Cholinergic pathways in CNS. In: L.L. Iverson, S.D. Iverson, and S.H. Snyder (Eds.), *Handbook of Psychopharmacology*, vol. 9. Plenum Press, New York, pp. 315-355.
Li, C.H., and Chung, D. (1976): Isolation and structure of an untreakontapeptide with opiate activity from camel pituitary glands. *Proc. Natl. Acad. Sci.* USA *73:* 1145-1148.
Li, C.H., Chung, D., Ramashiro, D., and Lee, C.Y. (1978): Isolation, characterization, and synthesis of a corticotropin-inhibiting peptide from human pituitary gland. *Proc. Natl. Acad. Sci.* USA *75:* 4306-4309.
Loh, H.H., and Li, C.H. (1977): Biologic activities of Beta-endorphin and its related peptides. In: D.T. Krieger, and W.F. Ganong (Eds.), *ACTH and Related Peptides: Structure, Regulation, and Action.* N.Y. Acad. Sci., New York, pp. 115-128.
Loh, Y.P. (1979): Immunological evidence for two common precursors to corticotropins, endorphins, and melanotropin in the neurointermediate lobe of the toad pituitary. *Proc. Natl. Acad. Sci.* USA *76:* 796-800.
Lucchesi, B.R., Schuster, C.R., and Emley, G.S. (1967): The role of nicotine as a determinant of cigarette smoking frequency in man with observations of certain cardiovascular effects associated with the tobacco alkaloid. *Clin. Pharmacol. Therap. 8:* 789-796.
Maas, J.W., Hattox, S.E., Landis, D.H., and Roth, R.H. (1976): The determination of a brain arteriovenous difference for 3 methoxy-4-hydroxyphenethyleneglycol (MHPG). *Brain Res. 118:* 167-173.
Mains. R.E., Eipper, B.A., and Ling, N. (1977): Common precursor to corticotropins and endorphins. *Proc. Natl. Acad. Sci.* USA *74:* 3014-3018.
Malizia, E., Andreucci, G., Cerbo, R., and Colombo, G. (1978): Effect of naloxone on the acupuncture-elicited analgesia in addicts. In: E. Costa and M. Trabucchi (Eds.), *Advances in Biochemical Psychopharmacology*, vol. 18. Raven Press, New York, pp. 361-362.
Margules, D.L., Moisset, B., Lewis, M.J., Shibuya, H., and Pert, C.B. (1978): B-Endorphin is associated with overeating in genetically obese mice (ob/ob) and rats (fa/fa). *Science 202:* 988-991.
Markley, H.G., and Mezey, E. (1978): Induction of alcohol withdrawal symptoms by nalorphine in chronic alcoholic patients. *Intl. J. Addict. 13:* 395-402.
Mausner, B., and Platt, E.S. (1971): *Smoking: A Behavioral Analysis.* Pergamon, New York.
Mayer, D.J., Price, D.D., and Rafii, A. (1977): Antagonism of acupuncture analgesia in man by the narcotic antagonist naloxone. *Brain Res. 121:* 368-372.
McKennell, A.C. (1970): Smoking motivation factors. *Br. J. Soc. Clin. Psychol. 9:* 8-22.
Meade, T.W., and Wald, N.J. (1977): Cigarette smoking patterns during the working day. *Br. J. Prev. Soc. Med. 31:* 25-29.
Myrsten. A.L., Post, B., Frankenhaeuser, M., and Johansson, G. (1972): Change in behavioral and physiological activation induced by cigarette smoking in habitual smokers. *Psychopharmacologia* (Berl.) *27:* 305-312.
Myrsten, A.L., Elgerot, A., and Edgren, B. (1977): Effect of abstinence from tobacco smoking on physiological and psychological arousal levels in habitual smokers. *Psychosom. Med. 39:* 25-38.
Olds, J. (1977): *Drives and Reinforcements.* Raven Press, New York.
Pelletier, G., and Desy, L. (1978): Localization of ACTH in the human hypothalamus. *Cell Tiss. Res. 196:* 525-530.
Pomeranz, B. (1978): Do endorphins mediate acupuncture analgesia? In: E. Costa and M. Trabucchi (Eds.), *Advances in Biochemical Psychopharmacology*, vol. 18. Raven Press, New York, pp. 351-359.

Pomeranz, B., and Chiu, D. (1976): Naloxone blockade of acupuncture analgesia: endorphin implicated. *Life Sci. 19:* 1757-1762.
Pradhan, S.N., and Bose, S. (1978): Interactions among central neurotransmitters. In: M.A. Lipton, A. DiMascio, and K.F. Killam (Eds.), *Psychopharmacology: A Generation of Progress.* Raven Press, New York, pp. 271-281.
Romano, C., and Goldstein, A. (1980): Stereospecific nicotine receptors on rat brain membranes. *Science 210:* 647-649.
Rossier, J., Battenberg, E., Pittman, Q., Bayon, A., Koda, L., Miller, R., Guillemin, R., and Bloom, F. (1979a): Hypothalamic enkephalin neurones may regulate the neurohypophysis. *Nature 277:* 653-655.
Rossier, J., Rogers, J., Shibasaki, T., Guillemin, R., and Bloom, F.E. (1979b): Opioid peptides and alpha-melanocyte-stimulating hormone in genetically obese (ob/ob) mice during development. *Proc. Natl. Acad. Sci. USA 76:* 2077-2080.
Rubin, R.P., and Warner, W. (1975): Nicotine-induced stimulation of steroidgenesis in adrenalcortical cells of the cat. *Br. J. Pharmacol. 53:* 357-362.
Russell, M.A.H. (1976): Tobacco smoking and nicotine dependence. In: R.J. Gibbons, Y. Israel, H. Kalant, R.E. Popham, W. Schmidt, and R.G. Smart (Eds.), *Research Advances in Alcohol and Drug Problems.* John Wiley, New York, pp. 1-47.
Russell, M.A.H., and Feyerabend, C. (1975): Blood and urinary nicotine in non-smokers. *Lancet i:* 179-180.
Russell, M.A.H., Wilson, C., Palel, V.A., Feyerabend, C., and Cole, P.V. (1975): Plasma nicotine levels after smoking cigarettes with high, medium and low nicotine yields. *Br. Med. J. 2:* 414-416.
Sauerbier, I., and Mayersback, H.V. (1977): Circadian variation of catecholamines in human blood. *Horm. Metab. Res. 9:* 529-530.
Schachter, S. (1977): Nicotine regulations in heavy and light smokers. *J. Exper. Psychol. 106:* 5-12.
Schachter, S., Silverstein, B., and Perlick, D. (1977): Psychological and pharmacological explanations of smoking under stress. *J. Exper. Psychol. 106:* 31-40.
Schechter, M.D., and Rosecrans, J.A. (1972): Nicotine as a discriminative stimulus in rats depleted of norepinephrine or 5-hydroxy-tryptamine. *Psychopharmacologia* (Berl.) *24:* 417-429.
Schildkraut, J.J., Meyer, R.E., Orsulak, P.J., Mirin, S.M., Roffman, M., Platz, P.A., Grab, E., Randall, M.E., and McDougle, M. (1975): The effects of heroin on catecholamine metabolism in man. In: B.K. Bernard (Ed.), *Aminergic Hypothesis of Behavior: Reality or Cliche?.* DHEW Pub. No. 78, pp. 137-145.
Schultzberg, M., Lundberg, J.M., Hökfelt, T., Terenius, J., Elde, R.P., and Goldstein, M. (1978): Enkephalin-like immunoreactivity in gland cells and nerve terminals of the adrenal medulla. *Neuroscience 3:* 1169-1186.
Segal, E., Dudai, Y., and Amsterdam, A. (1978): Distribution of an alpha-bungarotoxin-binding cholinergic nicotinic receptor in rat brain. *Brain Res. 148:* 105-119.
Shiffman, S.M., and Jarvik, M.E. (1976): Smoking withdrawal symptoms in two weeks of abstinence. *Psychopharmacology 50:* 35-39.
Smoking and Health: A Report of the Surgeon General (1979). U.S.D.H.E.W. Pub. No. 79-50066.
The Smoking Digest (1977). U.S.D.H.E.W.
Snyder, S.H., Pasternak, G.W., and Pert, C.B. (1975): Opiate receptor mechanisms. In: L.L. Iverson, S.D. Iverson, and S.H. Snyder (Eds.), *Handbook of Psychopharmacology,* vol. 5. Plenum Press, New York, pp. 329-360.

Stapleton, J.M., Lind, M.D., Merriman, V.J., and Reid, L.D. (1979): Naloxone inhibits diazepam-induced feeding in rats. *Life Sci. 24:* 2421-2426.

Stevens, H.A. (1976): Evidence that suggests a negative association between cigarette smoking and learning performance. *J. Clin. Psychol. 32:* 896-898.

Stolerman, I.P., Goldfarb, T., Fink, R., and Jarvik, M.E. (1973): Influencing cigarette smoking with nicotine antagonists. *Psychopharmacologia* (Berl.) *28:* 247-259.

Tucci, J.R., and Sode, J. (1972): Chronic cigarette smoking effect on adrenocortical and sympathoadrenomedullary activity in man. *J. Amer. Med. Assoc. 221:* 282-285.

Ulett, J.A., and Itil, T.M. (1969): Quantitative electroencephalogram in smoking and smoking deprivation. *Science 164:* 969-970.

Volle, R.L., and Koelle, G.B. (1975): Ganglionic stimulating and blocking agents. In: L.S. Goodman and A. Gilman (Eds.), *The Pharmacological Basis of Therapeutics.* MacMillan, New York, pp. 565-574.

Watts, D.T., and Bragg, A.D. (1956): Effects of smoking on the urinary output of epinephrine and norepinephrine in man. *J. Appl. Physiol. 9:* 275-278.

Wiedemann, E., Saito, T., Linfoot, J.A., and Li, C.H. (1979): Specific radioimmunoassay of human β-endorphin in unextracted plasma. *J. Clin. Endocrin. Metab. 49:* 478-480.

Wiegant, V.M., Gispen, W.H., Terenius, L., and DeWied, O. (1977): Acth-like peptide and morphine: interaction at the level of the CNS. *Psychoneuroendocrinology 2:* 63-69.

Winternitz, W.W., and Quillen, D. (1977): Acute hormonal response to cigarette smoking. *J. Clin. Pharmacol. 17:* 389-397.

Yanagida, H. (1978): Congenital insensitivity and naloxone. *Lancet ii:* 520-521.

4

Nicotine and the Regulation of Smoking Behavior*

R. Kuman
M. Lader

Cigarette smoking is one of the most persistent habits known to man; for several centuries he has been possessed by the bizarre but irresistible urge to inhale the smoke produced by burning the dried and shredded leaves of *Nicotiana tabacum*. The alternative methods of administration—sniffing and chewing—lost favour with the introduction of cheap cigarettes made from flue-cured tobacco. Unlike the smoking of cigars and pipes, absorption of nicotine from cigarette smoke mainly takes place in the lungs. Despite convincing evidence that life is shortened by about 12 minutes for every cigarette smoked, consumption continues unabated throughout the world.

If people are asked why they smoke, many reasons are given. In a national survey of adults conducted for the U.S. Public Health Service in 1966, questions were asked about smoking. Six factors were extracted from the data representing the following types of smoking: 1) habitual—the smoker smokes cigarettes because they are there; 2) addictive—he smokes to prevent the craving which withdrawal entails; 3) negative affect reduction—he smokes in order to cope with feelings of anxiety, tension, anger and aggression in difficult situations; 4) pleasurable relaxation—to "unwind;" 5) stimulation—to feel energized, alert and attentive; and 6) sensorimotor manipulation—to have something to do, lighting and handling the cigarette (Ikard, Green and Horn, 1969).

In a similar English study (McKennell, 1970), a checklist of the main occasions for smoking was administered to smokers and ex-smokers. Factor analysis

This chapter is based upon a manuscript originally written in 1979, that appeared in Current Developments in Psychopharmacology, *Vol. 6, Spectrum, New York, 1981.*

revealed seven factors. Five were related to within-individual aspects and comprised "nervous irritation," "relaxation," "smoking alone," "activity accompaniment," and "food substitution." Two covered social and social confidence smoking. Russell et al. (1974) mainly confirmed these findings but were unable to find a sedative factor.

Thus, smoking seems to be all things to all smokers. Indeed, it is probable that smokers smoke for different reasons or different combinations of reasons at different times. This raises the crucial issue as to whether these reasons reflect different pharmacological effects of tobacco smoke or whether complex behavioural factors govern smoking behaviour. Or, rather, what is the relative contribution of each? The active pharmacological principle in tobacco smoke is nicotine and it is generally presumed that smokers are self-administering nicotine.

In the following review, these questions are addressed in some detail from the point of view of the following:
1. The pharmacology of nicotine effects on the C.N.S. and the animal behaviour related to these effects.
2. The role of nicotine in smoking behaviour in man.
3. The reinforcing properties of nicotine and smoking.

The review is selective both in scope and depth as compendia on the nicotine and smoking literature exist (Larson and Silvette, 1961, 1968, 1971, 1975). The most recent review is that edited by Thornton (1978).

I. STUDIES IN ANIMALS

NICOTINE SELF-ADMINISTRATION

It is estimated that there are some 60 million smokers in the U.S.A. and 20 million in the United Kingdom. Each inhalation of tobacco smoke delivers a bolus of nicotine to the brain within about 7 seconds and a moderate/heavy smoker probably gives himself over 50,000 such doses of nicotine each year. Despite the immensity of the tobacco smoking habit there has been a disproportionately small amount of research into the psychopharmacology of smoking and into the role of nicotine. Several recent reviews have pointed to the fact that there is still no conclusive evidence about the very existence of reinforcing actions of nicotine (British Medical Journal, 1977; Kumar and Stolerman, 1977; Jaffe and Jarvik, 1978; Lader, 1978). Some idea of the size of the literature concerned with animal studies of drug self-administration can be obtained by a glance at some recent general reviews of the field (Thompson and Pickens, 1971; Proc. Bayer Symp., 1973; Proc. Symp. Control of Drug-Taking Behaviour by schedules of reinforcement, 1976; Kumar and Stolerman, 1977; Martin, 1977a, b; Pickens, Meisch and Thompson, 1978). The many hundreds of studies of the reinforcing properties of drugs, notably opioids, CNS stimulants such as the amphetamines and cocaine, sedative/hypnotics and ethanol, stand in stark contrast against the handful of reports of nicotine self-administration. In the case of the hallucinogens there is also a similar lack of hard evidence of self-administration by animals, but these drugs are misused relatively rarely and sporadically by man and it remains to be established whether in their case there results "a state which is characterized by a compulsion to take the drug on a continuous or periodic basis in order to experience its psychic effects, and sometimes to avoid the discomfort of its absence" (Eddy et al., 1964). This type of psychological state is, of course, well known to millions of habitual tobacco smokers although the evidence for a nicotine abstinence syndrome remains inconclusive (Jaffe and Jarvik, 1978).

Deneau and Inoki (1967) reported tests of intravenous self-administration in seven rhesus monkeys where they found that in most cases it was necessary to "prime" the subjects with repeated programmed injections before they would start responding (pressing a lever) for doses of nicotine (25 μg/kg nicotine base in saline); a lower dose was not self-administered. The average daily dose that was taken by different monkeys ranged between 0.7 and 1.7 mg/kg nicotine, but individual monkeys showed sharp variations. They often changed their intake by as much as 100% on consecutive days and they tended to take a large dose on one day followed by a small dose the next. In the second phase of the study by Deneau and Inoki (1967) doses were raised at approximately monthly intervals and although the monkeys responded on the lever less often, their total daily intake nevertheless increased. However, of six survivors, one refused to self-administer at the 50 μg/kg dose level and two stopped at 100 μg/kg. One monkey each stopped at the 500 μg/kg and 1000 μg/kg dose levels and only one monkey persisted in responding for 2 mg/kg doses; this last animal averaged a daily intake of just under 10 mg/kg and reached a maximum of 14 mg/kg. The maximum rates of responding in this study were seen at the lower doses (up to 68 responses per day); the patterns of responding were variable and the amounts of responding began to decrease as the concentration of nicotine was raised. Perhaps the reductions in response rates were due to the fact that doses of nicotine above 200 μg/kg produced increasingly severe effects such as yawning, piloerection, flushing and then pallor, mydriasis followed by miosis, dyspnoea, retching, vomiting and muscular weakness. In the light of such observations it is surprising that any animals continued to respond. Deneau and Inoki (1967) noted that even at high doses (1.0 and 2.0 mg/kg) these apparently unpleasant effects were very short lasting, disappearing completely by 20 minutes after the dose. They did not comment on the development of tolerance or lack of it.

There has been one further report of intravenous self-administration of nicotine by monkeys; Yanagita et al (1974) found that two out of three naive monkeys and all four "self-administration experienced" monkeys initiated and continued intravenous self-administration of nicotine (unit dose 20 µg/kg/injection). The monkeys responded only during the "lights on" period (8 a.m. to midnight) and the number of doses taken ranged from an average of 10/day to 100/day (i.e., a maximum daily total dose of 2 mg/kg/day). No toxic effects were seen. In another test there was some suggestion that monkeys would respond on a fixed-ratio schedule for large unit doses of nicotine (up to 0.2 mg/kg) but the rates of responding were far less than for cocaine reinforcement. Results of attempts to get monkeys to inhale tobacco smoke were inconclusive.

Clark (1969), in a preliminary report, described oral preferences for nicotine solutions in rats but the summarised data were of an anecdotal nature. He also reported that twelve rats learned to lever press for intravenous injections of nicotine (10 µg/kg base) after having received repeated programmed injections for a week beforehand. Halving the dose resulted in a 20 percent increase in rate of responding for 6 rats, but since data for the other 6 animals were not described it is not possible to conclude that there was evidence of dose-titration by the rats.

Sanger (1978) substituted solutions of nicotine bitartrate (0.05 mg/ml) for tapwater when measuring schedule-induced polydipsia in four rats. He found that the rats drank less, but nevertheless they consumed quite large doses by the oral route, up to 9.5 mg/kg per session. Although the experiment was not primarily concerned with nicotine dependence, it is worth noting that this type of nicotine ingestion does not necessarily reflect nicotine-seeking. A difficulty which is common to all tests of orally ingested doses of nicotine is that a substantial proportion of such doses is metabolised in the first pass through the liver.

Recently, Lang et al (1977) attempted tests in rats of the self-administration of intravenous doses of nicotine and they found that the animals would not respond for 0.05 and 0.1 mg/kg doses of nicotine bitartrate. If, however, the rats were food deprived and then given food pellets at 60 second intervals, i.e., the typical method for schedule-induced polydipsia, they responded more frequently for injections of nicotine than for saline. This interesting observation requires confirmation. It would be important to know what interactions occur between factors such as hunger, the behavioural consequences of the food delivery schedule and the putative reinforcing actions of nicotine. Could such a pattern of responding be blocked by mecamylamine and would the enhanced reinforcing action of nicotine persist in the absence of the food-delivery schedule?

Perhaps in an attempt to answer the criticism that human subjects do not "mainline" nicotine nor drink infusions of this drug, Jarvik (1967) reported some tests of tobacco smoking in monkeys. The animals seemed to puff more frequently at a tube connected to a lit cigarette than at an empty tube and they preferred cigarette smoke to hot air. There was, however, no evidence to suggest that they inhaled the smoke; the same criticism applies to the study reported by Glick et al (1970) where four thirsty monkeys were trained to puff at a tube in order to obtain water rewards. Stable rates of puffing were eventually achieved on a Fixed-Ratio 30 schedule where two tubes were available, one providing smoke from a permanently available cigarette and the other providing air. As in Jarvik's (1967) experiment, the monkeys preferred the smoke delivery tube. Their rates of puffing and preferences for smoke were then tested after intramuscular injections of mecamylamine, 0.8-3.2 mg/kg. At doses which varied from monkey to monkey, mecamylamine reversed the preferences for smoke without markedly affecting overall rates of puffing but given the lack of adequate controls such observations must remain tentative. The interpretation offered was that mecamylamine was blocking the actions of nicotine which was the rewarding component of the tobacco smoke; thus only the aversive components of smoke remained. Had there been evidence for actual inhalation of smoke, then, presumably, the putative aversive actions of nicotine would also have been liable to blockade. Such reversals were not confined to mecamylamine since hexamethonium also produced similar changes. Another puzzling feature of this study was that no increases in smoke preference were seen at low doses of mecamylamine; later tests in human volunteer subjects (Stolerman et al., 1973a) demonstrated increased smoking following medication with mecamylamine.

In summary, the few existing reports of nicotine self-administration by animals are largely of a preliminary nature and there is little or no systematic evidence about factors which might influence rates of self-administration nor about the ways, if any, in which the drug may be acting as a reinforcer. The remainder of this part of the review will therefore be concerned with behavioural studies in animals which may have some bearing upon questions about possible rewarding actions of nicotine: e.g.,–is nicotine rewarding indirectly because it improves alertness and hence learning and performance, or alternatively, is it reinforcing because it has some sort of tranquillising action and diminishes responses to stressors? Does nicotine use result in tolerance and abstinence phenomena and might the drug therefore be self-administered to alleviate or avoid abstinence? There seem to be marked individual differences described in studies of motives underlying smoking; are there analogous differences in animals' reactions to doses of nicotine?

TESTS OF SPONTANEOUS MOTOR ACTIVITY, LEARNING AND PERFORMANCE IN RODENTS

Nicotine affects the motor activity of rodents in complex ways and it has not been possible to arrive at descriptive generalisations about the mode of action of this drug in the way that attempts have been made to characterise other drugs such as amphetamine (e.g., Lyon and Robbins, 1975). Nicotine can apparently increase or diminish activity depending upon interactions between dose and factors such as species (Morrison and Armitage, 1967) strain and sex (Garg, 1969a; Bättig et al., 1976) or time of day that the tests were done (Bovet-Nitti and Bovet, 1966). Low doses typically increase levels of activity while higher doses have depressant effects. In general, it seems that animals showing low base-line (undruged) levels of activity are stimulated by nicotine while already active animals are either unaffected or are depressed (Morrison and Lee, 1968; Pradhan and Dutta, 1970), but there are some contradictory findings (Garg, 1969a). Attempts have been made to link the stimulant or depressant effects of nicotine with actions on fore-brain serotonin metabolism in rats showing high or low base-line levels of activity (Rosecrans, 1971) but since nicotine almost certainly exerts equally important effects on dopamine and noradrenaline as well as on acetylcholine, one is obliged, in the present state of knowledge, to agree with Jaffe and Jarvik (1978) that "effects on neurotransmitters do not provide significant insights into the ways in which nicotine reinforces smoking behaviour." Similarly, there is a temptation to draw parallels between the subtle and variable ways in which nicotine can modify learned and unlearned responses in animals and the variety of reasons that smokers give for smoking. Human typologies of smoking behaviour e.g., Tomkins (1966,) Ikard et al (1969), Russell et al (1974) characterise smokers in a number of overlapping ways (see also Introduction) but some other independent characteristics e.g. of a physiological nature, or in terms of responses to drugs other than nicotine should also be shown to co-vary with the different motivational types of "smoking personalities" that are derived from such studies.

In a test of bar-pressing by rats for water rewards Morrison et al (1969) found that, typically, injections of nicotine (0.4 mg/kg of the bitartrate) initially depressed responding and that about 30 minutes later there was a facilitation of the rate of bar-pressing. Mecamylamine blocked both effects of nicotine whereas atropine antagonised only the initial depressant action. It seemed therefore that in addition to producing muscarinic actions of acetylcholine, nicotine was also either stimulating (unidentified) nicotinic receptors or perhaps acting indirectly through some other mechanisms such as release of catecholamines. These possibilities were however not examined directly. In a similar study, Domino and Lutz (1973) have shown that tolerance develops rapidly to the initial suppressant actions of nicotine on responding by rats for water rewards. Although these workers did not demonstrate subsequent facilitation of behaviour, it would be interesting to compare the reactions of nicotine naive and tolerant rats on such tests when given drugs such as mecamylamine and atropine, and substances affecting other neurotransmitters.

In addition to differences in responsiveness related to time since medication (Morrison et al., 1969) other observations on the effects of nicotine on learned behaviour are also broadly consistent with tests of spontaneous activity in that the drug tends to increase low base-line rates of responding (Morrison, 1967, 1968; Pradhan and Dutta, 1970) while high rates are either unaffected (Morrison, 1967) or are reduced (Sitzer et al., 1970). Similarly, the acquisition of some behavioural responses, e.g., shuttle-box avoidance, is also facilitated in strains of animals that are normally "poor" avoiders (Bovet et al., 1966, 1967). In tests of the performance of pole-jump avoidance, Domino (1973) noted that with subcutaneous doses of nicotine base above 0.25 mg/kg there were consistent and selective depressions of avoidance while escape behaviour remained relatively unaffected. Such a differential effect was reminiscent of the profile of actions obtained with chlorpromazine, morphine and tetrahydrocannabinol. While recognizing that there was a hundredfold or more difference between the amounts of nicotine given by injection and those obtained by inhaling smoke, Domino (1973) wondered whether nicotine might not also have some "tranquillising" actions. The empirical nature of the pole-jump test and the varied actions of the reference drugs notwithstanding, this is an interesting speculation which is taken up in more detail elsewhere in this review.

An alternative possibility is that nicotine is a "stimulant" rather than a tranquilliser and in an experiement which aimed to mimic the sort of dose that is normally inhaled by taking a puff (equivalent to 1-2 μg/kg nicotine base given intravenously), Armitage et al (1968) showed that intermittent, small, intravenous doses of nicotine usually increased rates of bar-pressing by thirsty rats for water rewards. The speed of injection and the interval between injections were critical factors but it was felt that under selected conditions of dose and timing, these "smoking doses" of nicotine were producing some kind of central stimulant effects which, in turn, were responsible for the elevated rates of responding. Such an effect on performance might have some relevance to the facilitations of learning seen both in tests of avoidance behaviour (Bovet et al., 1966, 1967) or following post-trial injections of nicotine in maze-learning tasks (Garg, 1969b). Repeated intravenous injections of "smoking doses" of nicotine in anaesthetised cats resulted both in electrocortical desynchronisation and in an increase in the release of acetylcholine from the cortex (Armitage et al., 1968). It was suggested, therefore, that inhaled nicotine might be reinforcing because of its alerting actions. Such actions would depend critically upon the "base-line," i.e., concentration and efficiency might only improve if they were previously low. On the other hand a smoker who was over-aroused might seek a depressant effect of nicotine e.g., by increasing the dose inhaled. Armitage et al (1968) commented that "someone smoking a cigarette has literally finger-tip control of how much nicotine he takes into his mouth; by reducing the puff volume or inhaling less frequently he absorbs less nicotine." At first sight such an hypothesis seems very attractive; nicotine is a drug which has both depressant and stimulant effects on behaviour and on cortical activation, effects which depend critically upon dose and time. Since an individual's arousal level and efficiency are likely to fluctuate spontaneously as well as in response to environmental events, nicotine can be regarded as an all purpose modulator, by the use of which a smoker keeps his requirements for stimulation and sedation constantly tuned to perfection. It is, however, virtually impossible to prove or disprove such an all-embracing hypothesis which can easily adapt *posthoc* to accommodate almost any new data particularly if they do not extend to more than three or four points on a hypothetical inverted-U continuum.

NICOTINE, REINFORCEMENT AND "AROUSAL"

There are several studies in animals which bear directly on the question of arousal and nicotine reinforcement. Bradley and Elkes (1957) recorded electrical activity from different brain regions of various experimental preparations of cats and monkeys e.g., conscious, encephale isolé, cerveau isolé, or anaesthetised. They concluded that while cholinergic neurones were present throughout the brainstem activating system, nicotinic neurones were to be found only in the midbrain reticular formation. Yamamoto and Domino (1965) tested the effects of intravenous nicotine in cats with chronically implanted electrodes in the amygdala, hippocampus, posterior hypothalamus, mesencephalic reticular formation and on the surface of the somatosensory cortex. They compared the (+) and (-) isomers of nicotine and found that the (+) isomer was ineffective. (-) nicotine on the other hand, produced both behavioural and EEG arousal, followed a few minutes later by slow wave sleep. The first EEG sign of arousal was the emergency of hippocampal theta rhythm and this arousal-inducing action of nicotine was blocked by mecamylamine. Domino (1967), using mid, or high pontine preparations in several species, found that doses of nicotine ranging from 5-20 μg/kg intravenously resulted in EEG activation. In line with other speculations e.g., by Armitage et al (1968), he wondered whether these arousing effects were in any way relevant to the facilitations of learning seen in the acquisition of pole jump avoidance by "slow" rats.

Armitage and Hall (1968) calculated that when a smoker inhaled a puff he was probably taking the equivalent of an intravenous dose of the order of 1-2 μg/kg. These workers then delivered puffs of smoke which approximately mimicked human puffed doses into the tracheas of encephale isolé cats. After about 8 such puffs they observed signs of behavioural arousal, e.g., opening of eyes, reactions to visual stimuli, movements of ears and vibrissae, and, at the same time, desynchronisation of cortical activity.

Routtenberg (1968) proposed a "two-arousal" hypothesis in which the reticular formation and the limbic system were seen as functioning in a mutually inhibitory manner. The reticular formation was believed to be mediating non-specific or generalised arousal whereas the limbic structures were involved in the activation of goal-directed, incentive-oriented behaviours. Nelsen and her colleagues have reported a series of studies in which they link the effects of repeated medication with nicotine both with improvements in goal-directed responding (Nelsen and Goldstein, 1972) and with increasing dominance of the hypothesised limbic arousal mechanisms. A shift, it was argued, in the control of cortical arousal from the reticular formation to the hippocampus in rabbits (Bhattacharya and Goldstein, 1970), was consistent with their behavioural observations in rats that the subjects when injected repeatedly with nicotine, 100 μg/kg subcutaneously, made fewer inappropriate responses on a lever pressing task. In a later study, Nelsen et al (1975) reported that electrical stimulation of the reticular formation, via chronically implanted electrodes, disrupted performance of a lever-pressing task involving visual "attention" in rats. This effect was attenuated by acute subcutaneous medication with nicotine base, 100 μg/kg. The results of such experiments have not yet been confirmed and more detailed studies of chronic medication with nicotine are needed to test and refine hypotheses linking nicotine with arousal, incentive and performance. It is suggested, for example, that some smokers may not be inhaling to arouse or alert themselves (cf Domino, 1967; Armitage and Hall, 1968) but rather than by activating another brain system they damp down reticular activating mechanisms. In this context Friedman et al (1974) have suggested that smokers lower their arousal level by attenuating sensory input, but fuller comparisons are needed in man with intravenous or aerosol doses of nicotine which are obtained independently of smoking behavior before such interpretations are fully acceptable.

An extension of the arousal reduction hypotheses was put forward by Hall and Morrison (1973); these workers reported tests in which rats pressed levers in order to avoid electric shocks. Rats were trained either drugged with nicotine or with saline. Both groups learned the response and there was some early facilitation of responding by nicotine. However, when saline was substituted for the nicotine there were disruptions in performance and it was suggested that nicotine might be maintaining successful levels of performance because it diminished the subjects' response to stress. In support of the stress-relief hypothesis it was argued that since intravenous or intraventricular nicotine caused a release of noradrenaline from the hypothalamus (Hall and Turner, 1972) this in turn might inhibit the release of corticosteroids from the adrenal cortex (Van Loon et al., 1971). Subsequent reports (Balfour et al., 1975) have not supported the suggestion that nicotine might reduce corticosteroid secretion in stressed rats. Some further behavioural tests (Balfour and Morrison, 1975) have indicated that nicotine both facilitates avoidance responding and increases adrenal weight in rats. It is therefore not yet clear how nicotine acts on the pituitary-adrenal system in stressed or unstressed subjects. There are as yet no experimental findings to support the hypothesis that nicotine is self-administered in order to diminish responses to stressors.

NICOTINE AND BRAIN MECHANISMS OF REWARD

The amine releasing properties of nicotine are not well understood. Studies in animals indicate that nicotine can cause changes in turnover and release of both dopamine and noradrenaline from the brain (Sulser and Sanders Bush, 1971; Goodman, 1974; Westfall, 1974; Giorguieff et al., 1976; Lichtensteiger et al., 1976; De Belleroche and Bradford, 1978) and in addition to markedly altering the cortical release of acetylcholine (Armitage et al., 1969) nicotine also affects the turnover of serotonin (Rosecrans, 1971) as well as the uptake and release of both serotonin and noradrenaline by the hippocampus and hypothalamus (Balfour, 1973). The functional significance of such effects, e.g., in terms of consummatory responding (see Munster and Bättig, 1975) remains virtually unexplored and there have been very few studies of the effects of nicotine on intracranial self-stimulation behaviour (ICSS). It is well known that rats with electrodes placed either in the lateral or the posterior hypothalamus will respond for electrical stimulation and it has been shown that nicotine can facilitate ICSS (Wanner and Bättig, 1966; Olds and Domino, 1969; Pradhan and Bowling, 1971; Newman, 1972). Consistent with observations on responding for other types of reinforcers (see review by Sanger and Blackman, 1976), Pradhan and Bowling (1971) also found rate-dependent effects with ICSS; the lower the response rate, the more pronounced was the facilitating effect of nicotine. In rats which had high base-line rates of responding, it was found that nicotine could still exert facilitating effects if the rate was artificially lowered e.g., by reducing the intensity of the reinforcing current. The facilitation by nicotine was blocked by mecamylamine and also by pre-treatment with reserpine. It was therefore concluded (Pradhan and Bowling, 1971; German and Bowden, 1974) that nicotine was probably mediating its facilitatory effect on ICSS through the release of noradrenaline although other interpretations are possible for the effects of reserpine pre-treatment. Newman (1972) concurred with the idea that nicotine facilitated ICSS through actions on an activating noradrenergic "go" system and that the other part of the cholinergic influence on ICSS was a reciprocal, inhibitory "no-go" component, which was muscarinic in nature. Dose-dependent facilitating effects of nicotine were however not demonstrable as was the case with drugs such as amphetamine (Domino and Olds, 1972). There do not seem to have been further investigations of nicotine and ICSS and this apparent lack of interest is surprising in the light of recent general developments in this field relating to more specific identification of anatomical and chemical substrates of brain reward as well as refinements of hypotheses about incentive and reinforcement mechanisms (German and Bowden, 1974; Crow and Deakin, 1978; Wise, 1978).

COMMENTS ON STUDIES OF SITE OF ACTION OF NICOTINE IN THE CNS

Although there is general agreement that Renshaw cells in the spinal cord possess nicotinic receptors, very little is known about the presence and distribution of similar receptor sites elsewhere in the central nervous system. Recent binding studies using constituents of certain snake neurotoxins e.g., α-bungarotoxin (α-BT) and Naja naja toxin, have raised the possibility that sites analogous to peripheral nicotinic acetylcholine receptors can be mapped in the brain (Salvaterra et al., 1975; Speth et al., 1976; Morley et al., 1977; Moore and Brady, 1977; Hunt and Schmidt, 1978; Schechter et al., 1978). There are however some findings which suggest that central nicotinic receptors and toxin binding molecules may not be one and the same. For example, studies of ^{14}C-labelled nicotine accumulation in brain slice preparations (Goodman, 1974; Weiss and Alderdice, 1975; Alderdice and Weiss, 1975) suggest that there is some specific mechanism for sequestering nicotine and that mecamylamine competes with nicotine. However, the binding of α-BT to brain sites although diminished by acetylcholine, nicotine, curare, and decamethonium was not affected by atropine or mecamylamine (Morley et al., 1977). α-BT was found not to block the responses of Renshaw cells to acetylcholine (Duggan et al., 1976) and there was a similar lack of effect on sympathetic ganglia (Brown and Funagalli, 1977). On the other hand there is some anatomical correlation between brain regions which show the presence or absence of toxin binding and the occurrence or lack of "nicotinic" activity, e.g., the hippocampus and the caudate nucleus respectively (Schechter et al., 1978). Tests of stereospecific binding of nicotine itself (e.g., Martin et al., 1978) may help to clarify the nature and distribution of putative nicotinic receptors in the brain and thus lead to improved methods for studying the behavioural actions of nicotine.

NICOTINE AS A DISCRIMINATIVE STIMULUS

Morrison and Stephenson (1969) trained rats to make a saline-nicotine discrimination which they then showed could be blocked by a central antagonist (chlorisondamine). Very similar findings were later reported by Schechter and Rosecrans (1971) using a T-maze procedure. The nicotine cue waned over time after injection and it was found that 60 minutes after dosing, rats which had learned to respond correctly shortly after injections of nicotine or saline now responded randomly (Schechter and Jellinek, 1975). In a series of studies, using a two-lever operant task, similar to that described by Morrison and Stephenson (1969), Rosecrans and his colleagues have presented strong evidence that nicotine can assume stimulus control of operant behaviour, i.e., when drugged with nicotine the rats learn to respond on one lever only and when given saline they respond on the other (Hirschorn and Rosecrans, 1974). The nicotine cue was blocked in such tests by mecamylamine; other tests of the antagonism of the central nicotine cue showed that of a range of other possible antagonists or drugs which interfered with neurotransmitter functioning, e.g., hexamethonium, atropine, dibenamine, propranalol, α-methyl-paratyrosine and p-chlorophenylalanine, only α-methyl-paratyrosine had some blocking effect in one study but not in another. Such an action might well have reflected a more generalised effect and Rosecrans and Chance (1977) concluded that nicotine was acting on some specific cholinergic receptors independent from catechol and indoleamine systems. Other tests also summarised by Rosecrans and Chance (1977) have aimed to use more specific measures to deplete brain noradrenaline and dopamine. The effects of noradrenaline depletion in some ways suggested an increased sensitivity to nicotine while rats deficient in dopamine showed some impairments in their ability to respond to the nicotine cue.

STUDIES OF TOLERANCE TO NICOTINE

Morrison and Stephenson (1972) measured the locomotor activity of rats by an automated method and found that nicotine had an initial depressant effect followed by an increase above control levels. As the experiment progressed, it was found, following repeated medication, that the initial depression of activity became less and less apparent and, eventually, the action of nicotine became predominantly stimulant. Controls were incorporated for the effects of habituation to the apparatus. When animals were retested after an interval of 23 days there was still some tolerance evident to nicotine. Keenan and Johnson (1972) also tested the effects of repeated doses of nicotine on motor activity and their results were broadly consistent with those of Morrison and Stephenson (1972); in addition on cessation of nicotine treatment, they described a "rebound" increase in the amounts of rearing.

In a study of locomotor activity in rats, Stolerman et al (1973b) showed that ambulation and rearing were reduced in a dose-related way. When rats were injected repeatedly for three days and then "challenged" with nicotine the depressant action was greatly reduced. There were no signs of abstinence in nicotine pre-treated rats which were then tested with saline. Hatchell and Collins (1977) have subsequently demonstrated in mice that subjects' sex and strain can influence the development of tolerance. In the tests by Stolerman et al (1973b) it was also found that there was persisting evidence of tolerance 80 days after the end of the nicotine treatment. In a later experiment Stolerman et al (1974) showed that tolerance could be demonstrated even if repeated injections of nicotine were spaced widely apart, in this case at intervals of 3 days. The prolonged changes after repeated medication might be consistent with persistently altered metabolic responses which have been reported in human ex-smokers (Beckett and Triggs, 1967). Rosenthal and Slotkin (1977) have shown that a very large single dose of nicotine given to neonatal rats produces changes in catecholamine biosynthesis for up to 23 days. Studies in animals of the effects of chronic medication with nicotine (Bhagat, 1970a, b; Bhagat and Lind, 1971) have shown some gross changes e.g., increased adrenal weights and there are also indications of an increased turnover of brain noradrenaline and Westfall et al (1967) have reported variable changes in brain levels of serotonin.

Tests of learned behaviour have also been used to demonstrate the development of tolerance to the depressant effects of nicotine. Domino and Lutz (1973) found that a dose of 0.25 mg/kg nicotine base initially suppressed bar-pressing by rats for water rewards. With repeated daily tests, the rats began pressing after shorter and shorter delays following their injections but at no stage was there any facilitation of responding. There is no evidence for or against the notion that changes in such "depressant" actions of nicotine may parallel the development of tolerance to the aversive effects of the drug in man, especially nausea (Johnston, 1942; Rottenstein et al 1960; Beckett et al., 1971). There has been very little systemic research into the aversive properties of nicotine in spite of the fact that it is widely held that tolerance to such effects is a necessary step before smokers can go on to inhale increasing amounts of nicotine in the process of becoming dependent (see e.g., Russell, 1977).

Nelsen and Goldstein (1972) tested rats on an "attention" task based upon the procedure described by Kornetsky and Eliasson (1969) in which two types of error are recorded, those of omission and of commission. This is a difficult test in which animals must not only respond correctly in the presence of a given stimulus but they must also withold responses at other times. Acute doses of nicotine (100 μg/kg base) impaired performance generally but repeated testing against a background of chronic medication showed that while there were no systematic changes due to nicotine treatment on omission errors, errors of commission decreased and there was even a suggestion of improvement above base-line levels. The authors commented that "chronic nicotine treatment improved the efficiency of response to goal—or incentive-oriented stimuli without causing or being accompanied by a generalized increase in the level of activity." This particular study is important because it attempts to examine the effects of chronic nicotine treatment in relation to mechanisms of attention and arousal, although the findings have not yet been confirmed or extended.

Tolerance may develop at different rates to different actions of nicotine and experiments in rats suggest that tolerance can be detected to the effects of nicotine as a central cue. Schechter and Rosecrans (1972) using a T-maze task found that repeated, frequent injections of nicotine markedly impaired the ability of rats to make correct responses depending on whether they had just been given an injection of nicotine or saline.

"Acute" tolerance to nicotine: As distinct from possible metabolic disturbances after repeated or very large single doses of nicotine, some other physio-

logical changes may underlie the altered sensitivity to nicotine after single, relatively small doses. Stolerman et al (1973b) have shown a reduction in sensitivity to the locomotor depressant actions of "challenge" doses of nicotine, which reaches a peak by two hours after pre-treatment and then wanes over the next six hours. The time-course of acute tolerance on such behavioural tests cannot easily be reconciled with earlier observations e.g., by Domino (1967), who found that if intravenous doses of nicotine were spaced apart at intervals of greater than 30 minutes, then tolerance to the EEG activating effects of nicotine could not be detected. However, in a more recent study (Hubbard and Gohd, 1975) there was evidence of tolerance on measures of behavioural and EEG arousal after small doses of nicotine spaced one day apart. Very little seems to be known about the physiological changes which may underlie acute and prolonged tolerance after single or repeated doses of nicotine.

NICOTINE ABSTINENCE SYNDROME

The phenomena of tolerance and abstinence generally go hand in hand and form the basis for understanding some aspects at least of drug dependence (see review by Kumar and Stolerman, 1977). In their recent review, Jaffe and Jarvik (1978) observe that "a variety of psychological, behavioural and physiological disturbances have been reported to follow the discontinuation of smoking. Among the symptoms reported following the cessation of smoking, in addition to the craving for tobacco, are irritability, restlessness, dullness, sleep disturbances, gastro-intestinal disturbances, drowsiness, headache, amnesia, anxiety, and impairment of concentration, judgement, and psychomotor performance. The onset of such symptoms usually occurs within a matter of hours or days after smoking cessation, and have been reported to last from days to months." In spite of this impressive collection of symptoms and a variety of signs e.g., changes in EEG (Ulett and Itil, 1969; Vasquez and Toman, 1967) muscle tension (Hutchinson and Emley, 1973) weight gain (WHO, 1975), reliable animal models of the nicotine abstinence syndrome are conspicuous by their absence. Jaffe and Jarvik (1978) cite two studies in animals in one of which (Seevers, 1973) no significant signs of withdrawal were seen following abrupt cessation of nicotine medication in monkeys. Hutchinson and Emley (1973), however, found that monkeys became more irritable on being withdrawn from nicotine.

Larsson and Silvette (1975) in their comprehensive review cite Bernstein (1970) who commented that "there was no evidence from human studies to support the notion that a consistent, characteristic withdrawal syndrome occurs in all or even most individuals who discontinue smoking" and they then add that "had we the technique to measure the response of a neuron deprived of its once-containing nicotine milieu, we would possess visible evidence as striking as the convulsions which are part of the barbiturate abstinence syndrome." The paradox is that behavioural and physiological techniques are available which are highly sensitive in the case of other drugs and still the putative nicotine abstinence syndrome continues to elude definition and description.

II. STUDIES IN HUMANS

MEASUREMENT OF NICOTINE AND CARBOXYHAEMOGLOBIN CONCENTRATIONS

Nicotine

The study of nicotine and smoking behaviour in humans was long hampered by the inability to measure nicotine concentrations in biological fluids. Consequently, the pharmacokinetic and to some extent the pharmacodynamic aspects of nicotine actions in man were poorly understood. The development of gas chromatographic techniques for estimating nicotine (McNiven, 1965; Beckett and Triggs, 1966) has helped elucidate that role of nicotine in smoking. Using such a technique with a flame-ionization detector, Isaac and Rand (1972) attained a sensitivity of lng/ml of nicotine in a 2.5 ml sample. In six male habitual smokers plasma nicotine concentrations averaged 2.7 ng/ml before smoking (range 1-8) and 20.7 ng/ml (range 12-44) 30 minutes after smoking the last cigarette in a 6.5 hours *ad libitum* smoking session. Next, subjects refrained from smoking for 8 hours and then smoked one of their preferred brands of cigarettes at the rate of one puff/min. The amount of nicotine extracted from the smoke was calculated from the difference between the nicotine contents of exhaled and inhaled smoke and ranged from 0.86 to 3.12 mg. The maximal level to which the plasma nicotine rose was related to the amount of nicotine extracted ($r = 0.88$; $p < 0.02$). However, the amount extracted could differ greatly with a standard smoking machine. This illustrates the crude nature of nicotine yield as a relevant parameter in smoking experiments. Butt length and nicotine content are also only crude ways of estimating nicotine intake in a smoker.

The plasma half-life of nicotine was less than 30 minutes but cumulation quickly occurred in smokers smoking a cigarette every 30 minutes (Armitage, 1978). In spite of this, the rate of elimination is high enough for nicotine levels to drop substantially overnight so that day-to-day accumulation does not occur.

Russell's group have introduced almost routine monitoring of plasma nicotine concentrations in their various studies manipulating smoking behaviour (Feyerabenc, Levitt and Russell, 1975). They confirmed that smoking a single cigarette produces a rise in plasma nicotine concentration of about 25 ng/ml. Peak levels were higher in men (38 ng/ml) than in women (27 ng/ml) (Russell, Feyerabend and Cole, 1976).

In another study (Russell, Wilson, Patel, Feyerabend and Cole, 1975) 10 regular cigarette smokers continued to smoke their usual brand (mean yield 1.34 mg nicotine) or were switched to high-yield (3.2 mg) or low-yield (0.14 mg) cigarettes each for a day. Plasma nicotine levels 2 minutes after a normal cigarette in the mid-morning (before any switch) was 24.4 ng/ml with a range of 15.5-38.4 ng/ml among the smokers. Variation between days for each smoker was much less. There was no relation between the mid-morning nicotine level and the subjects' usual cigarette consumption or the nicotine yield of their usual brand of cigarette. When changed to a low nicotine cigarette for a day, consumption rose only slightly. However, significantly fewer high yield cigarettes were smoked on the test day (a fall from 10.8 to 6.7/day). Average afternoon levels of nicotine were no different from morning levels for normal cigarettes (30.1 cf. 24.4 ng/ml in the morning) or high yield ones (29.2 cf. 24.4 ng/ml). After switching to low nicotine cigarettes levels dropped to 8.5 ng/ml. Variation was great, especially after switch to high yield cigarettes, but it seemed that the adjustment was more in terms of the way the cigarette was smoked than the number, as the nicotine levels and number of cigarettes smoked stayed roughly the same. Again the nicotine yield of the cigarette as gauged from standard smoking machines was a misleading indication of potential smoking behaviour, showing no correlation to plasma nicotine peaks.

More recently, Russell and Feyerabend (1978) have reported on plasma nicotine concentrations during prolonged heavy smoking—three 1.3 mg nicotine cigarettes per hour for 7 hours. Concentrations rose over the first 3 hours but then reached a steady-state around 40-50 ng/ml. Even so, peaks and troughs associated with each cigarette were still identifiable. In another part of this study, plasma concentrations after repeated intravenous injections of nicotine were estimated. Nicotine peaks did not alter with repeated injections yet the concomitant tachycardias fell off markedly, suggesting a tachyphylactic effect.

Carboxyhaemoglobin Concentrations

Another blood estimation which has proved of value is the carboxyhaemoglobin level (COHb). The COHb level rose with every cigarette smoked by about 1.3 percent and fell between cigarettes but remained fairly constant otherwise throughout the day (Castleden and Cole, 1974). Therefore, a random COHb estimation was a fairly good indicator of the mean level of smoking maintained by a subject. One precaution is that an estimate should not be taken within 30 minutes of smoking a cigarette as it takes this time for the carbon monoxide to attain distribution equilibrium in the extravascular compartments of the body. COHb levels are consistently higher in smokers than non-smokers even during the night and are a fair reflection of the amount of cigarette smoke inhaled over an integral period of time.

Russell et al. (1973), in their study of subjects switching to high and low nicotine-yield cigarettes, found that COHb levels fell in both cases. The fall on switching to high yield cigarettes was attributed to the drop in the number of cigarettes smoked, the CO yield per cigarette remaining roughly the same. With the low-yield cigarettes, the CO delivery per cigarette was much lower also, which accounted for the drop in COHb levels.

Manufactured cigarettes vary greatly in the CO yield (Russell, Cole, Idle and Adams, 1975). For example, the mean increase after smoking a single cigarette was 1.45 percent for a standard-size brand (ten puffs) and 1.09 percent for a small-size brand (seven puffs). For extra-mild cigarettes, the increases were 0.64 and 0.75 percent, respectively, much more than the proportionate nicotine decrease (1.2 and 0.3 mg nicotine/cigarette) (Russell, Wilson, Cole, Idle and Feyerabend, 1973). Data such as these have led to calls that the CO yield of available brands of cigarettes be published as well as tar and nicotine yields. However, CO yields themselves depend on the puffing pattern and this varies greatly from individual to individual and with different types of cigarettes. Puffing-rate is highest at the beginning of a cigarette and then slows down, possibly because the nicotine and tar in the stub become more concentrated as the cigarette burns down. This is reflected in a rapid rise in COHb concentrations at the start of a cigarette followed by a levelling off or even a fall towards the end of the cigarette (Ashton and Telford, 1973).

Despite these problems, COHb blood concentration estimations provide a useful check on manipulations designed to reduce cigarette smoking in real-life conditions. With nicotine chewing-gums, for example, COHb levels dropped less than expected as recorded cigarette consumption fell off (table 3), suggesting a change in pattern of inhalation (Russell, Wilson, Feyerabend and Cole, 1976).

EFFECT OF NICOTINE ON SMOKING BEHAVIOUR

By Injection

In the earliest of these few studies, Johnston (1942) gave nicotine injections hypodermically to 35 volunteers. Some received single doses but most had multiple doses. Non-smokers after 1.3 mg nicotine termed the effects "queer," muzziness and light-headedness being commonly reported. Smokers, however, "invariably thought the sensation pleasant and, given an adequate dose, were disinclined for a smoke for some time thereafter." A dose of 1.6 mg usually produced toxic symptoms in non-smokers, whereas heavy inhalers or pipe smokers easily tolerated 6.5 mg injections. Intravenous injections of 0.14 to 0.21 mg of nicotine (? as the tartrate) closely simulated the subjective effects of a deep inhalation. The nicotine action was perceived in about 15 sec. both on inhalation of tobacco smoke and on intravenous injection of nicotine and lasted for 1 or 2 minutes. Johnston gave himself three to four daily subcutaneous injections of 1.3 mg nicotine for 20 days and found himself preferring these to smoking.

A study frequently cited as proving the crucial role of nicotine in smoking behaviour is that of Lucchesi et al. (1967). Subjects received nicotine via a slow intravenous infusion, but were unaware of the nature of the drug. They were allowed to smoke, the number and butt-weight of the cigarettes being measured. In the first experiment, 4 subjects received 1 mg of nicotine bitartrate over 20 minutes: smoking behaviour was not affected. Next, 5 subjects were given 2 mg of nicotine bitartrate in the first hour and 4 mg during each of the next 5 hours (totalling 22 mg over 6 hours which is equivalent to about 7 mg of nicotine base). There was a 27 percent reduction in the number of cigarettes smoked compared with saline infusion—from 10 down to 7.3 over the 6 hours ($p<0.001$). Butt weights increased 20 percent and they took fewer puffs. Finally, four subjects received 8 mg of nicotine bitartrate over 6 hours which increased heart rate but did not alter smoking behaviour. Thus, infusion rates of 4 mg/hour or so were needed to reduce smoking. The authors comments that "we should have observed a much greater reduction in the smoking frequency." But the infusion rate was only equivalent to about 1-2 cigarettes per hour and marked suppression was thus unlikely.

However, slow infusion does not mimic the repeated bolus effects which successive puffs and inhalations produces. In an attempt to simulate cigarette smoking more closely, we gave the nicotine in 10 bolus injections (Kumar, Cooke, Lader and Russell, 1977). First we established that "forced puffing" on a high or an average nicotine content cigarette, as compared with puffing on a nicotine-free herbal cigarette, produced a dose-related diminution in the number of puffs on a freely available lighted cigarette during the subsequent ten minutes (table 1). The volume per puff was also diminished and physiological effects were detected in the form of heart-rate increases and augmentation of the fast-wave (beta) activity in the EEG. In the second part of the experiment, nicotine bitartrate or saline were injected as 10 boluses to a total of 1.7 mg, 0.85 mg. and 0 mg/70 kg body weight of nicotine base over 10 minutes. Again, tachycardia and increase in EEG beta were produced in a dose-related manner. Surprisingly, no effect on the smoking behaviour was produced. This unexpected result suggests that, under the conditions of our experiment, nicotine was not the sole, or even the main, reinforcer of smoking. This study is being repeated with estimations of plasma nicotine as an additional and important measure.

By Inhalation

The most appropriate way to attempt to mimic the inhalation characteristics of the cigarette smoker is to administer nicotine by aerosol. There are problems in aerosol particle size, pH of the solution, rate of delivery and acceptability to the subject. That the approach is feasible is shown by a study in which two puffs from a nicotine aerosol (1.06 mg) seemed to compare with a single inhalation

TABLE 1. Effects of nicotine given by inhalation and by bolus injections at two dose-levels, as compared with placebo, on smoking behaviour and physiological activity during the ensuing 10 minutes.

	Mode of Administration					
	Inhalation Dose Level			Injection Dose Level		
Variable	0	Low	High	0	Low	High
Number of puffs/10 min.	8.0	6.7	4.8	10.0	8.8	9.5
Volume/puff (ml)	36.0	29.0	26.0	16.0	17.0	16.0
Heart rate/min.	75.9	77.2	79.3	73.5	76.0	78.2
Beta voltage (mV)	1.92	1.94	2.07	1.57	1.70	1.80

Abstracted from Kumar et al. (1977).

from a lighted cigarette (Herxheimer, Griffiths, Hamilton and Wakefield, 1967). In fact, similar increases in pulse rate and blood pressure were obtained in each instance. The mean pulse rate increase with the cigarette was 9.8 beats/min, with the aerosol 8.0; the corresponding figures for systolic and diastolic blood pressure were 5.2/3.2 and 6.7/7.9. The effects became apparent 1 or 2 minutes after the subject started to inhale nicotine but the peak effect was earlier with the aerosol. No systematic studies of aerosol nicotine effects on smoking behaviour have been reported.

By Mouth

This route of administration is ambiguously termed because it can refer to oral ingestion with absorption in the gastro-intestinal tract or to buccal absorption, the drug being retained in the mouth. Nicotine tartrate 10 mg in capsules or placebo capsules was administered 5 times a day on alternate days. On any given day all 5 capsules were either nicotine or placebo. The average number of cigarettes dropped marginally but significantly from a mean of 24.1 on placebo days to 22.4 on nicotine days. However, the average butt weight per cigarette and ratings of strength and quality of the cigarettes were not altered (Jarvik, Glick and Nakamura, 1970). Although the authors interpret the weak effect as pointing to the "important role played by secondary conditioning," there is no evidence that the nicotine was actually absorbed, or if absorbed that it was not extensively metabolised first-pass before reaching the systemic circulation.

Buccal absorption has the advantage of avoiding such metabolism and nicotine-containing chewing gums have been formulated (Fernö, Lichtnetkert and Lundgren, 1973) but proved disappointing in clinical trials as a smoking substitute (Brankmark, Ohlin and Westling, 1973). Using a similar preparation, Jarvik's group administered placebo, low-yield (1 mg) or high-yield (4 mg) nicotine gum to 56 undergraduate subjects and compared the effects on latency to lighting up the next cigarette and puff-time with those of nil, low (0.3 mg) and high (1.3 mg) nicotine content cigarettes (Koslowski, Jarvik and Gritz, 1975). The subjects were unaware that the experiment concerned smoking behaviour. The latency to lighting up the next standard cigarette was less after smoking low than high nicotine content cigarettes but was not affected by gum nicotine content (table 2). Conversely, the puff-times were unaffected by prior smoking of test cigarettes but were curtailed when a high nicotine gum had been chewed (table 2). There were complications in the design and execution of this experiment which render its interpretation difficult but the authors hazarded the opinion that pharmacokinetic differences in buccal and alveolar absorption were responsible for the differential effects on latency and puff-times. The lack of plasma nicotine levels is particularly unfortunate here.

TABLE 2. Effects of "pre-load" with nicotine gum or cigarette smoking on smoking behaviour

	Mode of Administration			
	Inhalation		Chewing-Gum	
	Dose Level		Dose Level	
Variable	Low	High	Low	High
Latency (minutes)	4.7	14.8	4.9	8.0
Total puff-time (sec)	22.0	15.0	28.0	14.0

N.B. Other controls were included.
Abstracted from Koslowski et al. (1975).

Nicotine gum has also been evaluated as an aid to giving up smoking but with pharmacokinetic controls sufficient to provide information about the role of nicotine in smoking behaviour (Russell, Wilson, Feyerabend and Cole, 1976). Forty-three smokers wishing to give up smoking were administered nicotine-containing gum (2 mg) or placebo gum in a repeated cross-over design. The subjects were first allowed to smoke freely and then encouraged to cut down and stop their consumption. A reduction of 31 percent was achieved on placebo gum, of 37 percent on the nicotine gum, even before the smokers tried to curtail their smoking (table 3). Substantial further reductions ensued when the smokers actively tried to give up. There was no difference between placebo and nicotine gums in this respect. COHb levels showed similar drops but there the differences between placebo and active gums were significant under both usual smoking ($p<0.01$) and trying to abstain ($p<0.02$) conditions (table 3). Nicotine levels were slightly lower on placebo gum than on nicotine gum but attained similar levels after smoking. When the subjects were trying not to smoke, nicotine levels were very much lower ($p<0.001$) but differences between the two gums were again not marked. It would seem that the nicotine gum does not substantially alter the number of cigarettes smoked as compared with placebo gum but does lessen the amount of inhalation as reflected by the COHb levels. Nicotine levels differed by only about 3 ng/ml between placebo and nicotine gum conditions probably because 2 mg/piece content is too low to produce nicotine levels comparable to smoking (4 mg is required).

TABLE 3. Mean values of cigarette consumption, COHb and nicotine levels in 43 smokers taking nicotine and placebo chewing gum

	Initial Levels Before Taking Gum	Smoking as Inclined		Trying to Stop	
		Placebo Gum	Nicotine Gum	Placebo Gum	Nicotine Gum
Daily cigarette consumption	33.3	23.0	20.9	3.9	4.1
COHb (%)	8.5	7.2	6.3	2.9	2.3
Nicotine	30.1	24.7	27.4	7.3	10.7

Abstracted from Russell et al. (1976).

Other Manipulations

A more indirect approach has comprised alteration of nicotine excretion by manipulating urinary pH. From the data of Beckett and Triggs (1966), it can be calculated that 35 percent of administered nicotine is excreted unchanged in an acidic urine, only 1 percent in an alkaline urine, and about 5-10 percent if the pH is uncontrolled. Based on the presumption that urinary pH manipulations would appreciably alter nicotine concentrations in the body, Schachter and his colleagues (1977) carried out the following series of experiments.

Records were kept of the amounts smoked by seven subjects during several 2-day periods when they were taking substantial amounts of either sodium carbonate, placebo or ascorbic acid.

TABLE 4. Mean number of cigarettes smoked and urinary pH values while subjects were taking sodium bicarbonate, placebo or ascorbic acid

Drug	Mean No. Cigarettes		Mean Urinary pH	
	First drug day	Second drug day	First drug day	Second drug day
Bicarbonate	37.2	35.7	6.8	7.4
Placebo	39.4	34.2	5.7	5.9
Ascorbic acid	38.4	42.1	6.2	5.7

Abstracted from Schachter et al. (1977).

The effects of these drugs on smoking are presented in table 4. Modest increases in smoking ($p<0.08$) occurred when the urine was marginally more acid, modest decreases ($p<0.05$) when alkalinisation was attempted. In a replication and extension of this study, cigarette consumption increased by a sixth when either ascorbic acid or glutamic acid were administered. This was rather surprising as the urinary pH dropped by only about 0.2 units.

Schachter and his team (1977) extended their observations to the effect of party-going on cigarette consumption. Social events were accompanied by a lowering of urinary pH averaging 0.4 units and cigarette consumption rose from a mean of 27.9 to 31.2. The decrease in urinary pH is presumably due to alcohol ingestion with its subsequent metabolism to acetic acid. Whether increased smoking at parties can be attributed to lowered urinary pH and more rapid excretion of nicotine is a question which awaits further study with monitoring of plasma nicotine levels.

The basic premise of these studies has been recently examined directly (Feyerabend and Russell, 1978). Urinary excretion of nicotine was influenced markedly by pH and the rate of urine flow, both factors being important. Plasma nicotine concentrations were about 30 percent higher under alkaline than under acidic urinary conditions although the urinary excretion rate was 30 times as slow.

A strategy stemming directly from classical pharmacology has been the use of nicotine antagonists (Stolerman, Goldfarb, Fink and Jarvik, 1973). The drugs administered were mecamylamine hydrochloride, a secondary compound which readily penetrates to the brain, and pentolinium tartrate, a quarternary derivative, which hardly crosses the "blood-brain-barrier." Doses were 7.5-17.5 mg and 100-150 mg respectively. Placebo controls were incorporated, each drug being given as a single dose. A battery of tests was administered including digit symbol substitution test, hand steadiness test, assessment of subjective state, and measurements of blood pressure and pulse rate. Smoking behaviour was monitored during the testing session.

TABLE 5. Mean number of cigarettes smoked and puffs on cigarettes during 2-h test sessions after drug administration.

Drug treatment	(mg)	N	Cigarettes after		Puffs after	
			drug	placebo	drug	placebo
Mecamylamine	7.5	8	4.4*	3.4	38.1	30.4
	12.5	14	4.8*	3.2	36.9*	26.1
	17.5	10	3.8	3.4	36.6	32.8
Pentolinium	100.0	10	3.6	3.8	32.9	35.4
	150.0	10	3.3*	4.3	36.6	37.5

*$p<0.05$
Abstracted from Stolerman et al. (1973).

Doses of mecamylamine, presumed to block the central cholinergic actions of nicotine, were associated with a significant increase in the number of cigarettes smoked and the number of puffs on the cigarettes (table 5). By contrast, pentolinium tended to decrease the number smoked, reaching significant levels after the higher dose. Mecamylamine but not pentolinium tended to reduce ratings of smoking satisfaction. Mecamylamine and pentolinium impaired performance on the digit symbol substitution test. Hand steadiness was improved by mecamylamine quite substantially but pentolinium had no effect. The cardiovascular measures, introduced as a check that physiological effects were being exerted, showed the expected changes—hypotension and tachycardia—after mecamylamine administration, but pentolinium yielded no clear-cut changes. Again, while interesting and sure to foster further research, this study is difficult to interpret in the absence of pharmacokinetic data from monitoring nicotine concentrations in the body. Chronic dosage would also be a useful development.

NICOTINE YIELD AND SMOKING BEHAVIOUR

A commonly-used approach has been to attempt to manipulate smoking by altering the amount of nicotine in the cigarette. From what has been discussed already, it will be appreciated that the nicotine yield can be a very poor indicator of the amount of nicotine extracted from the smoke and of plasma (and presumably brain) nicotine levels. Thus, number of cigarettes smoked, butt length and nicotine content may be inaccurate estimates of nicotine delivery. Puff frequency and depth are better, but still fall short of the ideal. With these reservations in mind, some studies on manipulating nicotine yield and observing behaviour are briefly reviewed.

An early study is also one of the more interesting from the point of view of nicotine delivery (Finnegan, Larson and Haag, 1945). Naturally low-content nicotine tobacco was treated with additional nicotine and both low-content and "spiked" tobacco were made up into cigarettes yielding 0.34 and 1.96 mg nicotine per cigarette. The latter was about normal for the time of the study. Twenty-four habitual cigarette smokers smoked their usual brands for a month to establish base-line cigarette consumption. They were then switched to the added nicotine cigarettes for about 2 weeks to accustom them to the rather inferior aroma and taste and then for 4 weeks on the low-nicotine cigarettes, with a final 2 weeks or so on the added nicotine preparation. The degree to which nicotine was missed was assessed by questioning and ranged from none to definite and prolonged lack of satisfaction with low nicotine cigarettes. The results are summarised in table 6. Although the smokers who increased their consumption when switched to low nicotine cigarettes apparently avoided dissatisfaction, it can be seen that the increase was far too small to maintain nicotine intake, unless the pattern of smoking and inhalation changed profoundly. Indeed, re-analysis of the published data shows that even the modest increase recorded was not really significant. The authors emphasise the protean nature of the smoking habit: in some smokers nicotine becomes a major factor, in others it seems irrelevant.

TABLE 6. Effect of nicotine yield on cigarette consumption and smoking satisfaction

Degree to which nicotine was missed	Yield (mg)	Standard brand 2.0	Average daily consumption		
			Nicotine added (first period) 1.96	Low nicotine 0.34	Nicotine added (second period) 1.96
Nil	N=6	26.9	26.6	30.9	26.8
Mild dissatisfaction	N=6	22.4	22.0	26.5	23.9
Definite temporary	N=3	23.6	28.3	28.6	27.6
Definite prolonged	N=9	25.0	24.7	24.6	24.9

Abstracted from Finnegan et al. (1945).

A similar conclusion can be drawn from the work of Cherry and Forbes (1972). On the basis of the butt analysis of nicotine, they reported that most smokers took in less nicotine when smoking a low-nicotine brand (yield 0.77 mg) than on a higher-nicotine brand (1.35 mg). However, a "minority" of smokers took in equal amounts of nicotine on both brands.

The smoking behaviour of 36 volunteer subjects with two types of cigarettes was noted (Ashton and Watson, 1970). The low nicotine cigarette had a filtertip so that only 1.0 mg nicotine was emitted in the smoke. The high nicotine cigarette yielded 2.1 mg. The subjects undertook two driving simulator tasks, easy and difficult, and smoked 2½ cigarettes during the task and during a rest period afterwards. The puff frequency was noted and the cigarette stub were analysed for nicotine content, allowing an estimate of the nicotine presented to the individual. During both tasks and the rest period, the puffs per minute and the time taken to smoke one cigarette were significantly different for the subjects on the two types of cigarettes. The nicotine delivered to the subject, however, was a little higher on the high-nicotine cigarette but only reached significance during the difficult task (table 7). These data seem to strongly support the hypothesis that smokers adjust their smoking rate and pattern to maintain nicotine intake constant, but it should be pointed out that the subjects were instructed to smoke at set times.

TABLE 7. Effect of nicotine content of cigarettes on some smoking variables during two tasks and a rest period.

Type of cigarette	Puffs per minute			Time per cigarette (min)		Nicotine deliverance (mg)		
	Easy	Difficult	Rest	Easy	Difficult	Easy	Difficult	Rest
Low nicotine N=17	1.74	1.87	2.44	7.58	7.58	173.0	179.0	214.0
	***	**	***	**	**	N.S.	*	N.S.
High nicotine N=19	0.98	1.02	1.94	9.11	8.89	179.0	184.0	222.0

$*p<0.05$ $**p<0.01$ $***p<0.001$
Abstracted from Ashton and Watson (1970).

Similar conclusions can be drawn from Frith's (1971) experiment. Nine subjects smoked three types of cigarettes delivering 1.0, 1.4 and 2.1 mg of nicotine respectively. The rate of puffing and volume per puff were registered on a special puffing machine over an 8-hour period. The number of cigarettes smoked decreased with increase in nicotine content and the time per cigarette increased. The subjects reported the high-nicotine cigarette to be stronger than the other two but were unable to distinguish between the latter.

The complexities of analysing smoking behaviour are well exemplified by the study of Turner, Sillett and Ball (1974). Ten volunteers smoked medium nicotine (1.4 mg) cigarettes for a week and then switched to low nicotine (0.8 mg) for the following week, the third week smoking very low nicotine (0.3 mg) cigarettes. Cigarette consumption, COHb percent, butt lengths and nicotine contents were measured. The number of cigarettes smoked daily rose with the switch to low nicotine cigarettes but rose no further when very low nicotine cigarettes were substituted (table 8). COHb levels did not alter from medium to low nicotine cigarette period but dropped significantly when on the very low nicotine cigarettes. The measured/expected filter nicotine ratio rose as the nicotine content dropped indicating greater extraction of nicotine from the cigarette and butt lengths were shorter. Six subjects found the medium brand too strong, eight initially rated the low nicotine brand too mild but by the end of the week all found them acceptable. All subjects rated the very low nicotine cigarettes weak and unsatisfying. From the calculated nicotine presentation per cigarette it can be estimated that in order to maintain nicotine intake constant an increase in daily consumption to 38 and 135 cigarettes respectively would have been required. Instead the daily nicotine intake dropped a little on the low nicotine cigarette and substantially on the very low one.

TABLE 8. Effect of nicotine contents of cigarettes on some smoking variables during ad libitum smoking

	Medium	Low	Very Low
Machine-smoked yield (mg)	1.4	0.8	0.3
Daily cigarette consumption	25.7	30.9	29.2
COHb percent	6.34	6.25	3.80
Ratio of measured nicotine butt content in study to that after machine smoking	0.62	0.77	1.23
Butt length (mm)	8.84	7.20	4.54
Calculated nicotine presentation per cigarette (mg)	0.89	0.60	0.17
Calculated nicotine presentation per day (mg)	22.9	19.2	5.0
Number of cigarettes required to maintain daily presentation		38	135

Abstracted from Turner et al. (1974).

Jarvik's group have carried out several studies in which cigarette lengths have been altered. In one study (Goldfarb and Jarvik, 1972), 18 subjects smoked cigarettes cut to half the original length for a week and for a second week smoked the distal half of regular length cigarettes down to a mark. The average number of the half-cigarettes smoked by the group as a whole did not differ from the number of whole cigarettes smoked in control weeks. However, 12 of the subjects did increase the number of half-cigarettes by an average of 7/day and of the marked cigarettes by 5/day, suggesting some attempt at compensation. The support for the titration of nicotine hypothesis is, however, very weak.

In a further study (Jarvik, Popek, Schneider, Baer-Weiss and Gritz, 1978), 28 subjects were given whole, half, quarter and eighth-length cigarettes in random order to smoke through a puffing device for 2 hour sessions. As table 9 shows, the number of cigarettes rises, the number of puffs decreases and satisfaction ratings drop as the cigarette length is decreased. The peculiar distribution of the number of puffs is unexplained and the problems of estimating nicotine presentation makes this study difficult to interpret. Although some partial compensation for nicotine content decrease has occurred, it is much less than the proportional decrease in cigarette length.

In the second part of this study, cigarette length and nicotine content were manipulated independently. Two strengths of cigarette, 2.0 and 0.2 mg, were smoked either full-length or quarter-length. Subjects smoked and puffed significantly more on the low nicotine than the high nicotine cigarettes (table 10). Subjects smoked significantly more quarter-length than full-length cigarettes but did not puff more. The number of puffs per cigarette was unaffected. Thus, again although there was some attempt to regulate nicotine intake, it fell far short of complete compensation, the number of cigarettes smoked with the low nicotine content increasing by only 20 percent instead of by 10 times.

TABLE 9. Effect of cigarette size and nicotine content on some smoking variables during a 2-h session.

	Nicotine content			
	High (2 mg)		Low (0.2 mg)	
Length:	1	¼	1	¼
Variable				
Number of cigarettes	5.7	11.7	7.0	14.0
Number of puffs	50.7	40.3	58.8	49.9
Puffs/cigarette	8.9	3.4	8.4	3.6
Satisfaction rating	3.6	4.0	3.7	3.9

Abstracted from Jarvik et al. (1978).

TABLE 10. Effect of cigarette size on some smoking variables during a 2-h session.

Variable	Size of cigarette			
	1	1/2	1/4	1/8
Number of cigarettes	5.4	8.2	10.3	15.2
Number of puffs	54.0	53.7	43.8	43.7
Puffs/cigarette	9.7	6.5	4.2	2.9
Satisfaction rating	5.2	4.9	3.6	2.7

Abstracted from Jarvik et al. (1978).

As nicotine and tar contents of cigarettes are closely related, tar could conceivably be the important factor in regulating smoking behaviour, the apparent effect of nicotine being artefactual. However, in one experiment, tar and nicotine contents were to some extent manipulated independently (Goldfarb, Gritz, Jarvik and Stolerman, 1976). The number of cigarettes smoked per day was unaffected by tar content whereas it decreased with increase in nicotine level; as with so many of these studies, this increase was insufficient to maintain nicotine intake constant. The smokers detected differences in the "strength" of the cigarettes, depending on nicotine and not tar content, but no systematic changes in "satisfaction" ratings were apparent.

NICOTINE AND AROUSAL

Nicotine has a wide range of physiological actions including a decrease in skeletal muscle tone, delay in gastric emptying, stimulation of salivary secretion and catecholamine release with ensuing secondary effects. Plasma cortisol and growth hormone concentrations are increased. Noradrenaline is released from peripheral noradrenergic endings. There is no evidence either supporting or refuting the hypothesis that one or more of such effects underlie the maintenance of smoking behaviour.

At a psychophysiological level, several attempts have been made to interpret the maintenance of smoking behavior (see Warburton and Wesnes, 1978). Eysenck (1963) has attempted to relate patterns of smoking with personality types and takes the view, for example, that individuals with extraverted personalities smoke in order to increase their level of arousal. These speculations are, however, based upon the assumption that extraversion and cortical arousal bear a recognisable relationship to each other. The concept of arousal can only be applied within narrow limits when physiological measures are involved. Furthermore, nicotine and smoking effects may involve the very physiological measures used as indicators of arousal.

Of several studies in this area, the most sophisticated, and the one which brings us full circle to the opening section on why people smoke, is that of Myrsten and co-workers (1975). A questionnaire was constructed which enables smokers to be divided into those who smoke primarily in high arousal situations —the presumption being that smoking is relaxing—and those who smoke mainly in low arousal situations, to combat boredom or to maintain alertness. Sixteen subjects, 8 high- and 8 low-arousal smokers, were selected from the 90 male light smokers screened. Two test conditions were used, a vigilance task which would induce low arousal, and a complex sensorimotor response task, requiring high alertness. Smoking two cigarettes during the test improved performance in the low-arousal test in the low-arousal smokers but slightly impaired it in the high-arousal smokers. In the high-arousal test, smoking had no effect in the low-arousal smokers but improved performance in the other group. Subjective reports tended to corroborate these differential effects of smoking in different types of smokers in different tasks. Nevertheless, such experiments are capable of very complex interpretations when the relationship between performance is entered into the equation. This relationship follows the classical inverted-U-shaped curves (Yerkes-Dodson Law). Accordingly several arousal points must be studied because with only two, it is impossible to say whether the performance/arousal points are on the ascending or descending limbs of the curve. Such a study would throw much light on arousal/smoking relationships but even so smokers may smoke for different reasons at different times.

Among similar experiments, one other may be mentioned. Fuller and Forrest (1973) reported that heavy smokers tend to puff more on their cigarettes under low-arousal than high-arousal conditions. However, nicotine extraction from the cigarettes was not altered suggesting perhaps that the behavioural but not the pharmacological factors could be manipulated by altering arousal conditions. This accords with the nicotine-substitution studies detailed earlier which suggested that cigarette smoking was rather more than just nicotine manipulation.

In spite of the widespread prevalence of the tobacco smoking habit and its continuing medical, commercial and political importance, research into the psychopharmacology of nicotine and other possible important constituents of tobacco has advanced relatively slowly. In this review we have paid particular attention to the pharmacological approach and to methodological issues as they apply to nicotine in tobacco smoking. The discussion of individual (constitutional) and environmental factors which may modify the putative reinforcing actions of nicotine in man has been intentionally restricted as this is a full topic in its own right. In summary, very little is known about the nature of the pharmacological rewards that are sought by novice smokers nor about the maintenance of the habit in established smokers. Similarly, the physiological changes which facilitate relapse in abstaining smokers also remain obscure.

REFERENCES

Alderdice, M.T. and Weiss, G.B. (1975): Effects of pharmacological agents on (14^C)–nicotine distribution and movements in slices from different rat brain areas. *Neuropharmacology 14:* 811-817.
Armitage, A.K. and Hall, G.H. (1968): Nicotine, smoking and cortical activation. *Nature 219:* 1179-1180.
Armitage, A.K., Hall, G.H. and Morrison, C.F. (1968): Pharmacological basis for the tobacco smoking habit. *Nature 217:* 331-334.
Armitage, A.K., Hall, G.H. and Sellers, C.M. (1969): Effects of nicotine on electrocortical activity and acetylcholine release from the cat cerebral cortex. *British Journal of Pharmacology 35:* 152-160.
Armitage, A.K. (1978): The role of nicotine in the tobacco smoking habit. In: R.E. Thornton (Ed.), *Smoking Behaviour.* Churchill Livingstone, Edinburgh, p. 229-243.
Ashton, H. and Telford, R. (1973): Smoking and carboxyhaemoglobin. *Lancet 2:* 857-858.
Ashton, H. and Watson, D.W. (1970): Puffing frequency and nicotine intake in cigarette smokers. *British Medical Journal 3:* 679-681.
Balfour, D.J.K. (1973): Effects of nicotine on the uptake and retention of noradrenaline and 5-hydroxytryptamine by rat brain homogenates. *European Journal of Pharmacology 23:* 19-26.
Balfour, D.J. and Morrison, C.F. (1975): A possible role for the pituitary adrenal system in the effects of nicotine on avoidance behaviour. *Pharmacology, Biochemistry and Behaviour 3:* 349-354.
Balfour, D.J., Khullar, A.K. and Longden, A. (1975): Effects of nicotine on plasma corticosterone and brain amines in stressed and unstressed rats. *Pharmacology, Biochemistry and Behaviour 3:* 179-184.
Bättig, K., Driscoll, P., Schlalter, J. and Uster, H.J. (1976): Effects of nicotine on the exploratory locomotion patterns of female Roman high- and low-avoidance rats. *Pharmacology, Biochemistry and Behaviour 4:* 435-439.
Beckett, A.H. and Triggs, E.J. (1966): Determination of nicotine and its metabolite, cotinine, in urine by gas chromatography. *Nature 211:* 1415-1417.
Beckett, A.H. and Triggs, E.J. (1967): Enzyme induction in man caused by smoking. *Nature 216:* 587.
Beckett, A.H., Garrod, J.W. and Jenner, P. (1971): The effect of smoking on nicotine metabolism *in vivo* in man. *Journal of Pharmacy and Pharmacology 23:* 62S-67S.
Bhagat, B. (1970a): Influence of chronic administration of nicotine on the turnover and metabolism of noradrenaline in the rat brain. *Psychopharmacologia 18:* 325-332.
Bhagat, B. (1970b): Effects of chronic administration of nicotine on storage and synthesis of noradrenaline in rat brain. *British Journal of Pharmacology 38:* 86-92.
Bhagat, B., Bayer, T. and Lind, C. (1971): Effects of chronic administration of nicotine on drug-induced hypnosis in mice. *Psychopharmacologia 21:* 287-293.
Bhattacharya, I.C. and Goldstein, L. (1970): Influence of acute and chronic nicotine administration on intra- and inter-structural relationships of the electrical activity in the rabbit brain. *Neuropharmacology 9:* 109-118.

Bovet-Nitti, F. and Bovet, D. (1966): Different action of nicotine during the day and night in spontaneous activity (running activity) of the rat. *Compte rendu de l'Academie des sciences 262:* 316-320.

Bovet, D., Bovet-Nitti, F., Oliverio, A. (1966): Effects of nicotine on avoidance conditioning of inbred strains of mice. *Psychopharmacologia 10:* 1-5.

Bovet, D., Bovet-Nitti, F., and Oliverio, A. (1967): Action of nicotine on spontaneous and acquired behaviour in rats and mice. *Annals of the New York Academy of Sciences 142:* 261-267.

Bradley, P.B. and Elkes, J. (1957): The effect of some drugs on the electrical activity of the brain. *Brain 80:* 77-117.

Brantmark, B., Ohlin, P. and Westling, H. (1973): Nicotine-containing chewing gum as an anti-smoking aid. *Psychopharmacologia 31:* 191-200.

British Medical Journal (1977): Editorial: Do people smoke for nicotine? *2:* 1041-1042.

Brown, D.A. and Fumagalli, L. (1977): Dissociation of α-bungarotoxin binding and receptor block in the rat superior cervical ganglion. *Brain Research 129:* 165.

Castleden, C.M. and Cole, P.V. (1974): Variations in carboxyhaemoglobin levels in smokers. *British Medical Journal 4:* 736-738.

Cherry, W.H. and Forbes, W.F. (1972): Canadian studies aimed toward a less harmful cigarette. *Journal of National Cancer Institute 48:* 1765-1773.

Clark, M.S. (1969): Self-administered nicotine solutions preferred to placebo by the rat. *British Journal Pharmacology 35:* 367.

Crow, T.J. and Deakin, J.F.W. (1978): Brain reinforcement centers and psychoactive drugs. In: Y. Israel, F.B. Glaser, H. Kalant, R.E. Popham, W. Schmidt and R.G. Smart (Eds.), *Research Advances in Alcohol and Drug Problems.* Plenum, New York, p. 25-76.

DeBelleroche, J. and Bradford, H.F. (1978): Biochemical evidence for the presence of presynaptic receptors on dopaminergic nerve terminals. *Brain Research 142:* 53-68.

Deneau, G.A. and Inoki, R. (1967): Nicotine self-administration in monkeys. *Annals of the New York Academy of Sciences 142:* 277-279.

Domino, E.F. (1967): Electroencephalographic and behavioural arousal effects of small doses of nicotine: a neuropsychopharmacological study. *Annals of the New York Academy of Sciences 142:* 216-244.

Domino, E.F. (1973): Neuropsychopharmacology of nicotine and tobacco smoking. In: W.L. Dunn (Ed.), *Smoking Behaviour: Motives and Incentives.* V.H. Winston, Washington, D.C. p. 5-31.

Domino, E.F. and Lutz, M.P. (1973): Tolerance to the effects of daily nicotine on rat bar pressing behaviour for water reinforcement. *Pharmacology, Biochemistry and Behaviour 1:* 445-448.

Domino, E.F. and Olds, M.E. (1972): Effects of d-amphetamine, scopolamine, chlordiazepoxide and diphenylhydantoin on self-stimulation behaviour and brain acetylcholine. *Psychopharmacologia 23:* 1-16.

Duggan, A.W., Hall, J.G. and Lee, C.Y. (1976): Alpha-bungarotoxin, cobra neurotoxin and excitation of Renshaw cells by acetylcholine. *Brain Research 107:* 166-170.

Eddy, N.B. et al., (1964): Evaluation of dependence-producing drugs. *W.H.O. Technical Report* No. 287.

Eysenck, H.J. (1963): Personality and cigarette smoking. *Life Sciences 3:* 777-792.

Fernö, O., Lichtneckert, S.J.A. and Lundgren, C.E.G. (1973): A substitute for tobacco smoking. *Psychopharmacologia 31:* 201-204.

Feyerabend, C., Levitt, T. and Russell, M.A.H. (1975): A rapid gas-liquid chromatographic estimation of nicotine in biological fluids. *Journal of Pharmacy and Pharmacology 27:* 434-436.

Feyerabend, C. and Russell, M.A.H. (1978): Effect of urinary pH and nicotine excretion rate on plasma nicotine during cigarette smoking and chewing nicotine gum. *British Journal of Clincial Pharmacology 5:* 293-298.
Finnegan, J.K., Larson, P.S. and Haag, H.B. (1945): The role of nicotine in the cigarette habit. *Science 102:* 94-96.
Friedman, J., Horvath, T. and Meares, R. (1974): Tobacco smoking and a "stimulus barrier." *Nature 248:* 455-456.
Frith, C.D. (1971): The effect of varying the nicotine content of cigarettes on human smoking behaviour. *Psychopharmacologia 19:* 188-192.
Fuller, R.G.C. and Forrest, D.W. (1973): Behavioural aspects of cigarette smoking in relation to arousal level. *Psychological Reports 33:* 115-121.
Garg, M. (1969a): Variation in effects of nicotine in four strains of rats. *Psychopharmacologia 14:* 432-438.
Garg, M. (1969b): The effect of nicotine on two different types of learning. *Psychopharmacologia 15:* 408-414.
German, D.C. and Bowden, D.M. (1974): Catecholamine systems as the neural substrate for intracranial self-stimulation: a hypothesis. *Brain Research 73:* 381-419.
Giorguieff, M.F., Le Floc'h, M.L., Westfall, T.C., Glowinski, J. and Besson, M.J. (1976): Nicotinic effect of acetylcholine on the release of newly synthesised (^{3}H) dopamine in rat striatal slices and cat caudate nucleus. *Brain Research 106:* 117-131.
Glick, S.D., Jarvik, M.E. and Nakamura, R.K. (1970): Inhibition by drugs of smoking behaviour in monkeys. *Nature 227:* 969-971.
Goldfarb, T., Gritz, E.R., Jarvik, M.E. and Stolerman, I.P. (1976): Reactions to cigarettes as a function of nicotine and "tar." *Clinical Pharmacology and Therapeutics 19:* 767-772.
Goldfarb, R.L. and Jarvik, M.E. (1972): Accommodation to restricted tobacco smoke intake in cigarette smokers. *International Journal of Addiction 7:* 559-565.
Goodman, F.R. (1974): Effects of nicotine on distribution and release of 14C-norepinephrine and 14C-dopamine in rat brain striatum and hypothalamus slices. *Neuropharmacology 13:* 1025-1032.
Hall, G.H. and Morrison, C.F. (1973): New evidence for a relationship between smoking, nicotine dependence and stress. *Nature 243:* 199-201.
Hall, G.H. and Turner, D.M. (1972): Effects of nicotine on the release of ^{3}H-noradrenaline from the hypothalamus. *Biochemical Pharmacology 21:* 1829-1838.
Hatchell, P.C. and Collins, A.C. (1977): Influences of genotype and sex on behavioural tolerance to nicotine in mice. *Pharmacology, Biochemistry and Behaviour 6:* 25-30.
Herxheimer, A., Griffiths, R.L., Hamilton, B. and Wakefield, M. (1967): Circulatory effects of nicotine aerosol inhalations and cigarette smoking in man. *Lancet 2:* 754-755.
Hirschhorn, I.D. and Rosecrans, S.A. (1974): Studies on the time course and the effect of cholinergic and adrenergic recptor blockers on the stimulus effect of nicotine. *Psychopharmacology 40:* 109-120.
Hubbard, J.E. and Gohd, R.S. (1975): Tolerance development to the arousal effects of nicotine. *Pharmacology, Biochemistry and Behaviour 3:* 471-476.
Hunt, S.P. and Schmidt, J. (1978): The electron microscopic autoradiographic localisation of α-bungarotoxin binding sites within the central nervous system of the rat. *Brain Research 142:* 152-159.
Hutchinson, R.R. and Ealey, G.S. (1973): Effects of nicotine on avoidance, conditioned suppression and aggression response measures in animals and man. In: W.L. Dunn (Ed.), *Smoking Behaviour: Motives and Incentives.* V.H. Winston, Washington, D.C. p. 171-196.

Ikard, F.F., Green, D.E. and Horn, D. (1969): A scale to differentiate between types of smokers as related to the management of affect. *International Journal of the Addictions 4:* 649-659.

Isaac, P.F. and Rand, M.J. (1972): Cigarette smoking and plasma levels of nicotine. *Nature 236:* 308-310.

Jaffe, J.H. and Jarvik, M.E. (1978): Tobacco use and tobacco use disorder. In: M.A. Lipton, A. DiMascio and K.F. Killam (Eds.), *Psychopharmacology: A Generation of Progress.* Raven Press, New York, p. 1665-1676.

Jarvik, M.E. (1967): Tobacco smoking in monkeys. *Annals of the New York Academy of Sciences 142:* 280-294.

Jarvik, M.E., Glick, S.D. and Nakamura, R.K. (1970): Inhibition of cigarette smoking by orally administered nicotine. *Clinical Pharmacology and Therapeutics 11:* 574-576.

Jarvik, M.E., Popek, P., Schneider, N.G., Bar-Weiss, V. and Gritz, E.R. (1978): Can cigarette size and nicotine content influence smoking and puffing rates? *Psychopharmacology 58:* 303.

Johnston, L.M. (1942): Tobacco smoking and nicotine. *Lancet 2:* 742.

Keenan, A. and Johnson, F.N. (1972): Development of behavioural tolerance to nicotine in the rat. *Experientia 28:* 428-429.

Kornetsky, C. and Eliasson, M. (1969): Reticular stimulation and chlorpromazine: An animal model for schizophrenic overarousal. *Science 165:* 1273-1274.

Kozlowski, L.T., Jarvik, M.E. and Gritz, E.R. (1975): Nicotine regulation and cigarette smoking. *Clinical Pharmacology and Therapeutics 17:* 93-97.

Kumar, R. and Stolerman, I.P. (1977): Experimental and clinical aspects of drug dependence. In: L.L. Iversen, S.D. Iversen and S.H. Snyder (Eds.), *Handbook of Psychopharmacology,* Vol. 7. Plenum Press, New York, p. 321-167.

Kumar, R., Cooke, E.C., Lader, M.H. and Russell, M.A.H. (1977): Is nicotine important in tobacco smoking? *Clinical Pharmacology and Therapeutics 21:* 520-529.

Lader, M.H. (1978): Nicotine and smoking behaviour. *British Journal of Clinical Pharmacology 5:* 289-292.

Lang, W.J., Latiff, A.A., McQueen, A. and Singer, G. (1977): Self-administration of nicotine with and without a food delivery schedule. *Pharmacology, Biochemistry and Behaviour 7:* 65-70.

Larson, P.S. and Silvette, H. (1961): *Tobacco: Experimental and Clinical Studies.* Williams and Wilkins, Baltimore. Supplements 1968, 1971, 1975.

Larson, P.S. and Silvette, H. (1975): *Tobacco: Experimental and Clincial Studies,* Suppl. III. Williams and Wilkins, Baltimore.

Lichtensteiger, W., Felix, D., Lienhart, R. and Hefti, F. (1976): A quantitative correlation between single unit activity and fluorescence intensity of dopamine neurones in zona compacta of substantia nigra, as demonstrated under the influence of nicotine and physostigmine. *Brain Research 117:* 85-103.

Lucchesi, B.R., Schuster, C.R. and Ealey, G.S. (1967): The role of nicotine as a determinant of cigarette smoking frequency in man with observations of certain cardiovascular effects associated with the tobacco alkaloid. *Clinical Pharmacology and Therapeutics 8:* 789-796.

Lyon, M. and Robbins, T.W. (1975): The action of central nervous system stimulant drugs: A general theory concerning amphetamine effects. In: W. Essman and L. Valzelli (Eds.), *Current Developments in Psychopharmacology,* Vol. 2, Spectrum, New York, p. 89-163.

Martin, W.R. (Ed.) (1977a): *Drug Addiction I. Morphine, Sedative/Hypnotic and Alcohol Dependence.* Springer Verlag, Berlin.

Martin, W.R. (Ed.) (1977b): *Drug Addiction II. Amphetamine, Psychotogen and Marihuana Dependence.* Springer Verlag, Berlin.

Martin, W.R., Aceto, M.D., Montgomery, J.L., May, E.L., Uwaydah, I.M. and Harris, L.S. (1978): Stereospecific binding of (-) -14$_C$ nicotine to rat brain. In: *Proceedings of 7th International Congress of Pharmacology,* Paris. p. 282.

McKennell, A.C. (1970): Smoking motivation factors. *British Journal of Social and Clinical Psychology 9:* 8-22.

McNiven, N.L., Raisinghani, K.H., Patashnik, S. and Dorfman, R.I. (1965): Determination of nicotine in smokers' urine by gas chromatography. *Nature 208:* 788.

Moore, W.M. and Brady, R.N. (1977): Studies of nicotinic acetylcholine receptor protein from rat brain. II. Partial Purification. *Biochemica Biophysica Acta 498:* 331-340.

Morley, B.J., Lorden, J.F., Brown, G.B., Kemp, G.E. and Bradley, R.J. (1977): Regional distribution of nicotinic acetylcholine receptor in rat brain. *Brain Research 134:* 161-166.

Morrison, C.F. (1967): Effects of nicotine on operant behaviour of rats. *International Journal of Neuropharmacology 6:* 229-240.

Morrison, C.F. and Armitage, A.K. (1967): Effects of nicotine upon the free operant behaviour of rats and spontaneous motor activity of mice. *Annals of the New York Academy of Sciences 142:* 268-276.

Morrison, C.F. (1968): The modification by physostigmine of some effects of nicotine on bar-pressing behaviour of rats. *British Journal of Pharmacology 32:* 28-33.

Morrison, C.F. and Lee, P.N. (1968): A comparison of the effects of nicotine and physostigmine on a measure of activity in the rat. *Psychopharmacologia 13:* 210-221.

Morrison, C.F. and Stephenson, J.A. (1969): Nicotine injections as the conditioned stimulus in discrimination learning. *Psychopharmacologia 15:* 351-360.

Morrison, C.F., Goodyear, J.M. and Sellers, C.M. (1969): Antagonism by antimuscarinic and ganglion blocking drugs of some of the behavioural effects of nicotine. *Psychopharmacologia 15:* 341-350.

Morrison, C.F. and Stephenson, J.A. (1972): The occurrence of tolerance to a central depressant effect of nicotine. *British Journal of Pharmacology 45:* 151-156.

Münster, G. and Bättig, K. (1975): Nicotine-induced hypophagia and hypodipsia in deprived and in hypothalamically stimulated rats. *Psychopharmacologia 41:* 211-217.

Myrsten, A.L., Andersson, K., Frankenhaeuser, M. and Elgerot, A. (1975): Immediate effects of cigarette smoking as related to different smoking habits. *Perceptual and Motor Skills 40:* 515-523.

Nelsen, J.M. and Goldstein, L. (1972): Improvement of performance on an attention task with chronic nicotine treatment in rats. *Psychopharmacologia 26:* 347-360.

Nelsen, J.M., Pelley, L., and Goldstein, L. (1975): Protection by nicotine from behavioural disruption caused by reticular formation stimulation in rats. *Pharmacology, Biochemistry and Behaviour 3:* 749-754.

Newman, L.M. (1972): Effects of cholinergic agonists and antagonists on self-stimulation behaviour in the rat. *Journal of Comparative and Physiological Psychology 79:* 394-413.

Olds, M.E. and Domino, E.F. (1969): Comparison of muscarinic and nicotinic cholinergic agonists on self-stimulation behaviour. *Journal of Pharmacology and Experimental Therapy 166:* 189-204.

Pickens, R., Neisch, R.A. and Thompson, T. (1978): Drug self-administration: An analysis of the reinforcing effects of drugs. In: L.L. Iversen, S.D. Iversen and S.H. Snyder (Eds.) *Handbook of Psychopharmacology,* Vol. 12. Plenum Press, New York. p. 1-37.

Pradhan, S.N. and Dutta, S.N. (1970): Comparative effects of nicotine and amphetamine on timing behaviour in rats. *Neuropharmacology 9:* 9-16.

Pradhan, S.N. and Bowling, C. (1971): Effects of nicotine on self-stimulation in rats. *Journal of Pharmacology and Experimental Therapy 176:* 229-243.

Proc. Bayer Symposium IV (1973): *Psychic Dependence,* edited by L. Goldberg and H. Hoffmeister, Springer Verlag, Berlin.

Proc. Symposium on Control of Drug Taking Behaviour by Schedules of Reinforcement (1976): *Pharmacological Reviews 27:* 291-446.

Rosecrans, J.A. (1971): Effects of nicotine on behavioural arousal and brain 5-hydroxytryptamine function in female rats selected for differences in activity. *European Journal of Pharmacology 14:* 29-37.

Rosecrans, J.A. and Chance, W.T. (1977): Cholinergic and non-cholinergic aspects of the discriminative stimulus properties of nicotine. In: H. Lal (Ed.) *Discriminative Stimulus Properties of Drugs.* Plenum Press, New York. p. 155-185.

Rosenthal, R.N. and Slotkin, T.A. (1977): Development of nicotinic responses in the rat adrenal medulla and long-term effects of neonatal nicotine administration. *British Journal of Pharmacology 60:* 59-64.

Rottenstein, H., Pierce, G., Russ, E., Felder, D. and Montgomery, H. (1960): Influence of nicotine on the blood flow of resting skeletal muscle and of the digits in normal subjects. *Annals of the New York Academy of Sciences 90:* 102-113.

Routtenberg, A. (1968): The two-arousal hypothesis: reticular formation and limbic system. *Psychological Review 75:* 51-80.

Russell, M.A.H., Wilson, C., Patel, U.A., Cole, P.V. and Feyerabend, C. (1973): Comparison of effect on tobacco consumption and carbon monoxide absorption of changing to high and low nicotine cigarettes. *British Medical Journal 4:* 512-516.

Russell, M.A.H., Wilson, C., Cole, P.V., Idle, M. and Feyerabend, C. (1973): Comparison of increases in carboxyhaemoglobin after smoking "extra-mild" and "non-mild" cigarettes. *Lancet 2:* 687-690.

Russell, M.A.H., Peto, J. and Patel, U.A. (1974): The classification of smoking by factorial structure of motives. *Journal of Royal Statistical Society 137:* 313-333.

Russell, M.A.H., Wilson, C., Patel, U.A., Feyerabend, C. and Cole, P.V. (1975): Plasma nicotine levels after smoking cigarettes with high, medium, and low nicotine yields. *British Medical Journal 2:* 414-416.

Russell, M.A.H., Cole, P.V., Idle, M.S. and Adams, L. (1975): Carbon monoxide yields of cigarettes and their relation to nicotine yield and type of filter. *British Medical Journal 3:* 71-73.

Russell, M.A.H., Feyerabend, C. and Cole, P.V. (1976): Plasma nicotine levels after cigarette smoking and chewing nicotine gum. *British Medical Journal 1:* 1043-1046.

Russell, M.A.H., Wilson, C., Feyerabend, C. and Cole, P.V. (1976): Effect of nicotine chewing gum on smoking behaviour and as an aid to cigarette withdrawal. *British Medical Journal 2:* 391-393.

Russell, M.A.H. (1977): Smoking problems: An overview. In: M.E. Jarvik, J.W. Cullen, E.R. Gritz, T.M. Vogt and L.J. West (Eds.) *Research on Smoking Behaviour.* NIDA Research Monograph No. 17, U.S. Government Printing Office, Washington, D.C. p. 13-34.

Russell, M.A.H. and Feyerabend, C. (1978): Cigarette smoking: A dependence on high-nicotine boli. *Drug Metabolism Reviews 8:* 29-57.

Salvaterra, P.M., Mahler, H.R. and Moore, W.J. (1975): Subcellular and regional distribution of ^{125}I-labelled α-bungarotoxin binding in rat brain and its relationship to acetylcholinesterase and choline acetyltransferase. *Journal of Biological Chemistry 250:* 6469-6475.

Sanger, D.J. (1978): Nicotine and schedule-induced drinking in rats. *Pharmacology, Biochemistry and Behaviour 8:* 343-346.

Sanger, D.J. and Blackman, D.E. (1976): Rate-dependent effects of drugs: A review of the literature. *Pharmacology, Biochemistry and Behaviour 4:* 73-83.

Schachter, S., Silverstein, B., Kozlowski, L.T., Perlick, D., Herman, C.P. and Liebling, B. (1977): Studies of the interaction of psychological and pharmacological determinants of smoking. *Journal of Experimental Psychology: General 106:* 3-40.

Schechter, M.S. and Rosecrans, J.A. (1971): CNS effect of nicotine as the discriminative stimulus for the rat in a T-maze. *Life Science 10:* 821-832.

Schechter, M.D. and Rosecrans, J.A. (1972): Behavioural tolerance to an effect of nicotine in the rat. *Archives Internationales de Pharmacodynamie 195:* 52-56.

Schechter, M.D. and Jellinek, P. (1975): Evidence for a cortical locus for the stimulus effect of nicotine. *European Journal of Pharmacology 34:* 65-73.

Schechter, N., Handy, I.C., Pezzementi, L. and Schmidt, J. (1978): Distribution α-bungarotoxin binding sites in the central nervous system and peripheral organs of the rat. *Toxicon 16:* 245-251.

Sitzer, M., Morrison, J. and Domino E. (1970): Effects of nicotine on fixed-interval behaviour and their modification by cholinergic antagonists. *Journal of Pharmacology and Experimental Therapy 171:* 166-177.

Speth, R.C., Chen, F.M., Lindstrom, J.M., Kobayashi, R.M. and Yamamura, H.I. (1977): Nicotinic cholinergic receptors in rat brain identified by (125^I) naja naja siamensis alpha-toxin binding. *Brain Research 131:* 350-355.

Stolerman, I.P., Goldfarb, T., Fink, R. and Jarvik, M.E. (1973a): Influencing cigarette smoking with nicotine antagonists. *Psychopharmacologia 28:* 247-259.

Stolerman, I.P., Fink, R. and Jarvik, M.E. (1973b): Acute and chronic tolerance to nicotine measured by activity in rats. *Psychopharmacologia 30:* 329-342.

Stolerman, I.P., Bunker, P. and Jarvik, M.E. (1974): Nicotine tolerance in rats: role of dose and dose interval. *Psychopharmacologia 34:* 317-324.

Sulser, F. and Sanders-Bush, E. (1971): Effects of drugs on amines in the CNS. *Annual Review of Pharmacology 11:* 209-230.

Thompson, T. and Pickens, R. (Eds.) (1971): *Stimulus Properties of Drugs.* Appleton-Centry-Crofts, New York.

Thornton, R.E. (Ed.) (1978): *Smoking Behaviour. Physiological and Psychological Influences.* Churchill Livingstone, Edinburgh.

Tomkins, S.E. (1966): Psychological model for smoking behaviour. *American Journal of Public Health and the Nation's Health 56:* 17-20.

Turner, J.A. McM., Sillett, R.W. and Ball, K.P. (1974): Some effects of changing to low-tar and low-nicotine cigarettes. *Lancet 2:* 737-739.

Ulett, J.A. and Itil, T.M. (1969): Quantitative electroencephalogram in smoking and smoking deprivation. *Science 164:* 969-970.

Van Loon, G.R., Scapagnigni, V., Cohen, R. and Ganong, W.F. (1971): Effect of intraventricular administration of adrenergic drugs on the adrenal venous 17-hydroxycorticosteroid response to surgical stress in the dog. *Neuroendocrinology 8:* 257-272.

Vasquez, A.J. and Toman, J.E.P. (1967): Some interactions of nicotine with other drugs upon central nervous function. *Annals of the New York Academy of Sciences 142:* 201-215.

Wanner, H.V. and Bättig, K. (1966): Wirkung von Nikotin und Amphetamin auf die Selbstreisung bei der Ratte. *Helvetica Physiologica Pharmacologica Acta 24:* 122-124.

Warburton, D.M. and Wesnes, K. (1978): Individual differences in smoking and attentional behviour. In: R.E. Thornton (Ed.) *Smoking Behaviour.* Churchill Livingstone, Edinburgh. p. 19-43.

Weiss, G.B. and Alderdice, M.T. (1975): Characterisation of (14-C) - nicotine accumulation and movements in slices from different rat brain areas. *Neuropharmacology 14:* 265-273.

Westfall, R.C., Fleming, R.M., Fudger, M.F. and Clark, W.G. (1967): Effect of nicotine and related substances upon amine levels in the brain. *Annals of the New York Academy of Sciences 142:* 83-100.

Westfall, R.C. (1974): Effect of nicotine and other drugs on the release of 3H-norepinephrine and 3H-dopamine from rat brain slices. *Neuropharmacology 13:* 693-700.

W.H.O. (1975): *Smoking—Its Effect on Health.* World Health Organisation Technical Report Series No. 568.

Wise, R.A. (1978): Catecholamine theories of reward: a critical review. *Brain Research 152:* 215-247.

Yamamoto, K.I. and Domino, E.F. (1965): Nicotine-induced EEG and behavioural arousal. *International Journal of Neuropharmacology 4:* 359-373.

Yanagita, R., Ando, K., Oinuma, N. and Ishida, K. (1974): Intravenous self-administration of nicotine and an attempt to produce smoking behaviour in monkeys. In: Report of the 36th Annual Scientific Meeting, Committee of Problems of Drug Dependence, National Academy of Sciences, Washington, D.C. p. 567-578.

5

Pharmacological Concepts in Learning and Memory Dysfunction

Walter B. Essman

INTRODUCTION

The consideration of dysfunction in the processes of learning and memory concerns at least two phases of a relationship between such processes and their clinical pharmacology. In one respect there are classes of drugs which may either facilitate the disruptive effect of given agents or events upon learning or memory in man, or, alternatively, may act to antagonize or attenuate such effects. In another regard, there are cognitive alterations upon which clinically utilized drugs may be superimposed and, as such, impaired memory or response acquisition may be benefitted or further impaired. Therefore, the cognitive dysfunction with which the present discussion is concerned relates to: (1) drug-induced dysfunction, and (2) drug effects upon organic- or state-induced dysfunction.

Drugs which affect either the performance of acquired behavior or the acquisition of new behaviors have generally included agents which may be considered as behaviorally facilitative or disruptive. The nature of such facilitation or disruption may be considered at the level of the response itself (secondary action) or in terms of action upon a mechanism contributing to the processes of learning or memory (primary action). Whereas the former may include peripheral as well as central nervous system sites of drug action (motor, neuromuscular, vascular, endocrine, or indirect visceral effects), the latter sites of drug effect usually concern the central nervous system, and involve either perikaryal or synaptic effects that can be regional, cellular, or subcellular in relation to the specificity with which pharmacological effects occur. To address oneself to primary actions of those agents which modify learning and/or memory processes, one must necessarily formulate a series of relationships by which either the electrophysiological, morphological or metabolic correlates of learning or memory are logically as well as empirically linked with parameters of behavioral change as mediated by drug action. The former two disciplines do not consistently succeed in satisfying such a stringent requirement, probably because of several limitations: (1) methodological limitations, (2) temporal variations, (3) limitations imposed by regional or cellular specificity, (4) the complexity of the learning situation or adequacy of response retrieval, (5) chronicity of the drug regimen required, and (6) the physiological approximation of drug dosage. Although not complete in its encompassment of all issues, empirical findings, and parameters of drug action (route, absorption, disposition, binding, metabolism, affinity, etc.) it appears that drug action, particularly as relevant for learning and memory, finds a more secure explanatory foundation in processes and events that can be correlated in terms of their metabolic action and for which such metabolic changes also constitute issues for learning and memory mechanisms.

Of course, at some levels metabolic effects of drugs are reflected electrophysiologically and to some degree, morphologically (*e.g.*, mitochondrial swelling, membrane changes, cytoplasmic inclusion bodies, etc.), although such changes have limited significance for either the mechanisms which underlie or the responses indicative of learning and/or memory.

The clinical pharmacology of learning and memory largely consists of a framework provided by a more basic pharmacology derived largely from animal studies, and to a more limited degree, the application of derivative findings to studies in man. Obviously a pharmacology of behaviorally facilitative agents has more direct clinical relevance than a pharmacology of disruptive agents, although the latter does provide insights into such phenomena as amnesic processes, documentation of cognitoxic agents, and the potential prevalence of specific behaviorally adverse drug interactions.

A further distinction between behaviorally active drug effects may be made on a clinical level between the facilitative or disruptive effects of a given agent in a "normal" human population as contrasted with a population characterized by a clinical entity involving a neurological, vascular, or metabolic lesion of the central nervous system. In the case of those agents for which facilitative effects are considered, there may well be differences in effect depending upon whether facilitation of learning or memory is defined as an improvement of normal performance, perception, or problem-solving ability, or as a reduced deficit in one or more responses from which learning or memory are inferred. The nature of the deficit as well as the mechanism of drug action are important in resolving such differences, particularly in those instances wherein a paradoxical effect of the drug may occur. For example, in children with so-called "minimal brain damage," barbiturates may act as stimulants and amphetamines as depressants; such effects can also be reflected in differences in drug effect in learning paradigms, where motivation, attention, and comprehension are important, and in responses reflecting memory (stored information, based upon acquired responses), that is subject to retrieval and may be discriminated from non-relevant, neutral, or other stimuli.

A problem that further complicates the analysis of a relationship between metabolic substrates for learning and memory processing and the effects of drugs upon these same metabolic events and associated behavioral alterations, lies in separating the peripheral effects of drug action from central effects. Peripheral effects of parenterally administered drugs occur at muscle and glandular sites, the response of which provides feedback as well as direct input to the central nervous system. Of course such effects may also occur secondary to direct central actions. These effects are not easily demonstrable in the clinical situation, but may be inferred from studies in which parenterally administered drugs that alter learning and/or memory actually consist of agents that do not traverse the blood-brain barrier and therefore exert no direct central effect.

DRUG AND STATE INTERACTIONS

The pharmacology of drugs affecting learning and memory involves agents that may be classed as psychoactive in the sense of their usual clinical application, as well as compounds that may have no direct clinical utility in the treatment of behavior disorders or altered affective states. There are a wide range of agents in clinical use for the management of behavior disturbances, hypertension, endocrine dysfunction, cardiac rhythm disturbances, obesity, etc., that are well known for their behavioral side effects, at least one of which is a disturbance of performance or motivation. These are important components of both learning ability or capacity and also of memory fixation, retrieval, and stability. These are not, however, agents the effects of which are directly upon learning or memory processes or upon the molecular events to which such processes may be related. Another aspect of this same issue is the interaction of both exogenous as well as endogenous molecules with drugs that may affect learning or memory processes. Previous or concurrent administration of agents such as phenytoin, phenobarbital, or steroids—capable of inducing hepatic enzymes for drug metabolism, may well shorten the duration of drug action, reduce its potency or minimize the degree to which it becomes capable of exerting an effective central molecular effect.

In another case, renal function, notably for those agents metabolized by this route, constitutes an endogenous basis for particular interactions. The elimination of drugs is, of course, altered by uremia in man and several factors of peripheral significance for central drug effects may be modified under such circumstances. For example, vitamin D oxidation is prolonged (Avioli et al., 1968), cortisol reduction is prolonged (Englert et al., 1958), p-aminosalicylate acetylation is prolonged (Ogg et al., 1968), insulin hydrolysis is prolonged (O'Brien and Sharp, 1967), and cholinesterase activity is slowed (Holmes et al., 1958). Urinary excretion of drugs that affect learning- and memory-related behaviors can be directly affected by several factors, but one basic parameter is the pH of the urine. Enhanced renal excretion of some acids, such as salicylic acid and phenobarbital, is brought about at high urinary pH, whereas at a low urinary pH, the excretion of such bases as amphetamine and quinidine is increased.

The alteration of drug action in liver disease may provide a basis upon which a number of pharmacological agents may actually contribute to severe learning and memory dysfunction by precipitating hepatic encephalopathy. A rapid alteration in the fluid and electrolyte balance can occur with the extensive use of diuretics in cirrhotic patients (Sherlock, 1968), leading to encephalopathy. Encephalopathy in patients with extensive liver disease may also be precipitated by sedatives, tranquilizers, and antidepressants (Schenker et al., 1974). This has been observed for monoamine oxidase inhibitors, benzodiazepines (Waldram et al., 1974), and phenothiazines (Maxwell et al., 1972). Certainly, a partial explanation for the cognitoxic effects of several of the agents mentioned in hepatic disease may find explanation in the cerebral molecular changes associated with hepatic encephalopathy (Zieve, 1966); several of these issues will be treated in further detail in a later section of this chapter.

Certainly a number of disease states also affect the disposition of several drugs that may have a role in their application to the study of learning and/or memory. This is a particularly relevant consideration inasmuch as one area to which pharmacological facilitation of learning or memory may hold considerable clinical relevance and applicability in the geriatric population, in which age-related and/or cerebrovascular or cellular change in cognition and affect, constitute consideration of altered learning or memory. Certainly in such a population disorders of learning and/or memory, even though separable from disorders of affect—both conceptually as well as therapeutically, are still subject to a number of coexisting disease states and their effect upon the disposition of potentially useful drugs. The development of an autonomic neuropathy in chronic renal failure reduces receptor sensitivity to atropine and related drugs (Lowenthal and Reidenberg, 1972), and in Bartter's syndrome there is an end-organ refractoriness to angiotensin (Bartter et al., 1962). Other alterations in drug disposition have also been described with renal dysfunction, and include such changes as vasopressin resistance (Tannen et al., 1969), carbohydrate dysmetabolism (Cerletty and Engbring, 1967), penicillin encephalopathy (Bloomer et al., 1967), increased barbiturate sensitivity and an elevation of free-drug level (Dundee and Richard, 1954), and increased erythropoiesis with androgens (Parker et al., 1972).

One group of agents that deserves some particular attention for their role in interaction with drugs related to the clinical pharmacology of learning and memory processes and their dysfunction are those compounds which affect the activity of monoamine oxidase (MAO). Aside from the direct regulation of putative neurotransmitters involved in learning and memory, MAO inhibitors appear capable of interacting with drugs that can influence learned behavior and memory. Several of such actions and interactions have been reviewed (Essman and Tagliente, 1978). In addition to the augmentation of pressor agents, the potentiation of hyperpyrexia produced by tricyclic compounds, and interaction with tyramine-containing foods, carbohydrate metabolism may be affected by MAO inhibitors; this effect can also constitute an interactive basis for learning and/or memory-active drugs. Specifically, hypoglycemia can occur from the administration of MAO inhibitors (Van Praag and Leijnse, 1963), as may the potentiation of the hypoglycemic effect of insulin (Adnitt, 1968). Certainly a compromise of carbohydrate tolerance and metabolism can alter the disposition of several cogniactive or cognitoxic agents. A notable instance for such an effect is diabetes mellitus, wherein cerebral respiration and blood flow are modified (Kety et al., 1948). Furthermore, the synthesis and degradation of brain serotonin is compromised in diabetes, and the cerebral uptake of digoxin was accelerated (Essman, 1977) altered carbohydrate metabolism, therefore, whether drug-induced or endogenously manifested, can affect the disposition of drugs that act upon the processes of learning and/or memory.

There appear to be endogenous factors characterizing some disease states, which may interact directly with a drug or drugs of potential use in the treatment of learning or memory disorders. For example, in Down's syndrome the response of the autonomic nervous system to atropine is greatly exaggerated and such hypersensitivity may reflect an endogenous alteration in autonomic threshold (Harris and Goodman, 1968). An autonomic imbalance in bronchial asthma has also been indicated as a basis for an abnormal response to epinephrine (Grieco et al., 1968).

There are numerous other endogenous factors that may constitute issues of clinical relevance for interaction with drugs that affect learning or memory processing or dysfunction. These may include endocrine factors such as altered thyroid activity (Doherty and Perkins, 1966), modified tissue response to drugs, as dependence upon parathormone (Schaaf and Payne, 1966), and modified drug metabolism through corticosteroids (Brooks et al., 1972); such factors may also involve plasma proteins, which when reduced, causes an elevation in the unbound fraction of most drugs, and when normal, may be competed for by concurrently administered drugs that are highly protein-bound. On the other hand, the increased availability of degradation products from plasma proteins, such as albumin degradation products, can decrease the central stimulant effects of some classic centrally-active stimulants (Buczko and Tarasiewicz, 1976).

One final point concerning drug interactions of relevance to the pharmacological issues relevant to learning and memory dysfunction deals with exogenous agents which may alter the availability of a particular drug at its site of action.

For example, blockade of the norepinephrine pump, by which norepinephrine is transported physiologically into the nerve ending, may be brought about by any of the tricyclic antidepressants (imipramine, desipramine, nortriptyline, amitriptyline, protriptyline, doxepin); such blockade can interfere with drugs that require access into the sympathetic nerve ending in order to effectively act; guanethidine, represents one such drug, which in the presence of a tricyclic antidepressant, cannot exert its blocking effect at the sympathetic nerve ending, and therefore fails to exert an effective antihypertensive action (Mitchell et al., 1970). Amphetamines, on the other hand, are transported, by a norepinephrine pump, into the nerve ending, thereby becoming capable of forcing guanethidine molecules out of the ending, and thus reversing the desired clinical effect. An example of increased drug availability at the receptor site may be found in the interaction between warfarin and drugs that alter protein binding, such as phenylbutazone; the latter displaces warfarin from albumin (Aggeler et al., 1967); another illustration is presented with chloral hydrate, the metabolite of which (trichloroacetic acid) displaces warfarin from albumin (Sellers and Koch-Weser, 1978). The clinical effects of warfarin under such circumstances are enhanced and its action prolonged.

It thereby should be emphasized that drug interactions or factors arising from either exogenous or endogenous sources may modify the action of pharmacological agents which alter the processes of learning or memory. Since such interactions, like the drugs themselves concerned, involve molecular events that can be related, at least indirectly, to similar effects upon learning and memory-related mechanisms that are altered by specific drugs, these are appropriate to consider in the present context. There is, of course, much more that needs to be known about drug interactions in learning and memory.

There are issues possibly related to the clinical pharmacology of learning and memory which are indirect or indistinct in present perspective. In any case, their clinical relevance may be in question. One such issue concerns so-called state-dependent learning, wherein accurate performance of an acquired response is contingent upon the drug state that is present during acquisition of the behavior. Barbiturates and cholinergic drugs have frequently been utilized to demonstrate such state-dependent properties, but several other classes of drug have also been implicated. It should be emphasized that state-dependent properties of drugs do not necessarily dispose their action to one of facilitation or impairment of either learning or memory.

Another issue concerns the controversial phenomenon of information transfer by brain tissue extracts. The experiments purporting to demonstrate this phenomenon have been carried out largely in mice and rats, and have been questioned by a failure of replicability as well as by the lack of any neurobiological mechanism that can satisfactorily explain the phenomenon. The molecular bases upon which such transfer of information studies have been founded rely upon ribonucleic acid (RNA) or proteins, or both, within the structure of which specific information may have been encoded. Indeed, there are some firm bases upon which RNA and protein occupy prominent roles in the mechanisms regulating learning and memory; direct or indirect inhibition of the synthesis of such macromolecules can impair learning or memory fixation and facilitation of learning or memory has been related to the central effects of certain peptides and nucleotide metabolites.

The ultimate significance of such issues for either learning and memory remains to be delineated on a much more detailed basis than presently available. There seems little doubt that the regional perikaryal and synaptic events of the central nervous system which are involved in the mediation of acquired behavior and the consolidation of the memory trace are also responsive to pharmacological agents which modify these processes.

MACROMOLECULES AND DRUG EFFECTS IN LEARNING AND MEMORY

The participation of macromolecular substrates in learning and memory processes has been based theoretically upon the view that frequency modulated inputs to the central nervous system alter the ionic equilibrium of the cell cytoplasm and modify the stability of the nitrogenous bases of the RNA molecule (Hydén, 1959). Altered molecular structure through base modification leads to the synthesis of new RNA-dependent proteins capable of interacting with molecules of complementary structure. The release of transmitter molecules from their presynaptic vesicular storage could follow as a result of such an interaction. The theory does hold considerable promise, even currently, but fails to resolve a number of issues that appear critical to an understanding of how learning and memory are affected by specific drugs. Namely, (1) the relationship between nuclear changes and synaptosomal effects remains unclear; (2) the protein interaction does not provide for a mechanism of reversibility to account for acquisition failure or retention deficits; (3) drug effects would have to involve either cytoplasmic ionic changes or alteration of vesicular release processes to be consistent with the overall concept; and (4) there is no adequate means of accounting for memory consolidation—a process that occupies a central conceptual role in dealing with drug effects upon memory fixation. To clarify the latter point, the preservation-consolidation hypothesis of memory fixation (Müller and Pilzecker, 1900) stated that the memory trace, a neural representation of an acquired stimulus, was actively perseverated in the neuron for a brief period beyond its initiation by an acquired stimulus. It was considered that once this perseverative activity was terminated, the memory trace was consolidated, the acquired stimulus was reproduced, and its retrieval from storage was possible. An agent or event capable of interfering with the onset, or progress of the perseveration phase (fixation), resulted in impairment in memory consolidation.

More recent experimental evidence has supported a memory consolidation process in both animals and man, and indeed the time-dependent nature of this process has made it a superb theoretical model by which drug effects upon memory have been evaluated.

The first suggestion that the interaction of an amnesic stimulus with a drug could be used to define the effect of the drug upon memory consolidation utilized electroconvulsive shock as the amnesic stimulus and a malononitrile derivative as the drug studied (Essman, 1965). These studies were based upon the use of a single-trial conditioning paradigm initially developed to study the temporal characteristics of memory consolidation (Jarvik and Essman, 1960; Essman and Alpern, 1964). These issues will be dealt with again in later sections of this chapter.

Another theoretical view of historical interest for a molecular approach to learning and memory is the position that a nucleoprotein lattice of regionally and experientially specific molecules constituted the basis for memory traces (Katz and Halstead, 1960). This view also offers considerable applicability for later investigations, notably those concerned with the use of inhibitors of protein synthesis as tools to study the stability or molecular-dependence of certain memories. For example such antibiotics as puromycin, which inhibit protein synthesis (Flexner and Flexner, 1968) are behaviorally disruptive (David, 1968). Although some, but not all, inhibitors of cerebral protein synthesis disrupt learning or interfere with memory formation or response retrieval, the fact that the same degree of inhibition without behavioral impairment places into question the validity of cerebral protein synthesis as generalized concept for learning and memory. The nature of specific proteins, their sites of activation and/or inhibition, endogenous factors by which such loci and effects are physiologically mediated remain to be more precisely defined. Such definition will have to be rather specific about the nature of those endogenous molecules which, when activated, bound, degraded, etc.,–either physiologically or pharmacologically, are capable of modifying the synthesis or disposition of proteins of possible significance for learning and memory.

A distinction should be made between macromolecular change as a dependent variable of learning and memory and macromolecular effect as a pharmacological variable in learning and memory. The former is highly relevant, conceptually and practically, to the latter, but it is the pharmacological aspect of this contingency that is of primary concern to this chapter. Macromolecular change, however, does deserve some comment. When rats were trained to reverse the use of their preferred forepaw to obtain food (reverse handedness) an increased incorporation of amino acid precursor into hippocampal nerve cell protein fractions was demonstrated (Hydén and Lange, 1970). A significant increase in the specific activity in two acidic protein fractions from the rat hippocampus (pyramidal cells from CA3 region) occurred, when reverse handedness was compared with an equal number of preferred handedness trials among control animals (Hydén and Lange, 1972). In highly inbred sublines or rats that differed in learning ability of an avoidance task, reversal of handedness training increased labeling of acidic proteins from the sensory-motor cortex, visual cortex, hippocampus, and entorhinal cortex occured for high-score learners, but no differences were observed for low-score learners (Hydén and Egyhazi, 1962, 1963, 1964), and significant changes in the base composition of RNA from nerve cells of the inferior temporal gyrus with a visual discrimination task in monkeys (Hydén et al., 1974); adenine was increased and cytosine was decreased. With a delayed-alternation type of learning the nerve cells of the gyrus principalis showed RNA base changes.

The issue of RNA base changes, its bearing upon the proteins synthesized regionally in nerve cells and their adjacent glia, and those drugs which may alter learning or memory has received some, but notably sparse attention in the experimental literature. It is interesting, however, that this issue was investigated experimentally after its rationale was derived from some clinical observations. Malononitrile, a central nervous system stimulant, was initially reported as having some success in the treatment of psychiatric patients. When tissue from the frontal lobes of malononitrile treated patients (post-lobotomy) was compared with untreated controls (accidental death) an increased production of nucleic acid and protein was measured (Hydén and Hartelius, 1948: Hartelius, 1950). This gave rise to other experiments in which the dimer of malononitrile, tricyanoaminopropene (TCAP), when parenterally administered, was shown to increase the RNA and nucleoprotein content of single neurons in the rabbit brain (Hydén and Egyhazi, 1961). Rabbits injected with 20 mg/kg of TCAP showed a 27 percent increase in nuclear protein and 26 percent increase in nuclear RNA in the Deiters' nerve cell one hour later; RNA from adjacent glia was decreased by 45 percent (Hydén, 1962). Drug-treated animals showed a significant decrease in nerve cell cytosine and glial cytosine was significantly increased. In contrast to this apparently reciprocal cellular base change following TCAP, a central nervous system stimulant, increased neuronal and glial cytosine occurred in the same region following the administration of tranylcypromine, a monoamine oxidase inhibitor and central stimulant that provides for the accumulation of those biogenic amines which depend upon this enzyme for their deamination.

Although somewhat preliminary to the issue of learning and memory, the molecular effects of central nervous system stimulants TCAP and tranylcypromine, do relate in several practical ways to learning and memory. Such relationships support not only a molecular relationship, but also suggest a basis for an interdependent role for nucleic acids and biogenic amines in the central nervous system.

The malononitrile derivatives represent one class of psychoactive agent which relates not only to brain nucleic acid metabolism and synthesis, but also to learning and memory. Although malononitrile and its derivatives are central stimulants, as defined by their electrophysiological activating effects and increase in locomotor activity produced, they have an anti-thyroid effect that apparently is not manifested either neurochemically or behaviorally upon acute administration. The behavioral effects of TCAP were noted as facilitatory, inasmuch as its acute administration enhanced the retention of a conditioned avoidance response in rodents (Chamberlain et al., 1963). In the behavioral situation, emotionality and the acquisition of maze behavior were unaffected by the drug.

A relationship between malononitrile derivatives and memory has been formulated on the basis of the interaction between the drug effect and the effect of an amnesic stimulus. The amnesic stimulus chosen was post-training electroconvulsive shock (ECS), which both in animals and in man acts to produce a temporally-dependent rate of retrograde amnesia; *i.e.*, as the interval between a learning experience and the administration of a single ECS (producing a full clonic-tonic convulsion with a post-ictal episode) is increased, the subsequent retrograde amnesia is less pronounced, in another respect, the shorter the time between behavioral acquisition and ECS, the greater the incidence of retrograde amnesia. One common denominator by which TCAP effects and ECS effects may be associated is that they affect the RNA content of cells in the brain. The RNA content of whole mouse brain was shown to be decreased by approximately 17 percent within 20 minutes after a single ECS. Under the same conditions, 72 percent of those mice trained to acquire a passive avoidance response and given ECS within 10 minutes after the training trial showed a retrograde amnesia for the avoidance response when they were tested 24 hours later. Mice treated with TCAP (20 mg/kg x 3 days) prior to training did not show any difference in acquisition or in susceptibility to ECS-induced convulsions, but only 27 percent of these animals showed a retrograde amnesia. The important point is that pre-treatment with TCAP blocked the RNA-depleting effect of ECS (Essman, 1965). The fact that TCAP produced such an effect without any anticonvulsant properties is of some methodological significance for the selection of presumed memory-facilitative drugs through the use of the consolidation-amnesia paradigm provided with the ECS model. Drugs that alter an ECS-induced convulsion may appear to be facilitatory if the amnesia is seizure-dependent. In this regard, then, drugs such as phenobarbital, phenytoin, carbonic anhydrase inhibitors, some benzodiazepines, some monoamine oxidase inhibitors, etc., might be expected to benefit the memory consolidation process since they act to reduce the electrical manifestation of seizure activity produced by ECS. In fact, none of these agents facilitates consolidation or reduces the amnesic affect of ECS. Neither the amnesic nor the biochemical effects of ECS were altered when the convulsion was blocked by pre-treatment with lidocaine hydrochloride; this local anesthetic and MAO inhibitor acts as a most effective anticonvulsant, but not as an antiamnesic (Essman, 1968). A similar effect was also observed with 2, 4-dichlorophenoxyacetic acid, a thermolytic drug that also acts as an anticonvulsant, but not as an anti-amnesic.

The regional and cellular effects of TCAP are of interest, and of possible relevance to a molecular view of memory consolidation. Those brain regions most apparently affected include the major structures comprising the limbic region and the corpus callosum; while the former is richly endowed with mixed cell populations, the latter lacks nerve cell bodies and contains only axons and glia (Essman, 1966). It was shown (Essman, 1965) that ECS reduced nerve cell RNA and increased glial RNA in cells isolated from the hippocampal cortex; TCAP increased nerve cell RNA and decreased glial RNA content for cells in this same region.

The enhancement of discrimination learning in rats (Daniel, 1967; Schmidt and Davenport, 1967) with TCAP has been reported, and the drug has also been shown to be without significant effect upon active avoidance and water maze learning (Brush et al., 1966), conditioned emotional response acquisition and extinction (Solyom and Gallay, 1966) maze learning (McNutt, 1967), passive avoidance learning (Gurowitz et al., 1969), or response rates during continuous avoidance performance (Stern and Heise, 1970). No effect upon brain RNA content or metabolism or upon antagonism of ECS-induced amnesia was found in mice (Buckholtz and Bowman, 1970). Elimination of the motor learning component of an acquisition task prior to the administration of TCAP (10 to 60 mg/kg x 3 days) provided for enhanced maze learning and a dose-related increase in whole brain RNA content (Lewis, 1967). The use of a trimer of malononitrile, tetracyanopropene (T4CAP), provided for facilitation of maze learning and habit reversal in mice (Lewis and Essman, 1967), but this effect was limited by the toxicity of this compound at doses above 30 mg/kg.

Learning capacity and memory function was tested using TCAP in 23 senile patients given the drug (600 mg/day, p.o.) without any evidence of drug benefit over that of a placebo (Talland et al., 1965). If, as suggested, this drug acts upon the memory consolidation process, either by minimizing molecular changes attendant upon amnesic stimuli that interfere with consolidation, or by accelerating the consolidation time, it may thereby act by reducing the interval within which amnesic stimuli may be active. It is not surprising that TCAP is ineffective in modifying multiple trial learning tasks or for memory and performance tasks in senile humans; the latter population, in particular, is one wherein pharmacological alteration of learning or memory becomes very difficult to define, it would appear more likely that a reduction of confusion and disorientation might be better achieved through the use of agents that favor increased attention and more consistent stimulation of the central nervous system. This topic is perhaps better relegated to a consideration of central nervous system stimulants and analeptics which will be discussed in a later section of this chapter.

A final word may be added regarding the anti-amnesic properties of T4CAP, which has been shown to facilitate memory consolidation in a dose-related manner (Essman and Essman, 1969). The results of these studies have led to the suggestion that a drug-induced facilitation of memory consolidation represents an action that involves both the interaction of RNA and serotonin. Whereas a number of amnesic agents or events such as ECS, audiogenic seizure, pentylenetetrazol convulsions, CO_2 inhalation, hypothermia, short chain fatty acid-induced coma, ether anesthesia, etc., reduce the regional content and metabolism of brain RNA, they also lead to an increased brain serotonin content or a reduction in its turnover.

SEROTONIN IN LEARNING AND MEMORY

The development of the concept of a serotonin-related basis for learning, memory consolidation, or amnesia has been based, not only upon a correlation of brain changes in this amine with amnesic agents or events, but also upon pharmacological studies (Essman, 1978). An early study (Wooley, 1965) found that mice in which brain serotonin was elevated with a combination of 5-hydroxytryptophan (60 mg/kg) and benzylmethoxy-tryptamine (15 mg/kg) had a 13 percent reduction in the average number of correct maze responses performed. A decrease in brain serotonin either with reserpine (1, 2 mg/kg) or oral DL-phenylalanine combined with L-tyrosine, increased correct maze responses by seven and nine percent, respectively.

A variety of agents that have been shown to exert a retrograde amnesic effect upon acquired behavior, such as barbiturates, anti-thermogenic phenoxyacetic acid derivatives, and general anesthetics (discussed in a later section of this chapter) have in common their ability to elevate regional concentrations of serotonin in the brain (Essman, 1970). Additionally, the serotonin increment associated with a shift from REM sleep to slow-wave sleep (Jouvet, 1969) has also been related to a time-related failure to demonstrate dream recall from the REM period. Agents that further reduce such recall, such as barbiturates also, as noted above, elevate brain levels of serotonin. Another finding which ties the elevation of brain serotonin level to an apparently dysfunctional memory consolidation is that the accumulation of short-chain fatty acids, such as occur in hepatic encephalopathy, lead to increased brain serotonin concentration (Baldessarini and Fischer, 1973); furthermore, such fatty acids as butyric acid, in elevating brain serotonin level, also bring about a significant retrograde amnesia and cause an appreciable inhibition of cerebral protein synthesis (Essman and Essman, 1977). Such inhibition of protein synthesis is most apparent in the hippocampus and appears to be mainly accounted for by the presynaptic nerve endings. This effect is very similar in site, magnitude, and course to that produced by other serotonin active amnesic conditions such as electroconvulsive shock (Essman, 1973).

A reduction in brain serotonin content with the tryptophan hydroxylase inhibitor, p-chlorophenylalanine (PCPA), produced a reduction in emotional reactivity in rats, an increased reactivity to painful stimuli, and increased acquisition of conditioned avoidance responses (Renen, 1967). The facilitation of a brightness discrimination response by rats, but not a position discrimination or reversal was caused by PCPA (Stevens et al., 1967). In mice PCPA did not facilitate passive avoidance response acquisition or reduce ECS-induced retrograde amnesia (it may be observed, however, that the maximum reduction in brain serotonin achieved with a 300 mg/kg dose of PCPA was only 39 percent, as contrasted with the approximate 90 percent depletion accomplished with a comparable dose of this drug in rats).

The clinical use of PCPA has been limited to experimental applications, not so much related to learning or memory, but to conditions wherein tissue or blood levels of serotonin are elevated and the drug has been utilized in an attempt to lower concentrations of this indole. This had found some limited usefulness in such conditions as carcinoid syndrome, medullary carcinoma of the thyroid, and mastocytosis, where some, but not all of the serotoninemia-related symptoms, such as diarrhea, pigmentation changes, and pruritus have been attenuated; the course of the clinical disorder, however, appears only minimally benefitted from this agent. In such conditions there is little evidence of a central serotonin excess or learning and memory changes, probably related to the poor transport of peripheral serotonin across the blood-brain barrier and the increased rate of peripheral catabolism and excretion.

RESERPINE EFFECTS

The reduced level of brain serotonin resulting from reserpine treatment (Pletscher et al., 1955) is difficult to directly relate to learning or memory in view of the multiple effects of this agent and its duration of action. In general, pharmacological doses of the *Rauwolfia* alkaloid impair performance and therefore it is methodologically relevant to separate performance measures from measures of learning and memory. There is a bearing of the serotonin depleting effects of reserpine upon the action and effects of other agents; this does relate to some of the methodological issues which concern learning and memory. For example, there is an interaction between reserpine and morphine (Shin and Cheon, 1973), such that the analgesic effects of morphine were eliminated, the hyperglycemic effects of morphine were augmented, and the elevated serum transaminase (SGOT, SGPT) activities induced by morphine were inhibited by reserpine. These findings strongly suggest that central as well as peripheral effects of other agents or the sites at which environmental stimuli act to produce such changes may be modified by reserpine. They also suggest, of course, that the central and peripheral effects of morphine may be serotonin dependent. This, although not the direct concern of this chapter, has been treated elsewhere, particularly as it concerns the analgesic effects of this narcotic (Samanin et al., 1970) and the effects of morphine upon myocardial metabolism (Essman,

1978). Aside from its clinical utility as an antihypertensive agent, the cardiovascular effects of reserpine cannot be overlooked (Luckens and Malone, 1973). Tachycardia produced by direct myocardial action is not blocked by reserpine, which only blocks catecholamine action at adrenergic receptors (Teoh and Cheah, 1973). These peripheral effects of reserpine are complex and may themselves contribute to altered performance in tests of learning or memory. Low doses of reserpine (0.05 mg/kg) facilitated avoidance learning in rats whereas at a higher dose (0.25 mg/kg), reduced pattern discrimination learning occurred; at a still higher dose (0.40 mg/kg) this drug impaired exploratory behavior (Walk et al., 1961).

The effects of reserpine upon avoidance learning and the consolidation of such responses have been varied. Conditioning of an emotional response was unaffected by reserpine (0.50 mg/kg), (Stein, 1956), but the performance of established conditioned emotional responses could be impaired with reserpine (Brady, 1956). Shuttle box escape behavior and avoidance response acquisition by mice were not affected by reserpine (2.5 mg/kg) and single-trial avoidance acquisition was also not affected (Essman, 1967). Reserpine also significantly attenuated the amnesic effects of ECS in mice (Essman, 1971). This latter effect might again be related to the serotonin-depleting effect of the drug and the failure of ECS to elevate brain serotonin in reserpine-treated animals. This finding holds some further significance in that reserpine acts as a proconvulsive agent; *i.e.*, it potentiates the seizure-producing effects of ECS and increases the intensity of the resulting convulsion. Again, as noted previously, there does not appear to be a relationship of amnesia to the absence of a convulsion, or the reduction in the amnesic potential of a convulsant to the intensity of the convulsion.

BARBITURATES AND SEDATIVES

The behavioral and molecular effects of two additional classes of psychoactive compound may be used as a further basis for relating neurometabolic changes to alterations in learning or memory. These sedative drugs include the barbiturates and the benzodiazepines. The regional effects of representative agents upon brain serotonin turnover have been studied and a generalized decrease in turnover was observed (Lidbrink et al., 1974). Sedative doses of a barbiturate produced a widely distributed reduction of brain serotonin turnover, whereas only serotonin turnover in the cerebral cortex as reduced by benzodiazepines. Brain serotonin content is also elevated during barbiturate sedation or anesthesia—an observation that is consistent with the reduction in turnover of this amine.

Pentobarbital has been rather generally applied to behavioral studies in animals and man with a variety of effects. In rats given pentobarbital (13 mg/kg) conditioned avoidance responses were acquired without any drug effect, but avoidance behavior after acquisition was reduced if drug administration was continued (Holmgren and Condi, 1964). It was also shown that conditioned motor reflexes could be developed in dogs under pentobarbital anesthesia (Teitelbaum et al., 1961). In the rhesus monkey lever pressing responses acquired to terminate painful stimulation were abolished by pentobarbital (Malis, 1962). Memory span in man was reduced by pentobarbital (100 mg/150 lb. body weight, IV) (Quarton and Talland, 1962). Running memory span was narrowed by pentobarbital (100 mg/68 kg, IV) when compared with a placebo in a double-blind study (Talland and Quarton, 1965).

The effect of at least one barbiturate, pentobarbital sodium, upon memory consolidation was evaluated in rats injected with this agent, as compared with controls given distilled water, following a daily trial for the acquisition of a maze response (Garg and Holland, 1968). The post-trial barbiturate-treated rats made significantly more errors in learning the maze response, suggesting that memory consolidation was impaired.

Increased response rates for learned responses have been reported as a result of phenobarbital treatment in rats (Kelleher et al., 1961) and pigeons (Bignami and Gatti, 1969). In contrast to the action of this long-acting barbiturate, an ultra-short acting agent, thiopental, produced an amnesic effect upon the recognition memory for pictures and the recall memory for word and letter associations (Osborn et al., 1967).

In general, except for some studies in which barbiturate state-dependency constitutes a possible basis for the effect of an agent upon learning or memory, barbiturates tend to impair acquisition and interfere with the retention of learned behavior. The effects of barbiturates upon the performance of learned responses that depends upon a motor component appear to be facilitated, whereas a verbal or associative component of acquired behavior appears impaired; the extent of impairment in the latter case seems to relate to blood levels of the barbiturate at those times that performance is measured.

Highly representative of the benzodiazepines is chlordiazepoxide, which has been shown (10 mg/kg) to impair conditioned escape behavior acquisition by rats (Cicala and Hartley, 1965). Both chlordiazepoxide and diazepam (5 mg/kg) increased a pedal-pressing response for electrical stimulation to the posterior hypothalamus of rats (Olds, 1966) and in rabbits, chlordiazepoxide impaired the acquisition of a two-way shuttle box avoidance response (Chisholm and Moore, 1970). In man, the performance of a digit-symbol substitution task was impaired by chlordiazepoxide (20 mg), with the maximum effect (approximately 12 percent reduction in the mean number of correct responses as compared with placebo treatment) observed 60 minutes after drug treatment. Some impaired performance was still apparent in drug-treated subjects by 180 minutes after the drug (Besser and Steinberg, 1967).

In several respects, the benzodiazepines thus far discussed may also be considered as minor tranquilizers, or even as mood alternates, depending upon the context within which and application for which they are clinically employed. In the following section the potentially amnesic properties of several benzodiazepine derivatives will be considered on a clinical level.

MOOD ALTERATIONS

Up to this point almost all of the psychoactive agents considered to affect learning or memory have included barbiturates and sedatives; some attention may also be given to agents that have been employed clinically as mood stabilizers. Among these are the tricyclic compounds commonly utilized for the treatment of depression. It may be recalled, as mentioned earlier, that at least one biochemical effect of agents in this class is to impair the norepinephrine pump, whereby catecholamines are actively transported into the presynaptic nerve ending. Aside from their ability to interact with drugs which depend upon an intact norepinephrine pump for pharmacological action, such as guanethidine, tricyclics such as imipramine also interact to potentiate the effect of drugs which also act upon the norepinephrine pump, such as the amphetamines. The stimulant effect of amphetamine (1 mg/kg, i.p.) upon the performance of a nondiscriminative avoidance task by rats was potentiated by imipramine (10 mg/kg, i.p.) (Weissman, 1961). Several studies have indicated that the effects of imipramine in animals can be generally viewed as sedative (Battig, 1961; Hanson, 1961; Herr et al., 1961; Maxwell and Palmer, 1961; Vernier, 1961; Sulser et al., 1962). Amitriptyline (0.1-1.0 mg/kg) and imipramine (0.05-3.00 mg/kg) did not alter the elaboration of conditioned defensive motor responses in cats to sequential auditory and visual stimuli that were reinforced by electric shock. Differentiation of the conditioned stimuli was not affected at higher drug doses (2.0 mg/kg), although there was an increased rate of interstimulus interval responding. Conditioned and unconditioned responses were decreased at higher doses (3.0-10.0 mg/kg) of the drugs (Vinogradov, 1969).

The effects of imipramine have also been studied for their possible role in memory consolidation, based upon the premise that amnesic effects associated with the elevation of brain serotonin might be blocked by tricyclics. Brain serotonin turnover, for example, is reduced after the administration of imipramine or chlorimipramine (Tissari and Suurhasko, 1972). A parallel observation has been made in the cerebrospinal fluid of depressed patients, wherein inhibition of 5-hydroxyindoleacetic acid efflux out of the CSF, lead to a reduced metabolite accumulation rate after treatment with amitriptyline and the imipramine (Post and Goodwin, 1974). These findings suggest that treatment with tricyclics decreased serotonin turnover in the central nervous system, possibly allowing for an accumulation of brain serotonin. A related observation that may, in part, account for the tricyclic-induced reduction in brain serotonin turnover is that *in vitro* studies have shown that imipramine and desipramine inhibit monoamine oxidase in rabbit brain (Roth and Gillis, 1974). This effect could also allow for an accumulation of non-deaminated brain serotonin.

The retrograde amnesic effects of ECS upon a passive avoidance response by mice was reduced by 14 percent when imipramine (20 mg/kg) was given one hour prior to the amnesic stimulus (Essman, 1970). Amitriptyline (10 mg/kg) reduced the acquisition of an active avoidance response in mice by 30 percent. The elevation of brain serotonin that followed the amnesic ECS stimulus was blocked in animals that had been treated by one of these tricyclics, thereby again favoring the view that interruption of memory consolidation by a rise of brain serotonin, could be blocked by drugs which prevent the brain serotonin rise after the amnesic stimulus is initiated.

There have been several reports regarding the amnesic effect of diazepam; this has been studied in rats (Soubrie et al., 1976) as well as in man. In the animal studies three benzodiazepines, diazepam, chlordiazepoxide, and lorazepam, were individually given to rats (0.6 to 40 mg/kg^{-1}) either 30 minutes prior to conditioned active avoidance trials or 30 minutes after. The benzodiazepines produced a dose-related reversal of behavioral inhibition for the avoidance task. Drugs given after the shock session did not affect shock-induced behavioral inhibition, thereby supporting the view that benzodiazepines interfere with the consolidation process (Soubrie et al., 1976). In man a possibly similar amnesic effect of diazepam has been reported (Mundow and Long, 1974). Verbal recall of visual, olfactory, or verbal stimuli presented to dental patients given 20 mg. diazepam (IV) was absent for the first stage of treatment. All 30 patients in this study were able to converse during the period for which subsequent amnesia became apparent (Foreman, 1974). There is some evidence that the peak amnesic effect of diazepam, occurs in the interval from 2 to 10 minutes following injection. In one series (Gregg et al., 1974), 7 male and 7 female patients were given an intravenous injection of diazepam (1 mg/7 lb. body weight, 1 mg/14 lb. body weight, or 1 mg/21 lb. body weight) or a placebo, and were then exposed to visual stimuli (line drawings of simple objects), auditory stimuli (common sounds), and painful stimuli (periosteal pressure applied to the clavicle, forehead, or ankle). Memory for the various stimuli, which were presented either immediately, 10, 20, or 30 minutes following drug injection, was tested 24 hours after each trial. All patients receiving the placebo indicated their recollection of the injection of the anesthetic (given 10 min. after placebo injection), whereas those patients receiving diazepam (mean dose = 7 mg, 11 mg, or 21 mg) showed only 57 percent, 50 percent, and 7 percent recall, respectively. A dose-related amnesia for all the sensory stimuli was apparent, with a peak effect when diazepam was given 10 min. prior to the stimuli. For the highest dose of diazepam (1 mg/1 lb. body weight), less than 30 percent of the stimuli were recalled, even when the interval between diazepam injection and stimulus presentation was 30 min. There was a statistically significant difference between the recall memory of male and female patients in this study, with the latter showing better recall after the intermediate and low dose of diazepam than males. This difference might best be attributed to sex-related differences in task motivation or attitude toward the experimenter (male). Inasmuch as the amnesic drug, diazepam, was presented prior to the stimuli for which subsequent amnesia was described, without any alteration of consciousness level or vital functions, it would seem most appropriate to consider the effect as an anterograde amnesia.

In 144 patients given diazepam (10 mg, i.m.) as a premedicant before surgery, 2 patients showed hazy memory of the trip to the operating room, 1 had no recollection of the IV injection, and 4 had only a hazy memory for this event. Four percent of the patients showed a partial amnesia (Pandit and Dundee, 1970). The diazepam premedication was given 60 to 90 minutes prior to anesthesia and memory testing was carried out at 6 and/or 24 hrs. after anesthesia.

Intravenous diazepam administered to patients prepared for oral surgery produced an anterograde amnesia on the day of surgery, for oral injections (53.9 percent), drilling (23.3 percent), chiseling (28 percent) and use of an oral elevator (40.3 percent). When tested during a one-week post-surgical follow-up visit, there was a 70.6 percent amnesia for the oral injection (Driscoll et al., 1972). Psychomotor performance was also measured in this study using a modified Bender-Gestalt test; a peak psychomotor deficit was observed after diazepam injection, with complete recovery by 1½ hours post-injection. This finding partially separates the psychomotor components of the cognitive task from the consolidation process involved with those stimuli present in operative situation.

The administration of diazepam in combination with other agents, which themselves may exert amnesic properties, has been studied. A considerable difference in the amnesic effect of such agents for events occurring prior to delivery to the operating room for minor gynecological surgery was noted depending upon whether they were given intravenously or intramuscularly as surgical premedication (Dundee et al., 1970). Diazepam alone (10 mg) caused a 3 percent incidence of anterograde amnesia when given i.m., but a 30 percent incidence when given IV. When the same dose of diazepam was combined with pethidine (100 mg), the i.m. route increased anterograde amnesia to 15 percent and IV to 92 percent. Pethidine alone provided for 5 and 25 percent anterograde amnesia, respectively for i.m. and IV routes. When combined with scopolamine methylbromide (hyoscine, 0.4 mg), the anterograde amnesic effect of diazepam was increased to 20 and 96 percent, respectively for i.m. and IV routes. Amnesia for the color of an object shown prior to the IV administration of a diazepam combination as well as amnesia for the color of an object shown 60 min. after recovery from anesthesia was tested and compared (Pandit et al., 1971). Diazepam (10 mg) alone produced 30 and 20 percent complete or partial amnesia, respectively pre-operatively and post-operatively. When combined with scopolamine methylbromide (0.4) pre-operative amnesia was increased to 90 percent and post-operative amnesia to 50 percent.

The exclusive amnesic property of scopolamine methylbromide (hyoscine) has been known for some time, and interest in this effect has been active since its initial description (Guass, 1906) as a pre-anesthetic medication in obstetrics and in surgical procedures (Thomson and Cotterill, 1909). In patients undergoing surgical procedures hyoscine was used as a pre-anesthetic medication, with morphine given for sedation. This was compared with atropine for the anterograde amnesic effect upon the post-operative recall of line drawings of simple familiar objects (Hardy and Wakely, 1962). Significantly more (7 percent) hyoscine-treated patients showed an amnesic effect, as compared with atropine-treated patients that showed no amnesia. An overall incidence of 13 percent for varying degrees of amnesic effect occurred with hyoscine. Hyoscine (0.4 and 0.6 mg) caused an anterograde amnesia for postcard pictures of familiar objects (35 and 50 percent) with a peak amnesic effect observed 50 to 80 min. after injection; this effect persisted for at least 2 hours (Dundee and Pandit, 1972b).

Apart from their use as pre-anesthetic medications and independent of other drug interactive effects, cholinergic agents do appear to play a relevant role in cognitive processes. Scopolamine (which blocks the synaptic acetylcholine receptor), methscopolamine bromide (which does not effectively cross the blood-brain barrier, and therefore acts on the peripheral cholinergic system), and physostigmine (which prolongs the action of acetylcholine by interfering with its hydrolysis by cholinesterase, the enzyme interfered with) were compared for their effects upon test performance for memory span, memory storage, and retrieval (Drachman and Leavitt, 1974). Scopolamine interfered with memory storage and retrieval without any alteration of memory span; methscopolamine bromide and physostigmine has no effects. A role for cholinergic neurons in memory/cognitive performance in man has been further supported by studies in which scopolamine impaired such functions; this effect could be reversed by the scopolamine antagonist, physostigmine, whereas amphetamine had no such effect (Drachman, 1977). A similar pattern of impaired cognitive function by central cholinergic blockade and that seen in normal aging has been observed and will be discussed in section 13 of this chapter.

The primary effect of scopolamine (5 to 10μg/kg., IV) upon the retention of word lists by normal volunteers was determined to be upon the acquisition of new material (Petersen, 1977). There was no effect of scopolamine (8 μg/kg) upon the recall of word lists learned prior to drug injection, but the acquisition of new information was impaired by this drug (Ghoneim and Mewaldt, 1977). Subjects given scopolamine followed by physostigmine (16 or 32 μg/kg., IV) showed significantly better immediate and delayed recall of word lists learned after drug treatment than subjects receiving scopolamine alone. This antagonism of the anterograde amnesic effect of scopolamine by physostigmine supports the role of the latter drug blocking the central anticholinergic effect of the former.

The amnesic effect of diazepam has also been studied in a non-operative situation with 12 young intelligent male volunteers, ranging in age from 20 to 34 years. A decision-making task, a vigilance task, and a list of words to be remembered were presented. Intravenous infusion of either saline (1 ml/min.) or diazepam (0.24 mg/kg, 5 mg/min) was then given for 3 to 4 min. There was only a slight reduction in the level of consciousness and accurate short-term processing of input was preserved within 20 min. of the diazepam injection (Clark et al., 1970). Recall of three word lists was impaired, as was their recognition, suggesting a diazepam-induced anterograde amnesia with peak efficacy within the first 10 minutes within diazepam administration.

The combined use of diazepam with morphine has been observed to exert amnesic effects, when this combination was employed in male surgical patients (Eisenberg and Kwan, 1971; Eisenberg et al., 1974). A similar intravenously administered combination (0.2 mg/kg morphine and 0.1 mg/kg diazepam), administered after delivery following cesarean section exerted both an anterograde and a retrograde amnesia (Abouleish and Taylor, 1976). A significant reduction in the incidence of the undesirable side effects of light anesthesia occurred. Only 1.9 percent of the 53 patients undergoing elective surgery had any awareness of pain and only 9 percent of the 68 patients in the study were able to recall the events prior to reaching the operating room.

A related benzodiazepine, lorazepam, has also been shown to impair memory in man (Heisterkamp and Cohen, 1975); the intravenous administration of this agent (3 and 5 mg) exerted a significantly greater retrograde amnesic effect for events in the 30 minutes prior to treatment than occurred with i.m. diazepam (5 and 10 mg). The use of lorazepam as a premedication in surgical patients has also provided evidence for the anterograde amnesic effects of this agent (Fragen and Caldwell, 1976), as compared with diazepam and placebo. Failure to recall events of the operative day occurred in about half of the lorazepam-treated patients with only minimal impairment observed for the diazepam group. A single picture shown to all patients 120 minutes after drug injection was recalled on the following day by only 7 of the 29 subjects receiving lorazepam, as compared with recall by 21 of the 29 subjects that received diazepam. The anterograde as well as the retrograde amnesic effects of lorazepam have also been studied at two dose levels in order to determine the time-effect relationship (Pandit et al., 1976). Intravenous lorazepam (2 mg, or 4 mg) was given to healthy subjects 5 to 240 minutes after being shown pictures of horses, flowers, or a dollar bill; recall of the pictures was tested the following day. With 2 mg. of lorazepam the anti-recall effect lasted only 30 min. with a 30 min. latency, whereas with 4 mg. the anti-recall effect occurred 15 min. after injection, for a duration of 4 hours, in 70 to 80 percent of the subjects.

Inherent in several of the studies discussed is the issue of the independence of pre-surgical medication-induced retrograde amnesia from an interaction contributing to that amnesia from the surgical anesthesia used. Whereas many studies have discounted the amnesic properties of surgical anesthesia, there is certainly evidence for the amnesic effects of such agents (Abt et al., 1961; Jarvik, 1964; Cherkin and Harroun, 1971). In comparing the amnesic effects of several pre-operative medications (atropine, pethidine, and pentobarbitone) with general anesthesia (thiopentone, halothane, and nitrous oxide), it was concluded that postoperative amnesia for auditory, visual, and painful stimuli was more dependent upon the general anesthetic than upon the pre-operative drug (Gruber and Reed, 1968). No anterograde amnesic effects of pethidine (50 mg) were observed in patients given this drug as a pre-anesthetic medication (Dundee and Pandit, 1972b). Stimuli shown from 1 to 60 min. after drug injection were recalled 6 hours after surgery.

Among the mood alterants there is at least one other agent that deserves mention for its effect upon memory processes; this is lithium carbonate. Although little appears to have been systematically investigated for the short-term memory effects of lithium salts, at least one study (Kusumo and Vaughan, 1977) has shown that patients taking this agent for affective disorders showed impaired short-term memory at 15 sec. delay intervals and enhanced long-term recall of difficult material.

GENERAL ANESTHETICS

The potentially amnesic effect of general anesthetics has been considered in a number of studies in both animals and man. One agent that has been considered is diethyl ether, which was shown to produce a retrograde amnesia for a conditioned response in mice (Essman and Jarvik, 1960). A similar effect of ether anesthesia upon the retention of an avoidance response in rats was also shown (Pearlman et al., 1961). A study of the time course over which diethyl ether, administered in an anesthetic dose to mice after acquisition of a one-trial avoidance response, was effective in producing a retrograde amnesia (Abt et al., 1961), indicated that virtually complete amnesia was produced by anesthesia given within 8 min. after a single training trial; between 16 and 20 min. after training, either produced amnesia in 50 to 60 percent of the animals. By 24 min. after training, ether anesthesia produced amnesia in only 20 percent of the mice. It was also shown (Essman and Jarvik, 1961) that ether anesthesia immediately after learning produced a complete retrograde amnesia for a passive avoidance response, when tested 24 hrs. after training. Anesthesia was ether, one hour after training had no effect upon the retention of the avoidance behavior. The finding that anesthesia with diethyl ether is capable of producing a time-dependent retrograde amnesia in rodents supports the view that changes associated with the effects of the anesthetic or of the anesthesia state are capable of interfering with the memory consolidation process. The result also stands as a contradiction of the view (Burns, 1958), that rapidly induced anesthesia does not produce retrograde amnesia.

In a clinical investigation (Artusio, 1955) with 135 patients, the effects of ether anesthesia upon memory was assessed during Plane 1 of anesthesia. In Plane 1 (the onset of anesthesia until some analgesia was achieved) of Stage 1 anesthesia there was no change in memory for recent or past events and simple problems could be solved. In Plane 2 of anesthesia there was some analgesia, although pain responses could still be elicited and simple instructions were followed. In post-operative memory testing there was total amnesia for all experiences during this Plane of anesthesia, although memory for recent and past events was intact. In Plane 3 there was complete anesthesia, although during this period the patients were still verbally responsive and special senses were intact. During Plane 3 of ether anesthesia there was diminution of memory for recent events and memory for past events, although ultimately reduced, was intact for a longer period than the former.

These studies in man and the concurrent animal investigations indicate that anterograde as well as retrograde amnesia may occur with diethyl ether anesthesia. It is also suggested that the duration of anesthesia or the actual loss of consciousness are not necessarily requisites for amnesia. Clinical studies in particular indicate that, like the amnesic effects of benzodiazepines, ether-induced amnesia is associated with analgesia. It is quite likely that those molecular changes that account for the disruption of memory consolidation or interfere with memory retrieval can be activated by either analgesia; this contradicts the long held view that loss of consciousness is a requirement for retrograde amnesia.

The issue of anesthesia-induced amnesia has not always been consistently supported. For example, for 26 healthy subjects to whom either halothane, Forane, thiopental, or nitrous oxide followed by halothane, was administered rapidly 30 seconds after a 10 second presentation of a visual stimulus, no retrograde amnesia was apparent when recall was tested 24 hours later (Bahlman et al., 1972). Such objects as a clock, camera, automobile, or beer can were described in great detail.

Nitrous oxide administered at subanesthetic doses, has also been cited as a potentially amnesic agent, however, its potential in this respect appears to be dose-related. Short-term memory or the input necessary to its fixation has been impaired by subanesthetic doses in man (Steinberg and Summerfield, 1957); the agent was given to volunteer subjects, instructed to acquire a rote learning task, at a Pa of 0.33—one-third of the partial pressure required for anesthesia. A concentration dependence for retrograde amnesia from nitrous oxide has been suggested (Parbrook, 1967), although at partial pressures between 0.2 to 0.5 Pa, no impairment of input or "short-term" recall (30 sec. after input) was found (Robson et al., 1960). An elevation of the partial pressure impaired later (2 to 5 min.) recall. The relationship between the concentration of nitrous oxide and its amnesic effect in man has not always been consistent between studies or within the same study. At a low partial pressure (0.2 Pa), nitrous oxide did not affect recall, but both short-term and long-term recall were reduced when 0.3 Pa was used (Parkhouse et al., 1960). Long-term recall was abolished at 0.4 Pa, and short-term recall was reduced.

The amnesic effects of general anesthetics upon memory functions in man have been considered (Adam, 1973) and it was observed that verbal memory was selectively affected by very low concentrations of fluroxene and halothane. High concentrations of fluroxene or halothane given to subjects for five hours affected newly acquired verbal stimuli but also impaired the search process in verbal memory (Adam, 1976). The latter effect was observed only for several hours after recovery from the anesthesia, but were no longer apparent on the next day or one week later.

The retrograde amnesic effect of four commonly used intravenous anesthetics was studied in healthy adult subjects, without any pre-anesthetic medications (Dundee and Pandit, 1972). Ten visual stimuli (pictures of familiar objects) were shown during a 15 min. period just prior to anesthesia with either thiopentone, propanidid, methohexitone, or diazepam. None of these intravenously injected agents produced any retrograde amnesia, consistent with an earlier discussion of the anterograde amnesic effect of anesthetic and/or pre-anesthetic agents. The duration of postoperative amnesia has also been related to a number of factors including age, type of general anesthetic used, and the time of day (Lambrechts and Parkhouse, 1961). Patients anesthetized with thiopentone nitrous oxide, and oxygen, under the age of 40 had the greatest percentage of amnesia for postoperative awakening of less than 8 hours, whereas amnesias for over 8 hours increased in frequency as a function of age. Ether and trichloroethylene produced the greatest incidence of post operative amnesia (49 percent and 50 percent respectively showing amnesias over 5 hrs.). Patients returned postoperatively between 6 A.M. and noon showed appreciably more (18 percent) amnesia of 8 hours or more. Such data warrant further consideration of the relationship between diurnal variations in the susceptibility to anterograde amnesic agents.

The use of a premedication with a general anesthetic also may contribute to the effect upon memory. The use of a narcotic as a preoperative medication in obstetric patients within six hours of general anesthesia (Wilson and Turner, 1969) reduced the frequency of unpleasant stimuli recalled during a cesarean section by 18 percent. Diazepam used as a premedication apparently increased (17.4 percent) the incidence of unpleasant stimulus recall associated with a cesarean section (Turner and Wilson, 1969). This finding contrasts with the studies cited earlier in support of diazepam as an anterograde amnesic agent—

even when used by itself in subanesthetic doses. When given intravenously (0.24 mg/kg) to healthy volunteers, recall was impaired for at least 30 minutes (Clark et al., 1970). This effect has been sufficiently well documented, so that in clinical use, for example, diazepam given several minutes prior to local anesthetic administration, reduced the recall of the latter to 16 percent with 10 mg and to 0 percent with a 30 mg dose (Keilty and Blackwood, 1969).

It is apparent that the potentiation as well as the antagonism of the memory effects of general anesthetics by other non-anesthetics depends upon the central interactions of these agents. General anesthetics elevate sensory thresholds and depress the reticular activity system of the brain. There is also some indication that neurotransmitter status is altered by general anesthetic agents, and such changes may reflect the central effect of the agent rather than the consequence of the anesthesia. In our own studies, we have observed an elevation of brain serotonin and a reduction of its turnover in the brains of animals exposed to diethyl ether or nitrous oxide. Serotonin utilization in rat brain as well as its synthesis has been shown to be delayed by both nitrous oxide and halothane anesthesia (Bourgoin et al., 1975). Partial inhibition of the active elimination of the acidic metabolite of serotonin from the brain also occurred. It is tempting to speculate that potentiation of antagonism of the amnesic effect of general anesthetics depends upon the molecular effect of the interactive agent. Studies are still required to delineate this possible mode of action.

ETHANOL

In considering the relationship between ethanol and the processes of learning and memory, a distinction between the acute and chronic effect of this agent becomes useful. It is well known that impairment of performance can occur with both acute and chronic ethanol administration (Weiss and Laties, 1962) and that chronic ethanolism can impair acquisition of responses and recall of recent experiences. There is some question, however, as to the degree to which such effects reside in: (1) the central physiological effect of ethanol, (b) a drug-induced cellular change approximating a neurological basis for a chronic brain syndrome, or (c) a metabolic lesion based upon a deficiency state wherein vitamin and/or electrolyte losses could independently contribute to altered sensory, motor, cognitive, intellectual, or performance functions. It should be apparent that if disturbances of memory are to be ascribed to ethanol, then there are probably several forms of ethanol amnesia. Two forms have been described (Ryback, 1970) and consist of (1) a state-dependent form, and (2) a "blackout" form. The former condition has been applied to a number of central nervous system depressants and cholinergic agents (Overton, 1966) in animals (Crow, 1966; Ryback, 1969) and in man (Storm and Caird, 1967; Goodwin et al., 1969) —and suggest that stimuli learned during a state following ethanol ingestion are best recalled in a similar subsequent ethanol-induced state. There is some controversy as to the genuine nature of universality of the state-dependent concept, particularly in view of the obvious fallacy that the ethanol state, wherein performance is maximally compromised, should confer a unique synaptic circumstance wherein memory is better recalled. To put state-dependency into a consolidation process that presumably occurred during ethanol intoxication, would argue itself against state-dependency. For example, we have shown that ethanol given to mice potentiates the amnesic effects of ECS given after avoidance conditioning. Such a potentiating effect is described by an increase in time after conditioning wherein ECS will produce a retrograde amnesia. Retention or amnesia was tested 24 hours after training where there was no longer an ethanol state. It would seem reasonable, therefore, on basic as well as clinical grounds, to question the validity of a state-dependent amnesic effect of ethanol. The experiment cited above may be taken as yet another example of an ethanol amnesia—a potentiated amnesia. One suggested basis for this effect is that ethanol, as well as ECS lead to an increase in brain serotonin content, and an elevation of brain serotonin can produce amnesia (Essman, 1970). Accumulative or additive effect of the two agents could increase the course of time over which memory consolidation occurs.

The "blackout" amnesia induced by ethanol refers to a profound short-term memory deficit associated with an acute elevation in the blood ethanol level (Ryback, 1969). Under these circumstances cues to the recent memory loss, ingestion of ethanol, or prompted recognition fail to provide for recall. There remains some question of the possible corollaries of a rapid, acute rise in blood level that could account for an apparently non-reversible and irretrievable memory loss. Hypoglycemia, hypomagnesemia, dehydration, pH change, etc., all represent possible factors that may result from the elevated blood ethanol and which may account, either individually or collectively, for the observed amnesia.

The combination of ethanol abuse and nutritional deficiency serve as a basis for Wernick's disease and Korsakoff's syndrome characterized, in addition to several neurological findings, by a disorder of memory. There is impairment of recent memory, a disorder in new learning, and intervals of retrograde amnesia. When recovery from these disorders has occurred, there is still a residual amnesia for the acute phase of the illness. Among those areas of the brain involving neuronal and myelin degeneration and gliosis, those structures probably most relevant to memory functions wherein structural changes occur in such ethanolic neuropathies are the mammillary bodies, formices, thalamic nuclei, and hypothalamus. It is apparent therefore, that memory disturbances resulting from the chronic effects of ethanol involve structural changes that are not apparent in those amnesias which result from acute ethanol treatment.

STIMULANTS

The action of central nervous system stimulants, such as the amphetamines, can be enhanced if the level of brain serotonin has been reduced. For example, interruption of the ascending serotoninergic pathways in the rat with lesions of the medical forebrain bundle, leading to a 60 to 84 percent decrease in telencephalic serotonin, produced a 3-fold enhancement of amphetamine effect (Green and Harvey, 1974). An increased rate of operant conditioning responding was observed. The effect of amphetamines upon learning or memory appear only indirectly related to their effect upon brain serotonin metabolism or dependency upon the level of brain serotonin. What appears more directly behaviorally relevant for the effect of amphetamines are the tasks upon which its potential effects on learning or memory are assessed. It may be noted, however, that amphetamine in doses exceeding 5 mg/kg release the extragranular stores of serotonin into the extraneuronal space, but the depletion of serotonin does not occur (Fuxe and Ungerstedt, 1968).

The effects of amphetamines upon performance have been critically assessed (Weiss and Laties, 1962) and it has been suggested that performance levels, lowered by fatigue, and work-performance decrements may be enhanced by these drugs. Such performance factors are often difficult to separate from the performance measurers in learning and memory tasks. Similarly, motivational components of learning or memory tasks may influence the effects of amphetamines upon such behaviors. Diamphetamine has been shown to increase the rate of conditioning in man (Franks and Trouton, 1958) and several tests of abstract reasoning, sentence completion, writing speed, and free association were enhanced by d-amphetamine (Nash, 1962). In a task involving the solution of arithmetic problems, a reduced error incidence, and a decreased performance decrement due to fatigue was also noted in subjects given a single oral dose of 10 mg of diamphetamine.

For tasks more directly related to memory processes, amphetamines have also been shown to exert a facilitative effect. Metamphetamine (15 mg/68 kg, IV) provided for an increased recall of a series of digits ranging from 8 to 20 items, when these were presented in different time sequences (Talland and Quarton, 1965). The acquisition of paired-associate verbal stimuli of low associative value was enhanced by d-amphetamine, but no effect upon the recall of these associated stimuli was found (Hurst et al., 1969).

The effects of metamphetamine upon short-term memory were investigated in subjects instructed to reproduce lists of digits after various delay times following their presentation (Crow and Bursill, 1970). Error rates for the drug-treated subjects exceeded those of the control at all delay intervals, although not significantly. There were also no differences between drug- and control-treated subjects for the changes in the error rate before and after treatment.

The effects of amphetamines have been observed to facilitate learning in hyperactive children (Conners and Eisenberg, 1963) and Porteus maze performance was improved by d-amphetamine in normal as well as in hyperactive children (Conners et al., 1964). A similar result was obtained when the quantitative score on the Porteus maze test was studied in children with an intercurrent lesion of the central nervous system (hyperkinetic) and in normal controls (Lasagna and Epstein, 1968). Non-organic subjects showed a 4.8 percent increase in maze test quotients after d-amphetamine, and the hyperkinetic (organic) groups showed a 23.8 percent increase for the same task after d-amphetamine.

Another group of central nervous system stimulants that has taken on possible significance for effects upon learning and memory processes includes the analeptics, with such drugs as strychnine, picrotoxin, and pentylenetetrazol. The use of strychnine tonics among the geriatric population as a remedy for, among other things, "memory loss," "forgetfulness," "memory lapses," and "improved concentration" were common applications called to one's attention on the labels of such products common to the pharmacist's shelves 75 years ago, and to some extent, available today. There have been various rationales upon which the presumed learning and memory facilitation by strychnine have been based. These include a drug-induced increase in brain excitability coincident with the learning experience (Lashley, 1917),–a premise by which improved maze acquisition by rats was explained, and, a drug-induced inhibition of cholinesterase activity (only demonstrated *in vitro*–Nachmansohn, 1938) used to account for a reduced incidence of maze acquisition errors by rats (McGaugh, 1961). There has also been the observation that 6 daily strychnine injections facilitated behavior in rats and led to an increase (27 percent) in the whole brain content of RNA (Carlini and Carlini, 1965).

There is rather consistent agreement regarding the central stimulant effects of strychnine, but some controversy regarding its efficacy in facilitating either learning or memory. The acceleration of visual acuity (Walsh, 1947), its effect upon appetitive behavior, its effect upon shock threshold, and seizure threshold —all introduce methodological problems that limit conclusions regarding strychnine as a facilitative drug. These limitations may all or individually apply to such studies in which the maze performance of rats was improved by strychnine given either before or after training (McGaugh et al., 1962; Petrinovich, 1963; McGaugh and Petrinovich, 1965; McGaugh, 1966, 1968). Another possibly important factor contributing to presumed behavioral facilitation by strychnine is the distribution of experience in learning trials. Rats given strychnine prior to massed trials required fewer trials and made fewer errors in acquiring a maze response, but no effect of the drug was apparent when the trials were spaced over longer intervals (Livecchi and Dusewica, 1969). This finding again supports the notion of an antifatigue effect of the drug upon maze acquisition with either massed or spaced trials (Dusewica and Livecchi, 1969). The absence of a post-trial effect of strychnine argues against its presumed pro-consolidation effect. Strychnine sulfate, in 8 doses ranging from 0.0005 to 0.60 mg/kg, failed to have any facilitative effect upon avoidance learning (Oglesby and Winter, 1973), again casting doubt upon the memory specific effect of strychnine as contrasted with its performance effects. The post-trial administration of strychnine sulfate to rats did not modify avoidance discrimination or task acquisition (Oglesby and Winter, 1974).

Another factor that may be important for the behavioral effects of strychnine concerns its neonatal administration and the variable of handling. Rat pups were given either strychnine or saline injections and either handled or non-manipulated between 2 and 5 days of age. Although strychnine had no effect upon active avoidance learning by the rats at 45 days of age, the handled animals showed significantly more avoidance behavior than the non-manipulated controls (Schaefer et al., 1974).

The view that behavioral facilitation by analeptics represents (1) an interaction with motivated behavior, (2) an anti-fatigue effect, or (3) an increased level of activation may, in addition to applying to strychnine, also apply to picrotoxin and pentylenetetrazol. The post-trial treatment of rats with picrotoxin has been reported to facilitate maze learning (Breen and McGaugh, 1961); the poorer learners among the rats showed facilitation (fewer errors) at a dose of picrotoxin (1.0 mg/kg) that did not alter the error incidence among the good learners. Semichronic post-trial administration of picrotoxin to rats (1.0 mg/kg) improved their maze-acquisition behavior (Garg and Holland, 1968), although this agent has also been shown to have no effect upon maze learning in other studies (Prien et al., 1963).

One basis for the action of picrotoxin may lie in its property as a central GABA receptor blocker (Curtis and Johnston, 1974), the brain GABA receptors appear to operate on the basis of hyperpolarization with increased permeability to chloride. There is some evidence that the GABA minergic may be critical for specific types of learning (Ishikawa and Saito, 1975).

On the basis of its selective reduction in short inhibitory post-synaptic currents and lack of effect upon long inhibitory post-synaptic current or excitatory post-synaptic currents, it has been suggested that pentylenetetrazol selectively blocks a cholinergic post-synaptic potential and acts postsynaptically (Wilson and Escueta, 1974). There have, in fact, been clinical applications of pentylenetetrazol for the treatment of memory disorders in geriatric patients with arteriosclerosis or associated chronic brain syndrome (Wolff, 1962), as well as for the treatment of senile attentional and social disorders (Goodhart and Helenore, 1963). The use of pentylenetetrazol in animal studies has yielded results which, on one hand, support its role as a facilitatory agent in subconvulsive doses (Loken, 1940, 1941; Irwin and Benuazizi, 1966; Hunt and Krivanek, 1966; McGaugh, 1966; Krivanek and McGaugh, 1968; Hunt and Bauer, 1969) and, on the other hand, have failed to find any facilitatory effect (Bunch and Mueller, 1941; Heron and Carlson, 1941; Kahan, 1966; Bovet et al., 1966; Pearl and McKean, 1967). It has been shown that rats given saline injections from 15 to 35 days of age and/or maturity prior to being tested for acquisition of a maze response, made more response errors than rats that were not injected; pentylenetetrazol (15 mg/kg) given during development or at maturity counteracted the disruptive effect of saline (Stein, 1974).

In convulsive doses, pentylenetetrazol has been shown to produce a retrograde amnesic effect; this may be accounted for by the convulsion as well as by the central effect of the drug, independent of the convulsion. A retrograde amnesic effect of pentylenetetrazol was produced when a convulsion occurred after an avoidance conditioning trial in rats (Pearlmen et al., 1961), the retrograde amnesic effect occurred even when the interval between training and drug treatment was as long as 8 hours. This profound effect may be accounted for by repetitive spontaneous seizure episodes following an initial drug-induced convulsion or may be precipitated by sensory stimuli, particularly auditory, that occur during the post-convulsive period. In mice pre-treated with lidocaine to block pentylenetetrazol induced convulsions, the drug still produced a retrograde amnesia for a passive avoidance response (Essman, 1968). These experiments did not support an RNA-related mechanism to account for the amnesic effect; a brain RNA decrement occurred when convulsions were precipitated, but when the convulsions were blocked, brain RNA concentration was not affected. Pentylenetetrazol convulsions also provide for a temporal gradient of retrograde amnesia if convulsive, but not excessively high, doses are given. The disruption of a conditioned taste aversion in rats has been shown for this agent (Millner and Palfai, 1974); the drug given within 5 seconds after conditioned taste aversion training disrupted the retention of the aversive behavior, whereas, when given 10 minutes before or after taste aversion training, has no effect upon the retention of the conditioned aversion.

It may be of further interest to note that a current standard compilation of prescribable approved drugs in the U.S. (Physician's Desk Reference, 1979) lists at least 6 preparations containing 100 mg of pentylenetetrazol, the indications for which have been variously given as "cerebral stimulant," to "enhance mental and physical activity," and "indicated in the treatment of memory defects."

The central action of pentylenetetrazol may relate to several biochemical mechanisms that are operative in learning and memory. Glutamic acid levels in brain are altered by pentylenetetrazol (Wiechert and Gollnitz, 1969a, b), and this probably bears upon the availability of precursor for brain GABA synthesis. Acetylcholine level is also modified by pentylenetetrazol (Richter and Crossland, 1949). It would certainly appear that such factors as dosage, duration of action, and site of cerebral excitation produced by this drug lie at the basis for its presumed effect upon learning and memory.

Another stimulant, probably in more common use, is caffeine, which certainly relates to the pharmacology of learning and memory. The action of this methyl xanthine upon learning and memory has, like other central stimulants, been dual in nature; some investigators (Lashley, 1917) have noted a dose-related retardation of maze learning in rats, or (Voronin and Napalkov, 1963) on inhibition of chains of alimentary reflexes. It was suggested (Pavlov, 1927) that negative conditioned reflexes are imapired by the drug, whereas positive conditioned reflexes are enhanced, depending upon a caffeine-induced reduction in internal inhibition. A caffeine-induced increase of locomotor activity has been noted in some studies (Dews, 1953); this effect could contribute to its action upon learning. In other studies (Greenblatt and Osterberg, 1961) the effects of caffeine upon locomotor activity appear dependent upon pre-drug baseline acitivity levels; if initially high, the drug exerts little locomotor stimulant effect. Caffeine given to mice during the nadir of their activity cycle (4 P.M.) significantly increased subsequent locomotor activity, but the same dose (25 mg/kg) given during the activity peak (4 to 8 A.M.) depressed locomotor activity level (Essman, 1971). Thus, there are several apparent variables, which, in animal studies, govern the direction in which the effects of caffeine alter behavior. These include: (1) the complexity of a choice task; (2) the active or passive nature of avoidance behavior; (3) the degree of locomotor activity effect; and (4) baseline or periodic variations upon which the drug effect is imposed.

In man, caffeine (1.5 gr.) given 2½ to 3 hours prior to the presentation of a list of nonsense syllables to be learned, provided for better learning of those stimuli for which there were pleasant associations and also an increase in the number of consonants learned (Tolman, 1917). There appear to be considerable inter-individual differences in the effects of the caffeine in coffee upon simple learning functions in man. Coffee given 20, 100, or 140 minutes prior to addition or memory span tasks, increased the accuracy of performance (Gililand and Nelson, 1939), but there was considerable variability in the magnitude of the effect. It would be difficult to generalize from such studies and speculate about the potentially facilitative effect of coffee consumption upon tasks requiring learning or depending upon the efficiency with which memory consolidation takes place. Just as there are wide variations in the caffeine content in different coffees, there are individual differences in the absorption, duration of effect, and magnitude of central action. Just as noted from animal studies, the central effects of caffeine and coffee appear to depend upon the activation and behavioral baselines upon which the drug is superimposed.

Performance of four measures on an automobile driving simulator was significantly enhanced by initial and supplemental doses of caffeine (Regina et al., 1974), suggesting that sustained task performance requiring motor learning can be facilitated by the drug. The reduction of drowsiness and increase in alertness produced by caffeine served as a basis for administering 300 mg of the drug to 60 volunteer college students then given the Paced Sequential Memory Task (Mitchell et al., 1974). A significant interaction was observed between the effects of caffeine and the placebo effect of the pill administration. It would appear that the placebo effect of the pill, which itself enhanced task performance, was further facilitated by caffeine. The use of stimulant drugs in hyperactive children, has been given some prior attention, but also has relevance for caffeine (Cole, 1975), particularly with a view toward its use in learning disorders manifested by hyperactive children. In doses equivalent to approximately two cups of coffee over a 4 to 5 hour period, caffeine did not benefit any of 25 hyperkinetic children tested (Gross, 1975). The behavior of most of the children was, in fact, worsened by caffeine, as compared with other stimulants such as methyphenidate and amphetamine. Such findings could again be in agreement with the view that baseline activation determines the extent to which the behavioral efficacy of caffeine may be provided; and, unlike other stimulants, caffeine does not produce a paradoxical effect upon a hyperexcited state.

As an example of how caffeine may exert dual effects in a learning-memory paradigm, mice were given the drug after one maze training trial and their performance was assessed on a testing trial given 24 hrs. later (Stripling and Alpern, 1974). A dose-dependent disruption of performance occurred on the 24 hour trial. When caffeine was given prior to a training trial, performance was facilitated. It was suggested that caffeine disrupted the long-term stores of memory for the initial training and also provided for proactive facilitation of maze learning. In the first circumstance it would appear that caffeine interferes with the memory consolidation process, whereas in the second condition memory consolidation may be facilitated as a result of drug-enhanced performance at learning.

A chemical relative of caffeine, uric acid, has also been implicated both behaviorally and biochemically in learning and memory processes. The endogenous level of uric acid has been suggested as mediating such functions as intellectual and cognitive behavior (Orowan, 1955), primarily on the basis of its potential as a central nervous system stimulant. One can certainly derive anecdotal evidence in support of a positive effect of uric acid from the clinical history of eminent persons who were hyperuricemic; a potent counterargument, however, is the question of whether the intellectual or cognitive ability of such persons was any different from that of normouricemic individuals who also achieved eminence. A low, but statistically significant correlation was found between the uric acid level of army recruits and their performance scores on a well standardized intelligence test (Stetten and Heron, 1959). A number of factors, other than a purely facilitative property of endogenous uric acid, may contribute to such a relationship; these include increased activation level, greater anti-fatigue potential and sustained alertness. These same fators may, in part, also account for the observations that academic achievement, defined by rank, publications, and prominence in one's discipline, is also associated with a higher level of uric acid (Brooks and Mueller, 1966).

The behavioral role of uric acid has been extensively reviewed (Essman, 1970b); in animal studies this agent has been shown to increase response times and decrease the incidence or errors made during the learning of a simple maze task by mice. Uricase, in a dose sufficient to reduce endogenous uric acid to allantoin (1.65 mg/kg), led to an increase in both maze response time and errors. Treatment with uric acid prior to single trial conditioning of an avoidance response, reduced the incidence of electroconvulsive shock-induced retrograde amnesia for that response. With ECS there was only a 20 percent incidence of response retention, however, in uric acid-treated mice, depending upon dose (0.5-20.0 mg/kg) there was from 47 to 73 percent retention of the conditioned avoidance response. These data suggested that uric acid, without affecting unconditioned behavior, seizure susceptibility, or response threshold to the unconditioned stimulus (foot shock), apparently facilitated memory consolidation either by (1) decreasing the consolidation time, thereby reducing the effective interval within which stimuli were capable of disrupting the consolidation process, or (2) reducing the central electrical and/or biochemical effect that accounts either for consolidation disruption or amnesia, (3) shifting the locus of central effect to a site where its memory disruptive effects are reduced, or (4) acting in competition with other molecules formed, released, or activated by the amnesic stimulus to reduce their effect.

There are two observations that have been made in conjunction with the possible pro-consolidation effect of uric acid which provide support for an effect on the molecular level. One such finding is that parenterally administered uric acid is capable of elevating brain RNA and able to block the RNA-reducing effect of at least one amnesic stimulus, ECS. Another finding is that the elevation of brain serotonin by ECS, another corollary of its amnesic effect, is attenuated if animals have been pretreated with uric acid. We have observed that the intracranial injection of serotonin in mice produces a retrograde amnesia (Essman, 1973) and that the site of maximal effect is the medial hippocampus. One of the effects that intrahippocampal serotonin injection shares in common with ECS, in addition to their effect as amnesic events, is their ability to produce a time-related, regional, cellular, and organelle specific inhibition of protein synthesis (Essman, 1972). Uric acid has been shown to (1) attenuate the amnesic effect of (a) ECS, (b) intrahippocampal serotonin injection, and (c) parenteral butyric acid injection, and (2) block the inhibition of protein synthesis normally produced by such treatments (Essman and Essman, 1977). The common denominator in those studies where uric acid facilitate memory consolidation by reducing the interfering effects of several amnesic treatments is that the elevation of brain serotonin (common to those amnesic stimuli considered) and the related inhibition of protein synthesis (the consequence of serotonin elevation) is attenuated or blocked by uric acid treatment. Whether this relationship also applies to endogenous uric acid remains in question and whether clinically utilized drugs (such as thiazides) which provide for increased uric acid levels, also relate to the proconsolidation effect of this agent, raises interesting questions that can possibly be partially answered in the clinical situation. Certainly, in this regard, antiuricogenic and uricosuric agents such as colchicine and allopurinal, also deserve examination for effects that may be relevant for learning and memory processes.

A related methyl xanthine, which like uric acid, acts to facilitate maze acquisition and reduces the amnesic effect of ECS in mice, is trimethyl uric acid (TMUA) (Essman, 1971). There is evidence that this agent stimulates brain RNA synthesis and reduces brain serotonin content—these effects being rather dose-specific (10 mg/kg) in mice. TMUA acts behaviorally like uric acid, but appears to be more specific for its selective neurochemical effects; its potential clinical utility remains, at present, undefined. Certainly its clinical applicability would appear warranted, if only its neurochemical effects were considered adequate to justify its use as a facilitative agent in learning and memory.

A stimulant that has been utilized clinically, at least partially on the basis of its reputed biochemical effects (stimulation of RNA polymerase activity in the rat brain) is magnesium pemoline (Glasky and Simon, 1966), although other groups have failed to replicate the biochemical observation (Morrison, 1967; Stein and Yellin, 1967). Behavioral facilitation in a series of animal studies was suggested for this drug (Plotnikoff, 1966a, b, c) where response acquisition was facilitated, more rapid task relearning after ECS was observed, and recovery of pre-ECS avoidance behavior occurred. The amnesic effect of ECS was reduced by magnesium pemoline in rats (Stein and Brink, 1969) and a similar effect was observed in man; patients given magnesium pemoline showed some facilitation of learning and memory tasks given after electroconvulsive therapy (Small and Small, 1967; Small et al., 1968).

With magnesium pemoline, as with other central nervous system stimulants, there is the possibility that sustained performance or attention are less compromised. Increased errors were noted, for example, under control conditions, for a non-motivated continuous attention task; magnesium pemoline, as well as caffeine and methylphenidate, prevented the error increase in these human subjects (Orzack et al., 1968). This agent, like other central stimulants, has been used in the treatment of childhood hyperkinesis (Page et al., 1974). Its efficacy in bringing about improved cognitive and perceptual functioning, as measured on test performance, without appreciable side effects with a single daily dosage, supports its clinical usefulness as an alternative to the amphetamines and methylphenidate for the management of hyperkinesis and associated learning problems.

Memory test performance among a geriatric population with documented memory defects was significantly improved by magnesium pemoline (Cameron,

1966). A 10 percent increase in memory score on the Wechsler Memory Quotient was achieved in subject given the drug (25 to 125 mg/day) for one month. The acute administration of magnesium pemoline (25, 37.5 mg, p.o.) to normal healthy males three hours before verbal and motor learning tasks did not affect learning, memory, or performance (Smith, 1967). Similarly, acute treatment of college students with magnesium pemoline (6.25 to 25.0 mg, p.o.) two and one-half hours prior to a learning task that depended upon the ability to discriminate light cues, failed to alter the rate at which the correct response was learned (Burns et al., 1967).

There has been the suggestion that magnesium pemoline increases the excitatory properties of a strong stimulus in a learning situation, without necessarily affecting performance (DiGiusto and King, 1972) in the absence of a discrete conditioned stimulus. This observation raises the interesting issue of sensory facilitation with stimulants such as magnesium pemoline and might possibly explain why for some subjects (senile geriatric, hyperactive children, intellectually defective, etc.) the effects, if due to a sensory enhancement, are more apparent than in a normal population where its anti-fatigue effects appear to be the most apparent. Random geriatric populations in whom there are no signs of organic brain pathology, intellectual deterioration, or perceptual dysfunction do not necessarily show any benefit on memory tasks from magnesium pemoline. In one such study (Gilbert et al., 1973) the performance of subjects given the drug did not differ from that of placebo-treated controls on the Wechsler Adult Intelligence Scale vocabulary subtest or the Guild Memory Test performance. From data obtained on a mood scale administered at the beginning and end of the study there was some indication that the drug increased depression and worrisomeness.

NICOTINE

The effects of nicotine upon behavioral responses and upon brain amines comprise major issues related to the clinical pharmacology of learning and memory. In animal studies nicotine (0.18 to 0.4 mg/kg, IV) increased locomotor activity levels (Bonta et al., 1960), whereas with chronic injection (0.5 to 0.1 mg/kg, s.c. or i.p.) a significant decrease in the running time of rats was observed (Eisenberg, 1948, 1954). In man, the effects of nicotine appear to reduce performance, but this effect may be related to a number of factors other than the central action of the drug, *per se*. The nicotine content of a single inhaled cigarette (estimated at approximately 1 to 2 µg/kg equivalents in the blood), given ten times over a six hour period, increased the onset of fatigue and did not affect vigilance or tracking behavior (Heimstra, 1962). Tracking performance was decreased by the inhalation of four cigarettes over a brief time period (Wenzel and Davis, 1961). A major deficiency in these studies is the absence of information regarding blood levels of nicotine at the time of performance evaluation; there are, however, other issues that render such results extremely difficult to interpret. There is no clear separation between the physiological or behavioral effects of the gas phase of cigarette smoke as distinguished from those of nicotine. There is also the question of the biological and/or behavioral effects of nicotine metabolites, formed by hepatic metabolism, upon the observed effects. Dosage, absorption, and elimination are subject to wide intra- as well as inter-individual variations and the cumulative dosage and cumulative effect over time remain unknown, still to be defined.

Animal studies of learning and memory provide some insights into both the effects of nicotine upon these processes as well as the neurochemical substrates of these processes affected by nicotine. The effects of nicotine upon learning in rodents has been shown to be related to the baseline behavior upon which the drug effect is imposed. Nicotine (0.1 mg/kg) administered prior to maze learning trials facilitated acquisition by younger rats (55, 61 days), that were better learners. Older rats (131, 158 days), that were poorer maze learners, did not show any drug-related alterations in their learning behavior (Linuchev and Michelson, 1965). In mice, nicotine (0.5 mg/kg) facilitated the learning of an avoidance response in strains that were poor learners, but in strains that were good avoidance learners, avoidance conditioning was impaired by the drug (Bovet et al., 1966). Other situations in which nicotine has been shown to facilitate learning include younger vs. older rats (Robustelli, 1966), task difficulty (Bovet-Nitti, 1966), younger vs. older mice (Olivero, 1967), morning vs. evening (Bovet et al., 1967) and in reactive vs. nonreactive rats (Garg and Holland, 1968).

Some of the results with nicotine have suggested that its central effect is mediated via a cholinergic mechanism. It was found that the facilitation of memory consolidation could be achieved by the post-training administration of atropine (Evangelista and Izquierdo, 1971), when atropine was given prior to a shuttle avoidance task, its stimulant effect upon performance added to the stimulant effect of nicotine (Evangelista and Izquierdo, 1972). In the same study the stimulant action of nicotine was antagonized by prolonged pre-treatment with atropine. The authors maintain that the drug effect, specific to the hippocampus, represents a probable electrical effect at that site. The interaction of nicotine and atropine in the hippocampus may be viewed as a cholinergic interaction. The ability of nicotine to reverse or block the cholinergic response to an amnesic stimulus could constitute another basis upon which the neurochemical effect of this drug could be related to memory consolidation. Nicotine sulfate (1.0 mg/kg) given to mice 15 min. prior to avoidance conditioning increased the amnesic effect of a post-training ECS (Essman, 1969). When given 60 minutes prior to training, the same dose of nicotine reduced the amnestic effect of a post-training ECS (Essman et al., 1968). ECS given to mice reduced the bound acetylcholine pool of the cerebral cortex by 88 percent and the acetylcholine content of the synaptic vesicles in this region by 30 percent within 10 minutes after convulsion. For mice that were treated with nicotine sulfate 45 minutes earlier, ECS did not significantly reduce the vesicular acetylcholine content (Essman, 1971). These findings support a cholinergic role in the action of nicotine upon memory consolidation since nicotine appears capable of reversing the cholinergic changes associated with retrograde amnesia.

An adrenergic mechanism to explain the action of nicotine upon learning has been proposed (Fulginiti and Orsingher, 1973) and is supported by some experimental data. Rats given nicotine showed facilitation of a conditioned response. This facilitative effect was significantly reduced if the animals were pre-treated with a-methyl-p-tyrosine, a tyrosine hydroxylase inhibitor that leads to reduced brain levels of catecholamines. The blockade of nicotine-facilitation of learning by a-methyl-p-tyrosine was abolished by nialamide, a monoamine oxidase inhibitor which provides for a sustained increase in brain catecholamines. The facilitative action of nicotine was thus shown to depend upon brain levels and/or metabolism of catecholamines.

A role for brain serotonin in the action of nicotine upon learning and memory has also been indicated. As previously noted, nicotine exerts a biphasic effect upon the amnesic effect of electroconvulsive shock, and this effect appears time-dependent. Coincident with the nicotine-induced antagonisn of the ECS-induced amnesia there was: (1) increased availability of centrally active peripheral metabolites of nicotine, (-) cotinine and 3-pyridylacetic acid; (2) blockade of the serotonin-elevating effect of ECS; and (3) an increase in brain serotonin turnover rate.

In addition to those factors mentioned there are others which have implications for the clinical pharmacology of nicotine in learning and memory. One of these is the rapid development of tolerance, which can persist for prolonged periods after withdrawal. This may be one condition that, in particular, may account for differences in the acute and chronic effects of nicotine upon learning and memory in man, and more generally to the issue of cigarette smoke and how it affects such processes. A possible mode applicable to man, that relates to this problem is the observation (Stolerman et al., 1973) that chronic tolerance produced in rats by nicotine injected, orally ingested with drinking water, or subcutaneously implanted, could persist for as long as 90 days after drug treatment. If facilitation of learning or memory were associated with either acute or chronic tolerance to nicotine, then maintenance of the tolerance state could constitute an important condition for such effects to be continued. In another respect, failure to maintain the tolerance state could itself be a basis for a secondary but real disruptive effect from nicotine.

In a clinical context of its broader psychoactive effects, nicotine is a mood alterant. As such, its subjective effect upon mood and affect, like that of any other psychoactive agent, can independently constitute a basis for its effect upon learning or memory in man. For example, smoking while involved in a learning or memory task may provide a subjective basis upon which cognitive performance is altered. For example, consideration of such factors as nicotine content of cigarettes, diurnal variations, and differences in puffing rate contributed to the subjective report of mood change in habitual smokers before and after smoking (Ague, 1973). Dose-dependent effects of nicotine on pleasantness, aggression, anxiety, and tension were observed. Such factors may well, depending upon the learning or memory conditions, serve as motivational states upon which response changes can be based.

The multiple ways in which several of the brain biogenic amines are involved in the clinical pharmacology of learning and memory offers interesting future prospects for agents that may provide further insight into the biochemical substrates of learning or memory or for the molecular relationships of specific drugs for these processes.

PROCAINE

The use of procaine hydrochloride or stabilized forms of this local anesthetic in geriatric populations as an agent to interrupt aging processes, reverse depression, and promote learning and memory has warranted some brief consideration of its place in the clinical pharmacology of learning and memory. Learning and memory was assessed in rats chronically treated with procaine, using a 13-choice maze (Aslan et al., 1965). Among control rats, 24-month-old animals made more errors per trial, had longer maze running times, and showed longer running times per trial than 10-month-old rats. Procaine-treated, 24-month-old rats, showed fewer maze errors than control rats, had shorter maze running times, and shorter running times per trial than non-drug treated control rats of the same age. These measures of learning and memory for the procaine-treated 24-month-old rat were comparable with those obtained from control rats of 10 months of age. The use of stabilized procaine hydrochloride (Gerovital H-3) in geriatric populations has been viewed as a possible route toward the use of this compound as an antidepressant or vehicle through which cognitive changes accompanying senility and arteriosclerotic brain disease might be modified (Smigel et al., 1960; Kral et al., 1962). Changes were observed in somatization and anxiety/depression by the third week of treatment with this agent in a group of depressed geriatric patients (Sakalis et al., 1974); no changes in memory were observed, however. One basis upon which the presumed mechanism of procaine action has been formulated is its inhibitory effect upon monoamine oxidase activity; it is particularly notable that the activity of this brain enzyme which regulates the catabolism of catecholamines and indole amines has been observed to increase with aging (Robinson et al., 1972). This increase was noted in human platelets and plasma and was correlated with an age-related increase in the hindbrain. Norepinephrine levels decreased with age, whereas serotonin content remained fairly uniform with age in the human hindbrain, but the serotonin metabolite, 5-hydroxyindoleacetic acid increased sharply after the age of 65; this latter observation could indicate a change in serotonin turnover in the hindbrain with aging. Procaine has been shown to be a monoamine oxidase inhibitor (MacFarlane and Besbris, 1974; MacFarlane, 1975). The drug was shown to be a reversible, competitive inhibitor of monoamine oxidase, suggesting that it may interfere with aging-related enzyme increments and favor the restoration of amine substrate and/or turnover rates characteristic of the pre-aging nervous system. This action of procaine as an MAO inhibitor contrasts with the mode of inhibitor action of other, more traditional agents such as pargyline and phenylzine which are irreversible inhibitors and tranylcypromine, which is a partially reversible inhibitor. It is a matter of conjecture as to whether the efficacy of an MAO inhibitor as an antidepressant in clinical use or its effect upon learning and memory processes depends upon the reversibility of enzyme inhibition. In particular, these findings do raise the question of the extent to which clinically utilized MAO inhibitors serve to modify either learning or memory.

A difference in the effects of iproniazid and tranylcypromine upon a dark-avoidance conditioned response was demonstrated in mice (Bucci and Bovet, 1974). Iproniazid (25.5 and 100 mg/kg) decreased the percentage of conditioned responses, whereas tranylcypromine (2.5 and 5.0 mg/kg) caused a marked increase in the percentage of conditioned responses five hours after administration. The point in time at which maximal facilitation of conditioned response performance after tranylcypromine treatment occurred, was coincident with a maximal increase in brain norepinephrine after MAO inhibition. It may be of interest to consider that iproniazid-induced conditioned response impairment relates well in time to maximal elevation in brain serotonin. The difference in time course in the change in these brain amines by different MAO inhibitors in different concentrations could constitute a determinant of the outcome upon learned behavior. This view is further supported in studies demonstrating a biphasic effect of tranylcypromine on learned behavior in rats (Bucci, 1974). An initial depressant effect of the drug upon both spontaneous motor activity and the acquisition of a learned conditioned response was observed, but, by 5 hours after drug treatment, conditioned avoidance behavior and locomotor activity were stimulated. The initial substrate of MAO to increase following enzyme inhibition is serotonin, and by 5 hours brain norepinephrine has maximally increased. The biphasic behavioral effect of tranylcypromine may be related to those brain amines which are elevated at those times where learned behavior is measured.

In man, the effects of tranylcypromine have been studied upon conditioning and learning in an attempt to relate possible effects of this MAO inhibitor to its arousal effect (Weckowicz et al., 1974). No significant difference in eyelid conditioning were observed between drug- and placebo-treated subjects, except for a relationship, in the placebo group only, between eyelid conditionability and anxiety score. Paired-associate learning among placebo-treated subjects was facilitated in those subjects with a higher anxiety score. The apparently facilitative effects of anxiety level upon eyelid conditioning and paired-associate learning appeared to be eliminated by tranylcypromine which, regardless of differences in noted depression or anxiety, did not facilitate conditioning or learning. An issue of some importance in this study is the anticipated time course over which the action of tranylcypromine may occur. There could well be a considerable disparity in time between the antidepressant effects of this agent and its effects upon either learned behavior—which is most probably an effect upon performance, and its effects upon the acquisition or retention of behavior.

Like the time course and central effects of clinically utilized MAO inhibitors, some further definition of these parameters for procaine is indicated. As a weak inhibitor of MAO, that is reversible and competitive, procaine probably avoids some of the toxic and untoward effects encountered with other MAO inhibitors; it is not immediately apparent, however, if the possibly unique mode of MAO inhibition and the associated stimulant-like effect of procaine is adequate to account for possibly facilitative effects upon learning or memory.

Another consideration that applies to procaine is the degree to which its action may depend upon smooth muscle effects or cerebral vascular resistance. In this regard some comparisons with such agents as vasodilators and mediators of altered cellular metabolism may be warranted.

DRUGS IN DEMENTIA AND AGING

A partial basis for the use of specific drugs to improve the learning and/or memory dysfunction associated with dementias and aging lies in the presumed modification of cerebral change which presumably accounts for such disorders. Such changes include those associated with cerebral blood flow, cerebral vascular resistance, cerebral glucose utilization, and cerebral oxidative metabolism. To some extent all of these have been given consideration in previous sections of this chapter, although not necessarily with specific attention to the cognitive defects of the dementias or of aging.

Increased cerebral blood flow and decreased cerebral-vascular resistance result from the administration of the non-specific smooth muscle relaxant, papaverine. This agent has been employed with varied success in the treatment of a variety of symptoms in the geriatric patient, including mental confusion (La Brecque, 1966), chronic brain syndrome secondary to cerebral arteriosclerosis (Stern, 1970; Ritter et al., 1971; McQuillan et al., 1974), and response defects in psychological and psychophysical test performance (Smith et al., 1968). Some studies (Bazo, 1973) have indicated that papaverine has little effect upon intellectual function or cognition when given for 12 weeks to a population with cerebral arteriosclerosis with cerebrovascular insufficiency, however, other studies (Bambasova et al., 1974) have indicated that the drug did improve intellectual functions and verbal communication and reduced anxiety and depression in patients with arteriosclerotic dementia.

Similar disorders of cognition, relevant to learning and memory, have been treated in patients with senile dementia or compromised cerebral circulatory functions using the dihydrogenated ergot alkaloid, hydergine. This agent has been reported to have varied cognifacilitory success, but appears to compare favorably with and even provide for more effective therapeutic promise than papaverine (Gerin, 1969; Banen, 1971; Rao and Norris, 1972). In a double-blind study in which hydergine and papaverine were compared the former drug provided significantly better enhancement of cognitive and intellectual function (Bazo, 1973). A combination of hydergine with thiridazine proved to be beneficial in the treatment of several pathological states characteristic of senescence and cerebral atherosclerosis (Predescu et al., 1974); these findings suggest that hydergine therapy may provide a favorable baseline upon which to superimpose the potentially beneficial effects of other central stimulants in the elderly. Hydergine was found to be markedly more beneficial than papaverine in the treatment of a number of selected symptoms associated with aging (Rosen, 1975). On rated symptomatology there was twice the improvement noted with hydergine than with papaverine., in particular—mental alertness, which appears to be a significant factor underlying the motivational as well as persistence aspects of performance on tasks that require new learning or the retrieval of recent memory. A partial basis of the rationale for the clinical use of papaverine and ergot alkaloids, particularly for decreased learning ability and compromised memory functions in aging, is the possibility that cerebral vasodilatation and altered cerebral blood flow will permit the access of endogenous as well as exogenous substances to the central nervous system, where they may exert a positive effect. Aside from one suggestive study (Predescu et al., 1974) where the presumed transport and central action of a stimulant was enhanced by combination with an ergot preparation, there has been little use made clinically of this approach to the pharmacotherapy of geriatric cognitive dysfunction. It would appear that considerable merit lies in the use of such an approach. A possibly related issue and one for which some preliminary comment may be offered concerns the effects of proteins, peptides, and amino acids upon learning and memory. An increased cerebral blood flow could make these selectively, or as an aggregate, more readily available for central transport and provide for effects, either directly or secondary to their availability which account for improved cognitive functions.

One agent that has been given some attention as a potential "activator" of memory functions in geriatric patients is meclofenoxate (2-diethylaminoethyl-4-chlorophenoxyacetate hydrochloride)—a compound that has been purported to enhance alternate glycolytic pathways in cerebral hypoxic states. This agent, given to elderly, mildly demented patients, in a well controlled study, significantly improved the learning performance of the treated group, as compared with placebo (Gedye et al., 1972). No effect of meclofexate, however, was observed under controlled administration to intellectually deteriorated geriatric patients, when they were tested on a battery of 8 tests (Oliver and Restell, 1967). The consolidation of newly acquired data appeared to be facilitated in a healthy geriatric population by meclofexate, but recall of other information appeared unaffected (Marcer and Hopkins, 1977). Increased mental alertness was also reported by those subjects that received this drug.

An agent studied extensively in a wide variety of animal studies is piracetam, a compound structurally similar to a-amino butyric acid, which has been employed in studies of cognitive function in man. Some improved performance has been observed when this drug was administered to healthy subjects (Dimond, 1975; Mindus et al., 1975), whereas in memory dysfunction and cognitive defects associated with such clinical entities as cardiac pacemaker patients (Lagergren and Levander, 1974; Lagergren, 1974), cognitively compromised chronic alcoholics (Binder, 1974) and senile geriatric patients (Delwaide, 1975; Eckmann, 1975) memory was benefited. It is difficult to assess the precise cogni-specific role of piracetam since most of the studies advocating its benefits lack the double-blind, placebo cross-over type of design rigor that might factor out some of the contributory variables.

A topic of some current interest concerns the therapeutic approach to the treatment of the memory dysfunction and dementia characteristic of Alzheimer's disease. Supplemental dietary allocations of lecithin (phosphatidyl choline), a precursor of cerebral as well as peripheral choline, and possible accelerant of cerebral acetylcholine synthesis, has been suggested as a preventive modality in the dementia of Alzheimer's disease (Perry et al., 1977). No changes in cognitive performance were measured in patients with Alzheimer's disease given choline chloride (Boyd et al., 1977), although behavioral improvement was noted. Choline bitartrate given to patients with Alzheimer's disease produced improved cognitive changes in one out of three subjects (Etienne et al., 1978), and the beneficial effect of this agent was suggested as perhaps being more apparent in a younger age group with the same dementia. Similarly limited cognitive benefit of choline was observed in a group of similar age (Smith et al., 1978), but in early Alzheimer's disease (patients age 59 to 64, with 2 to 5 years evolution of disease) cognitive performance was benefited by choline citrate (9 g/day for 21 days). Thirty pictures and a word association, a motor learning task, and vigilance tests were evaluated for learning, relearning, and recall. Initial learning in this group was improved by choline (33 percent), as were relearning (22 percent), and recall (24 percent). Severe amnesia in patients under the age of 65 appears to be somewhat improved by dietary supplementation with choline (Signoret et al., 1978).

It might be appropriate at this point to comment further on the role of choline in learning and memory within the perspective of the cholinergic system more generally relevant to cognitive processes. A parallel between memory dysfunction in aging (Drachman and Leavitt, 1972) and the memory disorder induced in normal subjects with scopolamine has been suggested (Drachman and Leavitt, 1974). These parallels possess as common denominators of the memory storage and retrieval defects—(a) their nonspecificity, (b) a "neuronal fallout"-like phenomenon; *i.e.,* a loss of functional cholinergic neurons, (c) defects in cholinergic synthesis, release, or receptor action. A number of similarities between the disruptive effects of scopolamine (cholinergic receptor blockade at the synapse) upon memory functions and those observed in aging have been identified. Delayed recall of digits was profoundly impaired by scopolamine (Safer and Allen, 1971), and this drug similarly interfered with performance on subtests of the Wechsler Memory Scale (Ostfeld and Arguente, 1962). Whether the reactivation of functionally inactivated cholinergic receptors is feasible by pharmacological or dietary means remains a question to be answered by careful, well designed experimental studies. One approach to this issue has been made in normal volunteer subjects given a single oral dose (10g) of choline chloride and tested for its effects upon serial learning (Sitaran et al., 1978); the premise underlying this study was that choline, by increasing plasma and brain levels, and by providing sufficient substrate quantities for acetylcholine, might improve cholinergically related cognitive processes. Choline significantly increased the recall of serially learned, unrelated words and also selectively enhanced the storage and recall of low imagery words without affecting the response to high imagery words. A possible clinical application of these findings could be in the treatment of dementia associated with Huntington's disease, which appears to be conditional upon effective cholinergic functions, and in which impaired serial learning and altered recall probability for high- and low-imagery words has been observed (Caine et al., 1977).

The potential significance of other neurotransmitter-like substances for the pharmacological management of the learning and memory dysfunctions in aging and the dementias of neurological disorders may relate, in part, to some of the observations discussed earlier in this chapter. The increased activity of brain MAO activity in aging (Robinson et al., 1972) poses the very interesting question of whether greater deamination of specific neurotransmitters alters the synaptic and/or receptor processes required for the efficient maintenance of cognitive functions in aging.

It remains for some consideration to be given to the potential role of exogenous peptides as facilitative agents for cognitive processes. In several respects this topic relates to the present one in terms of its potential clinical applicability to geriatric cognitive dysfunction, but also may provide insight into some of the molecular processing which underlies the stability of information storage.

PEPTIDES

Analogs of ACTH or MSH have been used to investigate changes in learned behavior and the retrieval of acquired responses. Several studies in animals have indicated that ACTH facilitates shuttle box avoidance in rats (Beatty et al., 1970) conditioned with a high intensity foot shock. Other studies (Stratton and Kastin, 1974) found that at a low level of foot shock in a shuttle box avoidance rats given MSH showed improved acquisition. Positively reinforced learned behavior has also been facilitated by the administration of ACTH (Guth et al., 1971) or MSH (Stratton and Kastin, 1975).

Some limited data for the effects of one analog of ACTH, consisting of the amino acids 4 - 10, are available from studies in man. In subjects treated with $ACTH_{4-10}$ greater attention was rendered to stimuli presented in a visual discrimination paradigm (Sandman et al., 1975). The attention requirements of subjects for a continuous reaction time task was improved for subjects given $ACTH_{4-10}$ (Gaillard and Sanders, 1975). A failure to observe any effect of $ACTH_{4-10}$ upon the serial learning of paired associate stimuli or short-term memory for numbers has been noted; these tasks may be less dependent upon attentional factors, which in other studies with this peptide appear to be maximally affected.

Studies performed with healthy, normal human volunteers have indicated the $ACTH_{4-10}$ administration is capable of altering attention (Miller et al., 1975) as well as cognitive function (Marx, 1975). In psychiatric patients receiving electroconvulsive therapy (ECT) the polypeptide appeared to possess an antiamnesic effect for memory of a paired associate word list and picture recall affected by ECT (Small et al., 1977). Memory dysfunction after multiple ECTs was not affected by $ACTH_{4-10}$. A battery of memory-related tasks given to healthy adult volunteers was also affected by the administration of $ACTH_{4-10}$ (Miller et al., 1976). Significantly better scores were obtained as a consequence of drug treatment, on the Wechsler Memory Scale; specifically, digit recall and visual reproduction scores were higher for peptide-treated subjects (5 and 12 percent, respectively).

The central effects of synthetic ACTH analogs have been considered and relate in a most interesting way to some of the points considered in earlier discussions. After chronic peptide administration to the rat it was found that midbrain gamma amino butyric acid (GABA) and serotonin concentrations were reduced, norepinephrine turnover was increased, and serotonin turnover was decreased (Leonard, 1974).

There are many more questions about peptide-induced facilitation of learning and memory processes, particularly in man, that remain to be answered. Notable among these are issues of disposition, absorption, transport, and stability of parenterally administered compounds, the amino acid composition and/or sequence of which appears to make them quite specific as activators of cognitive functions. Again, as previously discussed for other agents, effects upon fatigue, vigilance, attention, and motivation are all issues that limit the specificity of peptides for the enhancement of learning and/or memory. The chronicity of treatment, the dose regimen, and the indirect contributions of peptides to the hormonal status of the adrenal, particularly after chronic administration, all represent factors which can affect the outcome of behavior studies, especially those in which task performance requires complex responses to stimuli of low associative value or situations of little failure risk. The major difference between the requirements for peptide administration in man and other agents used to affect learning or memory is that the former must be injected rather than ingested. This introduces not only a more potent placebo effect, greater inter-subject variability, and a difference in the time course of presumed maximal action, but also limits the subject population wherein this route of administration becomes acceptable or is tolerated. A motivational variable clearly emerges for the subject willing to tolerate a series of injections with a goal of improved cognitive performance, as compared with those subjects that are either not risk-takers or view the goal as not worth the treatment. These considerations place limitations upon the extent to which the clinical use of peptides for the enhancement of learning and memory may be relevant to sufficiently compete for further evaluation.

SOME CONCLUDING OBSERVATIONS

There have been numerous other pharmacological agents which have been considered to possess a role in the mediation of learning and memory processes and as such could have clinical applicability in man. These include such compounds as niacin, glutamic acid, thyroxine, pyridoxine, trace metals, etc. A major consideration in the application of these agents as well as others to learning or memory processes is the behavioral baseline upon which effects are superimposed and against which effects are evaluated. Differences in drug effect between a control population and one with arteriosclerotic changes, mental deficiency, learning disabilities, perceptual disorders, etc., may not always represent the best basis for clinical evaluation. The separation of performance effects (motor acceleration, anti-fatigue, etc.) from sensory effects (lowered sensory threshold, increased vigilance, etc.) from behavioral effects (increased motivation, interest, attention, etc.) essentially constitutes the most fundamental requirement for defining a clinical pharmacology of learning and memory. The need for such a pharmacology exists on several levels of function and dysfunction, but it appears more apparent that drug effects upon learning and memory processes depend upon the central biochemical action of the drug and the central mechanism to the cognitive function are tied. Several of these interdependencies of drug action and underlying mechanisms have been either proposed or experimentally supported but others still wait such definition. It is through such definition that a clinical pharmacology of learning and memory will evolve and its pharmacopae will increase.

REFERENCES

Abouleish, E., and Taylor, F.H. (1976): Effect of morphine-diazepam on signs of anesthesia, awareness, and dreams of patients under N_2O for Cesarean section. *Anesth. Analgesia* 55: 702-705.

Abt, J.P., Essman, W.B., and Jarvik, M.E. (1971): Ether induced retrograde amnesia for one trial conditioning in mice. *Science 133:* 1477-1478.

Adam, N. (1973): Effects of general anesthetics on memory functions in man. *J. Comp. Physiol. Psychol. 83:* 294-297.

Adam, N. (1976): Effects of general anesthetic on search in memory. *T.I.T.J. Life Sci. 6:* 29-34.

Adnitt, P.I. (1968): Hypoglycemic action of monoamine oxidase inhibitors (MAOI's) *Diabetes 17:* 628-633.

Aggeler, P.M., O'Reilley, R.A., and Leong, L. (1967): Potentiation of anticoagulant effects of warfarin by phenylbutazone. *New Engl. J. Med. 276:* 496-501.

Ague, C. (1973): Nicotine and smoking; Effect upon subjective changes in mood. *Psychopharmacologia* (Berlin) *30:* 323-328.

Aslan, A., Vrabiescu, A., Domilescu, C., Campeanu, L., Costiniu, M., and Stanescu, S. (1965): Long-term treatment with procaine (Gerobital H3) in albino rats. *J. Gerontol. 20:* 1-8.

Artusio, J.J., Jr. (1955): Ether analgesia during major surgery. *JAMA 157:* 33-36.

Avioli, L.V., Birge, S., Lee, S.W., and Slatopolsky, E. (1968): The metabolic fate of vitamin D_3-^3H in chronic renal failure. *J. Clin. Invest. 47:* 2239-2252.

Bahlman, S.H., Eger, E.I., II, and Cromwell, T.H. (1972): Anesthetics and amnesia. *Anesthesiol. 36:* 191.

Baldessarini, R.J., and Fischer, J.E. (1973): Metabolism in rat brain after surgical diversion of portal venous circulation. *Nature* (New Biol.) *245:* 25-27.

Bambasova, E., Bilkova, J., and Budinska, K. (1974): Papaverin in the treatment of psychiatric patients. *Activit. Nerv. Sup.* (Praha) *16:* 192-193.

Banen, D. (1971): An ergot preparation (Hydergine) for relief of symptoms of cerebrovascular insufficiency. *J. Amer. Geriatr. Soc. 20:* 22-29.

Bartter, F.C., Pronove, P., Gill, J.R., Jr. (1962): Hyperplasia of the juxtaglomerular complex with hyperaldosteronism and hypokalemic alkalosis: a new syndrome. *Amer. J. Med. 33:* 811-828.

Battig, K. (1961): Die Wirkung pharmakologisher Stoffe auf verschiedene Funktionen des Verhaltens der Ratte. *Pfulger's Arch. Ges. Physiol. 274:* 59.

Bazo, A. (1973): An ergot alkaloid preparation (Hydergine) versus Papaverine in treating common complaints of the aged: double-blind study. *J. Amer. Geriatr. Soc. 21:* 63-71.

Beatty, D.A., Beatty, W.A., Bowman, R.E., and Gilchrist, J.C. (1970): The effects of ACTH adrenalectomy and dexamethasone on the acquisition of an avoidance response in rats. *Physiol. Behav. 5:* 939-944.

Besser, G.M., and Steinberg, H. (1967): L'interaction du chlordiazepoxide et du dextroamphetamine chez l'homme. *Thérapie 22:* 977-990.
Bignami, G., and Gatti, G.L. (1969): Analysis of drug effects on multiple fixed ratio 33-fixed interval 5 min. in pigeons. *Psychopharmacologia 15:* 310-332.
Binder, S. (1974): Die Wirkung des Nootropikums Piracetam aud die KortiKale Leistungsféhigkeit chronische alkoholiker. *Münch. Med. Wsch. 116/48:* 2127-2130.
Bloomer, H.A., Barton, L.J., and Meddock, R.K., Jr. (1967): Penicillin-induced encephalopathy in uremic patients. *J.A.M.A. 200:* 121-123.
Bonta, I.L., Delver, A., Simons, L., and deVox, C.J. (1960): A newly developed motility apparatus and its applicability in two pharmacological designs. *Arch. Int. Pharmacodyn. Therap. 129:* 381-394.
Bovet, D., McGaugh, J.L., and Oliverio, A. (1966): Effects of posttrial administration of drugs on avoidance learning of mice. *Life Sci. 5:* 1309-1315.
Bovet-Nitti, F. (1966): Facilitation of simultaneous visual discrimination by nicotine in the rat. *Psychopharmacologia 10:* 59-66.
Bovet, D., Bovet-Nitti, F., and Oliverio, A. (1967): Action of nicotine on spontaneous and acquired behaivor of rats and mice. *Ann. N.Y. Acad. Sci. 142:* 261-267.
Boyd, W.D., Graham-White, J., Blackwood, G., Glen, I., and McQueen, J. (1977): Clinical effects of choline in Alzheimer senile dementia. *Lancet 2:* 711.
Breen, R.A., and McGaugh, J.L. (1961): Facilitation of maze learning with posttrial injections of picrotoxin. *J. Comp. Physiol. Psychol. 54:* 498-501.
Brooks, G.W., and Mueller, E. (1966): Serum urate concentrations among university professors; relation to drive, achievement, and leadership. *JAMA 195:* 415-418.
Brooks, S.M., Werk, E.E., Ackerman, S.J., Sullivan, I., and Thrasher, K. (1972): Adverse effects of phenobarbital on corticosteroid metabolism in patients with bronchial asthma. *New Engl. J. Med. 286:* 1125-1126.
Brush, F.R., Davenport, J.W., and Polidora, V.J. (1966): TCAP: Negative results in avoidance and water maze learning and retention. *Psychon. Sci. 4:* 183-184.
Bucci, L. (1974): The biphasic effect of small doses of tranylepromine on the spontaneous motor activity and learned conditioned behavior in rats. *Pharmacol.* (Basel) *12:* 354-361.
Bucci, L., and Bovet, D. (1974): The effect of iproniazid and tranylcypromine studied with a dark-avoidance conditioned schedule. *Psychopharmacologia 35:* 179-188.
Buckholtz, N.A., and Bowman, R.E. (1970): Retrograde amnesia and brain RNA content after TCAP. *Physiol. Behav. 5:* 911-924.
Buczko, W., and Tarasiewicz, S. (1976): The influence of albumin degradation products (ADP) on the central action of caffeine. *Acta Med. Pol. 17:* 111-117.
Bunch, M.E., and Mueller, C.G. (1941): The influence of metrazol upon maze learning ability. *J. Comp. Psychol. 32:* 569-574.
Burns, B.D. (1958): *The Mammalian Cerebral Cortex.* Edward Arnold, London. p. 90.
Burns, J.T., House, R.F., Fensch, F.C., and Miller, J.G. (1967): Effects of magnesium pemoline and dextroamphetamine on human learning. *Science 155:* 849-851.
Caine, E.D., Ebert, M.H., and Weingartner, H. (1977): An outline for the analysis of dementia. The memory disorder of Huntington's disease. *Neurology 27:* 1087-1092.
Cameron, D.E. (1966): Presidential address. Society of Biological Psychiatry meeting, Washington, D.C.
Carlini, G.R.S., and Carlini, E.A. (1965): Effects of strychnine and *Cannabis Sativa* (Marihuana) on the nucleic acid content in brain of the rat. *Med. Pharmacol. Exp. 12:* 21-26.
Cerletty, J.M., and Engbring, N.H. (1967): Azotemia and glucose intolerance. *Ann. Int. Med. 66:* 1097-1108.
Chamberlain, R.J., Rothschild, G.H., and Gerard, R.W. (1963): Drugs affecting RNA and learning. *Proc. Nat. Acad. Sci. 52:* 918-924.

Cherkin, A., and Herroun, P. (1971): Anesthesia and memory processes. *Anesthesiology 34:* 469-474.

Chisholm, D.C., and Moore, J.W. (1970): Effects of chlordiazepoxide on the acquisition of shuttle avoidance in the rabbit. *Psychon. Sci. 19:* 21-22.

Cicala, G.A., and Hartley, D.L. (1965): The effects of chlordiazepoxide on the acquisition and performance on a conditioned escape response in rats. *Psychol. Rec. 15:* 435-440.

Clarke, P.R., Eccersley, P.S., Frisby, J.P., and Thornton, J.A. (1970): The amnesic effect of diazepam (Valium). *Brit. J. Anaesth. 42:* 690-697.

Cole, S.O. (1975): Hyperkinetic children: the use of stimulant drugs evaluated. *Amer. J. Orthopsychiat. 45:* 28-37.

Conners, C.K., and Eisenberg, L. (1963): The effects of methylphenidate on symptomatology and learning in disturbed children. *Amer. J., Psychia. 120:* 458-464.

Conners, C.K., Eisenberg, L., and Sharpe, L. (1964): Effects of methylphenidate (Ritalin) on paired-associate learning and Porteus maze performance in emotionally disturbed children. *J. Consult. Psychol. 28:* 14-22.

Crow, T.J., and Bursill, A.E. (1970): An investigation into the effects of metamphetamine on short-term memory in man. In: E. Costa and S. Garattini (Eds.) *Amphetamines and Related Compounds.* Raven Press, New York. pp. 889-895.

Crow, L.T. (1966): Effects of alcohol on conditioned avoidance responding. *Physiol. Behav. 1:* 89-91.

Curtis, D.R., and Johnston, G.A.R. (1974): Amino acid transmitters in the mammalian central nervous system. *Ergeb. Physiol. 69:* 97-188.

Daniels, D. (1967): The effect of TCAP on acquisition of discrimination learning in the rat. *Psychonom. Sci. 7:* 5-6.

Davis, R.E. (1968): Environmental control of memory fixation in goldfish. *J. Comp. Physiol. Psychol. 65:* 72-78.

Delwaide, P. (1975): Etude contrôlée d'un nootrope chez des déments séniles. *Int. Congr. Psychosom. Med.,* 3rd Congress. Rome.

Dews, P.B. (1953): The measurement of the influence of drugs on voluntary activity in mice. *Brit. J. Pharmac. Chemother. 8:* 46-48.

DiGiusto, E.L., and King, M.G. (1972): Magnesium pemoline: enhancement of performance. *Psychol. Rep. 30:* 863-866.

Dimond, S.J. (1975): The effects of a nonotropic substance on the capacity for verbal memory and learning in normal man. *Int. Congr. Psychosom. Med.,* 3rd Congress. Rome.

Doherty, J.E., and Perkins, W.H. (1966): Digoxin metabolism in hypo-and hyperthyroidism. *Ann. Int. Med. 64:* 489-507.

Drachman, D.A. (1977): Memory and cognitive function in man: does the cholinergic system have a specific role? *Neurology 28:* 783-790.

Drachman, D.A., and Leavitt, J. (1972): Memory impairment in the aged: Storage versus retrieval deficit. *J. Exp. Psychol. 93:* 302-308.

Drachman, D.A., and Leavitt, J.A. (1974): Human memory and the cholinergic system. A relationship to aging? *Arch. Neurol. 30:* 113-121.

Driscoll, E.J., Smilack, Z.H., Lightbody, P.M., and Fiorucci, R.D. (1972): Sedation with intravenous diazepam. *J. Oral Surg. 30:* 332-343.

Dundee, J.W., Haslett, W.H.K., Keilty, S.R., and Pandit, S.K. (1970): Studies of drugs given before anesthesia. XX. Diazepam-containing mixtures. *Br. J. Anesth. 42:* 143-150.

Dundee, J.W., and Pandit, S.K. (1972a): Studies on drug-induced amnesia with intravenous anesthetic agents in man. *Brit. J. Clin. Pract. 26:* 164-166.

Dundee, J.W., and Pandit, S.K. (1972b): Anterograde amnesic effects of pethidine, hyoscine and diazepam in adults. *Brit. J. Pharmacol. 44:* 140-144.

Dundee, J.W., and Richard, R.K. (1954): Effect of azotemia upon the action of intravenous barbiturate anesthesia. *Anesthesiology 15:* 333-346.
Dusewicz, R.A., and Livecchi, S.G. (1969): The effects of posttrial administration of strychnine upon maze learning. *Psychol. Rec. 19:* 461-463.
Eckmann, F. (1975): Mise en évidence par la méthode en double aveugle des propertés des nootropes dan les syndromes psycho-organique séniles. *Int. Congr. Psychosom. Med.,* 3rd Congress. Rome.
Egyhazi, E., and Hydén, H. (1961): Experimentally induced changes in the base composition of the ribonucleic acid of isolated nerve cells and their oligodendroglial cells. *J. Biophys. Biochem. Cytol. 10:* 403-410.
Eisenberg, J.M. (1948): The effect of nicotine on maze learning ability of albino rats. *Fed. Proc. 7:* 31-32.
Eisenberg, J.M. (1954): The effect of nicotine on maze behavior of albino rats. *J. Psychol. 37:* 291-295.
Eisenberg, L., and Kwan, A.M. (1971): Neuroleptanesthesia with diazepam-morphine in poor-risk surgical patients. *Can. Anesth. Soc. J. 18:* 465-472.
Eisenberg, L., Taub, H.A., and Burana, A. (1974): Memory under diazepam-morphine neuroleptanesthesia in male surgical patients. *Anesth. Analgesia 53:* 488-495.
Englert, E., Brown, H., Willardson, D.G., Wallach, S., and Simons, E.L. (1958): Metabolism of free and conjugated 17-hydroxycorticosteroids in subjects with uremia. *J. Clin. Endocr. 18:* 36-48.
Essman, W.B. (1965): Facilitation of memory consolidation by chemically induced acceleration of RNA synthesis. *Proc. XXIII Internat. Congr. Physiol. Sciences* 470.
Essman, W.B. (1967): Facilitation of maze acquisition by mice with Tricyanoaminopropene (TCAP) given during early postnatal development. *Psychon. Sci. 9:* 51-52.
Essman, W.B. (1968): Retrograde amnesia in seizure-protected mice: Behavioral and biochemical effects of pentylenetetrazol. *Physiol. Behav. 3:* 549-552.
Essman, W.B. (1968): Electroshock-induced retrograde amnesia in seizure-protected mice. *Pyschol. Rep. 22:* 929-935.
Essman, W.B. (1969b): Mediation of memory consolidation: Behavioral and biochemical effects of nicotine and nicotine metabolites. *Proc. 4th Int. Congr. Pharmacol.* Basel. 289.
Essman, W.B. (1970): The role of biogenic amines in memory consolidation. In: G. Adám (Ed.) *The Biology of Memory.* Akad. Kiado Publ., Budapest. p. 213-238.
Essman, W.B. (1970b): Central nervous system metabolism, drug effects, and higher functions. In: W.L. Smith (Ed.) *Drugs and Cerebral Function.* Chas. Thomas, Springfield, IL. p. 151-175.
Essman, W.B. (1971): Drug effects and learning and memory processes. *Adv. Pharmacol. Chemother. 9:* 241-330.
Essman, W.B. (1971): Some neurochemical correlates of altered memory consolidation. *Trans. N.Y. Acad. Sci.*
Essman, W.B. (1972): Metabolic and behavioral consequences of nicotine. In. W.L. Smith (Ed.) *Cerebral Function Development and Drug Action.* Chas. Thomas, Springfield, IL. p. 273-287.
Essman, W.B. (1972): Retrograde amnesia and cerebral protein synthesis: Initiation and inhibition by 5-Hydroxytryptamine. *Totus Homo 4:* 61-67.
Essman, W.B. (1973): Neuromolecular modulation of experimentally induced retrograde amnesia. *Confinia Neurol. 35:* 1-22.
Essman, W.B. (1973). *Neurochemistry of Cerebral Electroshock.* Spectrum Publ., New York.

Essman, W.B. (1977): Non-drug factors in the evaluation of psychotropic drugs. In: A. Bertelli, G.B. Cassano, P. Castro Giovanni, J. Levine, and J.R. Wittenborn (Eds.), *Evaluation of New Drugs in Clinical Psychopharmacology.* J.R. Prous, Barcelona. pp. 107-114.

Essman, W.B. (1978): Morphine action in myocardial metabolopathies. In: M.L. Adler, L. Manara, and R. Samanin (Eds.) *Factors Affecting the Action of Narcotics.* Raven Press, New York. p. 681-701.

Essman, W.B. (1978): Serotonin in learning and memory. In: W.B. Essman (Ed.) *Serotonin in Health and Disease, Vol. III. The Central Nervous System.* Spectrum Publ., New York. p. 69-143.

Essman, W.B., and Alpern, H. (1964): Single trial learning: Methodology and results with mice. *Psych. Rep. 15:* 731-740.

Essman, W.B., and Essman, S.G. (1977): Amine regulation of protein synthesis in retrograde amnesia. In: J.M.R. Delgado, and F. DeFeudis (Eds.) *Behavioral Neurochemistry.* Spectrum Publ., New York. p. 25-61.

Essman, W.B., and Jarvik, M.E. (1960): The retrograde effect of ether anesthesia on a conditioned avoidance response in mice. *Amer. Psychol. 15:* 498.

Essman, W.B., and Jarvik, M.E. (1961): Impairment of retention for a conditioned response by ether anesthesia in mice. *Psychopharmacologia 2:* 172-176.

Essman, W.B., Steinberg, M.I., and Golod, M.I. (1968): Alterations in the behavioral and biochemical effects of electroconvulsive shock with nicotine. *Psychonom. Sci. 12:* 107-108.

Essman, W.B., and Tagliente, T. (1978): Monoamine oxidase and serotonin regulation. In: W.B. Essman (Ed.) *Serotonin in Health and Disease, Vol. I. Localization and Disposition.* Spectrum Publ., New York. p. 301-362.

Etienne, P., Gauthier, S., Johnson, G., Collier, B., Mendis, T., Dastoor, D., Cole, M., and Muller, H.F. (1978): Clinical effects of choline in Alzheimer's disease. *Lancet 1:* 508-509.

Evangelista, A.M., and Izquierdo, I. (1971): The effect of pre- and posttrial amphetamine injections on avoidance responses of rats. *Psychopharmacologia* (Berlin) *20:* 42-47.

Evangelista, A.M., and Izquierdo, I. (1972): Effects of avoidance or avoidance conditioning: interaction with nicotine and comparison with N-methylatropine. *Psychopharmacologia* (Berlin) *27:* 241-248.

Flexner, L.B., and Flexner, J.A. (1968): Intercerebral saline: Effect on memory of trained mice treated with puromycin. *Science 159:* 330-331.

Foreman, P.A. (1974): Control of the anxiety/pain complex in dentistry. *Oral Surg. Med. Pathol. 37:* 337-349.

Fragen, R.J., and CAldwell, N. (1976): Lorazepam premedication: lack of recall and relief of anxiety. *Anesth. Analgesia 55:* 792-792.

Franks, C.M., and Trouton, D. (1958): Effects of amobarbital sodium and dexamphetamine sulfate on the conditioning of the eyeblink response. *J. Comp. Physiol. Psychol. 51:* 220-222.

Fulginiti, S., and Orsingher, O.A. (1973): Further evidence in support of a common adrenergic mechanism for the facilitatory action on learning of amphetamine and nicotine in rats. *J. Pharmacol. 25:* 580-581.

Fuxe, K., and Ungerstedt, U. (1968): Histochemical studies on the effect of (+) amphetaamine, drugs of the imipramine group and tryptamine on the central catecholamine and 5-hydroxytryptamine neurons after intracranial injections of catecholamines and 5-hydroxytryptamine. *Eur. J. Pharmacol. 4:* 135-144.

Gaillard, A.W.K., and Sanders, A.F. (1975): Some effects of ACTH 4-10 on perfromance during a serial learning task. *Psychopharmacologia* (Berlin) *42:* 201-208.

Garg, M., and Holland, H.C. (1968): Consolidation of maze learning: The effects of posttrial injections of a stimulant drug (Picrotoxin). *Psychopharmacologia 12:* 96-103.
Garg, M., and Holland, H.C. (1968): Consolidation of maze learning: A further study of posttrial injections of a stimulant drug (Nicotine). *Int. J. Neuropharmacol. 7:* 55-59.
Gauss, C.J. (1906): Geburten in kunstlichem dammerschlaf. *Arch. Gynekol. 78:* 579.
Gedye, J.L., Exton-Smith, A.N., and Wedgewood, J. (1972): A method for measuring mental performance in the elderly and its use in a pilot clinical trial of meclofenoxate in organic dementia. *Age Ageing 1:* 74-80.
Gerin, J. (1969): Symptomatic treatment of cerebrovascular insufficiency with Hydergine. *Curr. Therap. Res. 11:* 539-546.
Ghoneim, M.M., and Mewaldt, S.P. (1977): Studies on human memory: The interactions of diazepam, scopolamine, and physostigmine. *Psychopharmacol. 52:* 1-6.
Gilbert, J.G., Donnelly, K.J., Zimmer, L.E., and Kubis, J.F. (1973): Effect of magnesium penoline and methylphenidate on memory improvement and mood in normal aging subjects. *Int. J. Aging Hum. Dev. 4:* 35-51.
Gililand, A.R., and Nelson, D. (1939): The effects of coffee on certain mental and physiological functions. *J. Gen. Psychol. 21:* 339-348.
Glasky, A.J., and Simon, L.N. (1966): Magnesium pemoline: Enhancement of brain RNA polymerases. *Science 151:* 702-703.
Goodhart, R.S., and Helenore, J.C. (Eds.) (1963): *Modern Drug Encyclopedia and Therapeutic Index, 9th Ed.,* Rueben H. Donnelley, New York.
Goodwin, D.W., Powell, B., and Brenner, D. (1969): Alcohol and recall: state-dependent effects in man. *Science 163:* 1358-1360.
Green, T.K., and Harvey, J.A. (1974): Enhancement of amphetamine action after interruption of ascending serotonergic pathways. *J. Pharmacol. Exp. Thera. 190:* 109-117.
Greenblatt, E.N., and Osterberg, A.C. (1961): Effect of drugs on the maintenance of exploratory behavior in mice. *Fed. Proc. 20:* 397.
Gregg, J.M., Ryan, D.E., and Levin, K.H. (1974): The amnesic actions of diazepam. *Oral Surg. 32:* 651-664.
Grieco, M.H., Pierson, R.N., Jr., and Pi-Sunyer, F.X. (1968): Comparison of the circulatory and metabolic effects of isoproterenol, epinephrine, methoxamine in normal and asthmatic subjects. *Amer. J. Med. 44:* 863-872.
Gross, M.D. (1975): Caffeine in the treatment of children with minimal brain dysfunction or hyperkinetic syndrome. *Psychosomatics 16:* 26-27.
Gruber, R.P., and Reed, D.R. (1968): Postoperative anterograde amnesia. *Br. J. Anesth. 40:* 845-849.
Gurowitz, E.M., Lubar, J.F., Ain, B.R., and Gross, D.A. (1967): Disruption of passive avoidance learning by magnesium pemoline. *Psychonom. Sci. 8:* 19-20.
Guth, S., Levine, S., and Seward, J.P. (1971): Appetitive acquisition and extinction with exogenous ACTH. *Physiol. Behav. 7:* 195-200.
Hanson, H.M. (1961): The effects of amitriptyline, imipramine, chlorpromazine and nialamide on avoidance behavior. *Fed. Proc. 20:* 396.
Hardy, T.K., and Wakely, D. (1962): The amnesic properties of hyoscine and atropine in pre-anesthetic medication. *Anaesth. 17:* 331-336.
Harris, W.S., and Goodman, R.M. (1968): Hyperreactivity to atropine in Down's syndrome. *New Engl. J. Med. 279:* 407-410.
Hartelius, H. (1950): Further experiences of the use of malononitrile in the treatment of mental illness. *Amer. J. Psychiat. 107:* 95-101.
Heimstra, N.W. (1962): Social influence on the response to drugs. II. Chlorpromazine and iproniazid. *Psychopharmacologia 3:* 72-78.

Heisterkamp, D.V., and Cohen, P.J. (1975): The effect of intravenous premedication with lorazepam (ativan), pentobarbital and diazepam on recall. *Br. J. Anesth. 47:* 79-81.
Heron, W.T., and Carlson, W.S. (1941): The effects of metrazol shock on retention of the maze habit. *J. Comp. Physiol. Psychol. 32:* 307-309.
Holmes, J.H., Nakamoto, S., and Sawyer, K.C. (1958): Changes in blood composition before and after dialysis with the Kolff turn coil kidney. *Trans. Amer. Soc. Artif. Int. Organs 4:* 16-23.
Holmgren, B., and Condi, C. (1964): Conditioned avoidance reflex under pentobarbital. *Boletin del Instituto de Estudios Medicos y Biologicos 22:* 21-38.
Hunt, E.B., and Bauer, R.H. (1969): Facilitation of learning by delayed injections of pentylenetetrazol. *Psychopharmacologia 16:* 139-146.
Hunt, E.B., and Krivanek, J. (1966): The effects of pentylenetetrazol and methylphenoxypropane on discrimination learning. *Psychopharmacologia 9:* 1-16.
Hurst, P.M., Radlov, R., Chubb, N., and Bagley, S.K. (1969): Effects of d-amphetamine on acquisition, persistence, and recall. *Amer. J. Psychol. 82:* 307-319.
Hydén, H. (1959): In: Proc. IVth Int. Cong. Biochem., Vienna. London: Pergamon Press, Vol. 3.
Hydén, H. (1962): A molecular basis of neuron-glia interaction. In: F.O. Schmitt (Ed.), *Macromolecular Specificity and Biological Memory.* The M.I.T. Press, Cambridge, Mass. p. 55-69.
Hydén, H., and Egyhazi, E. (1962): Nuclear RNA changes of nerve cells during a learning experiment in rats. *Proc. Nat. Acad. Sci.* (Wash.) *48:* 1366-1373.
Hydén, H., and Egyhazi, E. (1963): Glial RNA changes during a learning experiment in rats. *Proc. Nat. Acad. Sci.* (Wash.) *49:* 618-624.
Hydén, H., and Egyhazi, E. (1964): Changes in RNA content and base composition in cortieal neurons of rats in learning experiment involving transfer of handedness. *Proc. Nat. Acad. Sci.* (Wash.) *52:* 1030-1035.
Hydén, H., and Hartelius, H. (1969): Stimulation of the nucleo-protein production in the nerve cells by malononitrile and its effect on psychic functions in mental disorders. *Acta Psychiat. (Suppl.) 48:* 117 pages.
Hydén, H., and Lange, P.W. (1970): Brain-cell protein synthesis specifically related to learning. *Proc. Nat. Acad. Sci.* (Wash.) *65:* 898-904.
Hydén, H., and Lange, P.W. (1972): Protein synthesis in hippocampal nerve cells during reversal of handedness in rats. *Brain Res. 45:* 314-317.
Hydén, H., Lange, P.W., Mihailovic, L.J., and Petrovic-Minic, B. (1974): Changes of RNA base composition in nerve cells of monkeys subjected to visual discrimination and delayed alternation performance. *Brain Res. 65:* 215-230.
Hydén, H., Lange, P.W., and Seyfried, C. (1973): Biochemical brain protein changes produced by selective breeding for learning in rats. *Brain. Res. 61:* 446-451.
Irwin, S., and Benuazizi, A. (1966): Pentylenetetrazol enhances memory functions. *Science 152:* 100-102.
Ishikawa, K., and Saito, S. (1975): The possible role of GABA on rats discrimination learning. *Abstr. 6th Int. Congr. Pharmacol.,* 369.
Jarvik, M.E. (1964): The influence of drugs upon memory. In:H. Steinberg, A.V.S. De-Reuck, and J. Knight (Eds.), *Animal Behavior and Drug Action.* Little Brown, Boston, p. 44-61.
Jarvik, M.E., and Essman, W.B. (1960): A simple one-trial learning technique for mice. *Physhol. Rep. 6:* 290.
Jouvet, M. (1969): Biogenic amines and the states of sleep. *Science 163:* 32-41.

Kahan, S.A. (1966): The effects of metrazol on operant response rates. *Physiol. Behav. 1:* 117-123.
Katz, J.J., and Halstead, W.C. (1960): Protein organization and mental function. *Comp. Psychol. Monogr. 20:* 1-38.
Keilty, S.R., and Blackwood, S. (1969): Sedation for conservative dentistry. *Brit. J. Clin. Prac. 23:* 365-367.
Kelleher, R.T., Fry, W., Deegan, J., and Cook, L. (1961): Effect of meprobamate on operant behavior in rats. *J. Pharmacol. Exp. Therap. 133:* 271-280.
Kety, S.S., Polls, B.D., Nadler, C.S., and Schmidt, C.F. (1958): The blood flow and oxygen consumption of the human brain in diabetic acidosis and coma. *J. Clin. Invest. 27:* 500-510.
Kral, V.A., Cahn, C., Deutsch, M., Mueller, H., and Solyom, L. (1962): Procaine (Novocaine) treatment of patients with senile and arteriosclerotic brain disease. *Canad. Med. Assoc. J. 87:* 1109-1113.
Krivanek, J., and McGaugh, J.L. (1968): Effects of pentylenetetrazol on memory storage in mice. *Psychopharmacologia 12:* 303-321.
Kusumo, K.S., and Vaughan, M. (1977): Effects of lithium salts on memory. *Brit. J. Psychiat. 131:* 453-457.
Lagergren, K. (1974): The effect of exogenous change in heart rate upon mental performance in patients treated with artificial pacemakers for complete heart block. *Brit. Heart J. 36:* 1126-1132.
Lagergren, K., and Levander, S. (1974): A double-blind study on the effects of Piracetam (1-acetamide-2 pyrrolidone) upon perceptual and psychomotor performance at varied heart rates in patients treated with artificial pacemakers. *J. Pharmacol.* (Paris) 5, Suppl. 2: 55-56.
Lambrechts, W., and Parkhouse, J. (1961): Postoperative amnesia. *Brit. J. Anaesth. 33:* 397-404.
Lasagna, L., and Epstein, L.C. (1968): The use of amphetamines in the treatment of hyperkinetic children. *J. Nerv. Ment. Dis. 146:* 136-146.
Lashley, K.S. (1917): The effect of strychnine and caffeine upon rate of learning. *Psychobiol. 1:* 141-170.
LeBrecque, D.C. (1966): Papaverine hydrochloride as therapy for mentally confused geriatric patients. *Curr. Therap. Res. 8:* 106-111.
Leonard, B.E. (1974): The effect of two synthetic ACTH analogues on the metabolism of biogenic amines in the rat brain. *Arch. Int. Pharmacodyn. 20:* 242-253.
Lewis, S. (1967): Maze acquisition and nucleic acid metabolism: Effects of two malononitrile derivatives. Paper presented at meeting of Eastern Psychological Assn., Boston.
Lewis, S., and Essman, W.B. (1967): Maze acquisition and RNA material: Effects of two malononitrile derivatives. Unpublished material.
Lidbraink, P., Corrodi, H., and Fuxe, K. (1974): Benzodiazepines and barbiturates: turnover changes in central 5-hydroxytryptamine pathways. *Eur. J. Pharmacol.* (Amsterdam) *26:* 35-40.
Linuchev, M.N., and Nichelson, M.J. (1965): Action of nicotine on the rate of elaboration of food motor conditioned reflexes in rats of different ages. *Activ. Nerv. Sup. 7:* 25-30.
Livecchi, S.G., and Dusewicz, R.A. (1969): Effects of pre-trial strychnine on maze learning. *Psychol. Rep. 24:* 735-736.
Loken, R.D. (1940): The influence of metrazol upon maze behavior. *Psychol. Bull. 37:* 592.
Loken, R.D., (1941): Metrazol and maze behavior. *J. Comp. Psychol. 32:* 11-16.
Lowenthal, D.T., and Reidenberg, M.M. (1972): The heart rate response to atropine in uremic patients, obese subjects before and during fasting, and patients with other chronic illnesses. *Proc. Soc. Exp. Biol. Med. 139:* 390-393.

Luckens, M.M., and Malone, M.H. (1973): Cardiovascular effects of reserpine, yohimbine, and reserpine-yohimbine mixtures on intact anesthetized dog. *J. Pharm. Sci. 62:* 1268-1290.
MacFarlane, M.D. (1975): Procaine HCl (Gerovital H3): A weak, reversible fully competitive inhibitor of monoamine oxidase. *Fed. Proc. 34:* 108-110.
MacFarlane, M.D., and Besbris, H. (1974): Procaine (Gerovital H3) therapy: mechanism of inhibition of monoamine oxidase. *J. Amer. Geriatr. Soc. 22:* 365-371.
Marcer, D., and Hopkins, S.M. (1977): The differential effects of meclofenoxate on memory loss in the elderly. *Age Ageing 6:* 123-131.
Marx, J.L. (1975): Learning and behavior. I. Effects of pituitary hormones. *Science 190:* 367-370.
Maxwell, J.D., Carrella, M., Parkes, J.D., Williams, R., Mould, G.P., and Curry, S.H. (1972): Plasma disappearance and cerebral effect of chlorpromazine in cirrhosis. *Clin. Sci. 43:* 143-151.
McGaugh, J.L. (1961): Facilitative and disruptive effects of strychnine sulphate on maze learning. *Psychol. Rep. 8:* 99-104.
McGaugh, J.L. (1966): Time-dependent processes in memory storage. *Science 153:* 1351-1358.
McGaugh, J.L. (1968): Drug facilitation of memory and learning. In: D.H. Efron (Ed.), *Psychopharmacology: A Review of Progress, 1957-1967.* U.S. Gov't. Printing Office, Washington, D.C.
McGaugh, J.L., and Petrinovich, L. (1965): Effects of drugs on learning and memory. *Int. Rev. Neurobiol. 8:* 139-196.
McGaugh, J.L., and Thomson, C.W. (1962): Facilitation of simultaneous discrimination learning with strychnine sulphate. *Psychopharmacologia 3:* 166-172.
McGaugh, J.L., Thomson, C.W., Westbrook, W.H., and Hudspeth, W.J. (1962): A further study of learning facilitation with strychnine sulfate. *Psychopharmacologia 3:* 352-360.
McNutt, L. (1967): 1,1,3-Tricyano - 2 amino - 1-propene; a pharmacological attempt to enhance learning ability. *Proc. 75th Ann. Conv. Amer. Psychol. Assn. 2:* 77-78.
McQuillan, L.M., Lapec, C.A., and Vibal, S.R. (1974): Evaluation of EEG and clinical changes associated with Pavabid therapy in chronic brain syndrome. *Curr. Therap. Res. 16:* 49-58.
Miller, L.H., Harris, L.C., Jr., Kastin, A.J., and Van Riezen, H. (1975): A neuroheptapeptide influence on attention in man. *4th Int. Congr. Int. Soc. Psychoneuroendocrinol.,* Aug. 22-26, Aspen, Col.
Miller, L.H., Harris, L.C., Van Riezen, H., and Rastin, A.J. (1976): Neuroheptapeptide influence on attention and memory in man. *Pharmacol. Biochem. Behav. 5:* Suppl. 1, 17-21.
Millner, J.R., and Palfai, R. (1974): Metrazol disrupts conditioned aversion produced by L_1Cl: a time dependent effect. *Research Rpts.,* NIMH, No. MH12125.
Mindus, P., Cronholm, B., Levander, S., and Schalling, D. (1975): Piracetam and mental performance in aging people. *Ann. Mtg. Amer. Psychol. Assn.,* Los Angeles.
Mitchell, J.R., Cavanaugh, J.H., Arias, L., and Oates, J.A. (1970): Guanethidine and related agents. III. Antagonism by drugs which inhibit the norepinephrine pump in man. *J. Clin. Invest. 49:* 1596-1604.
Mitchell, V.E., Ross., S., and Hurst, P.M. (1974): Drugs and placebos: effects of caffeine on cognitive performance. *Psychol. Rep. 35:* 387-883.
Morrison, C.F. (1967): Effects of nicotine on operant behavior or rats. *Int. J. Neuropharmacol. 6:* 229-240.

Müller, G.E., and Pilzecker, A. (1900): Experimentalle Beitraege zur Lehre vom Gedächtnis. *Z. Psychol. 1:* 1-188.
Mundow, L.S., and Long, S.V. (1974): The amnestic value of diazepam at forceps delivery. *Irish J. Med. Sci. 143:* 101-104.
Nachmansohn, D. (1938): Sur l'action de la strychnine. *Seanc. Soc. Biol. 129:* 941-943.
Nash, H. (1962): Psychologic effects of amphetamines and barbiturates. *J. Nerv. Ment. Dis. 134:* 203-217.
O'Brien, J.P., and Sharp, A.R. (19647): The influence of renal disease on the insulin (I^{131}) disappearance curve in man. *Metabolism 16:* 76-83.
Ogg, C.S., Toseland, P.A., and Cameron, J.S. (1968): Pulmonary tuberculosis in patient on hemodialysis. *Brit. Med. J. 2:* 283-284.
Oglesby, M.W., and Winter, J.C. (1973): Post-trial strychnine: lack of effect on conditioned avoidance learning. *Fed. Proc. 32:* 818.
Oglesby, M.W., and Winter, J.C. (1974): Strychnine sulfate and piracetam: lack of effect on learning in the rat. *Psychopharmacologia* (Berlin) *36:* 163-173.
Olds, M.E. (1966): Facilitatory action of diazepam and chlordiazepoxide on hypothalamic reward behavior. *J. Comp. Physiol. Psychol. 62:* 136-140.
Oliver, J.E., and Restell, M. (1967): Serial testing in assessing the effect of meclofenoxate on patients with memory defects. *Br. J. Psychiat. 113:* 219-222.
Oliverio, A. (1967): Analysis of the "anti-fatigue" activity of amphetamine. *Role of Central Adrenergic Mechanisms* II Farmaco (Milan) *6:* 441-449.
Orowan, E. (1955): The origin of man. *Nature 175:* 683-684.
Orzack, M.H., Taylor, C.L., and Kornetsky, C. (1968): A research report on the antifatigue effects of magnesium pemoline. *Psychopharmacologia 13:* 413-417.
Ostfeld, A.M., and Arguente, A. (1962): The central nervous system effects of hyoscine in man. *J. Pharmacol. Exp. Therap. 137:* 133-139.
Overton, D.A. (1966): State-dependent learning produced by depressant and atropine-like drugs. *Psychopharmacologia 10:* 6-31.
Page, J.G., Janicki, R.S., Bernstein, J.E., Curran, C.F., and Mitchell, F.A. (1974): Pemoline (Cylirt) in the treatment of childhood hyperkinesis. *J. Lng. Disabil. 7:* 498-503.
Pandit, S.K., and Dundee, J.W. (1970): Pre-operative amnesia. *Anaesthesia 24:* 493-499.
Pandit, S.K., Dundee, J.W., and Keilty, S.R. (1971): Amnesia studies with intravenous premedication. *Anesthesia 26:* 421-428.
Pandit, S.K., Heisterkamp, D.V., and Cohen, P.J. (1976): Further studies of the anti-recall effect of lorazepam: a dose-time-effect relationship. *Anesthesiology 45:* 495-500.
Parbrook, G.D. (1967): The levels of nitrous oxide analgesia. *Brit. J. Anaesth. 39:* 974-982.
Parker, J.P., Beirne, G.J., and Desai, J.N. (1972): Androgen-induced increase in red cell 2, 3-diphosphoglycerate. *New Engl. J. Med. 287:* 381-383.
Parkhouse, J., Henrie, J.R., and Duncan, G.M. (1960): Nitrous oxide analgesia in relation to mental performance. *J. Pharmacol. Exp. Therap. 128:* 44-54.
Pavlov, I.P. (1927): *Conditioned Reflexes.* Oxford Univ. Press, London.
Pearl, S., and McKean, D.B. (1967): Pentylenetetrazol: failure to improve memory in mice. *Science 157:* 220.
Pearlman, C.A., Jr., Sharpless, S.K., and Jarvik, M.E. (1961): Retrograde amnesia produced by anesthetic and convulsant agents. *J. Comp. Physiol. Psychol. 54:* 109-112.
Perry, E.K., Perry, R.H., and Tomlinson, B.E. (1977): Dietary lecithin supplements in dementia of Alzheimer type? *Lancet 2:* 242-243.
Petersen, R.C. (1977): Scopolamine induced learning failures in man. *Psychopharmacol. 52:* 283-289.
Petrinovich, L. (1963): Facilitation of successive discrimination learning by strychnine sulfate. *Psychopharmacologia 4:* 103-113.

Physician's Desk Reference (1979): 3rd. Ed., Medical Economics Co., Oradell, N.J.
Pletscher, A., Shore, P.A., and Brodie, B.B. (1955): Serotonin release as a possible mechanism of reserpine action. *Science 122:* 374-375.
Plotnikoff, N.M. (1966a): Magnesium pemoline: Enhancement of learning and memory of a conditioned avoidance response. *Science 151:* 703-705.
Plotnikoff, N.M. (1966b): Magnesium pemoline: Antagonism of retrograde amnesia in rats. *Fed. Proc. 25:* 262.
Plotnikoff, N.M. (1966c): Magnesium pemoline: Enhancement of memory after electroconvulsive shock in rats. *Life Sci. 5:* 1495-1598.
Post, R.M., and Goodwin, F.K. (1974): Effect of amitriptyline and imipramine on amine metabolites in the cerebrospinal fluid of depressed patients. *Arch. Gen. Psychiat. 30:* 234-239.
Predescu, V., Giureze, T., Tudorache, D., Nica, St., Ionescu, R., Nicholschi, L., Hiturad, A., Popovici, E., and Curelaru, S. (1974): Hydergine-thioridazine combination in the treatment of psychopathological states in old age. *Activ. Nerv. Sup.* (Praha) *16:* 237-238.
Prien, R.F., Wagner, J.J., Jr., and Kahn, S. (1963): Lack of facilitation in maze learning by picrotoxin and strychnine sulfate. *Amer. J. Psychol. 204:* 448-492.
Quarton, G.C., and Talland, G.A. (1962): The effects of methamphetamine and pentobarbital on two measures of attention. *Psychopharmacologia 3:* 66-71.
Rao, D.B., and Norris, J.R. (1972): A double-blind investigation of Hydergine in the treatment of cerebrovascular insufficiency in the elderly. *Johns Hopkins Med. J. 130:* 317-324.
Regina, E.G., Smith, G.M., Keiper, C.G., and McKelvey, R.K. (1974): Effects of caffeine on alertness in simulated automobile driving. *J. Appl. Psychol. 59:* 483-489.
Richter, D., and Crossland, J. (1949): Variation in acetylcholine content of brain with physiological state. *Amer. J. Physiol. 159:* 247-254.
Ritter, R.M., Nail, H.R., Tatum, P., and Blazi, M.L. (1971): The effect of papaverine on patients with cerebral arteriosclerosis. *Clin. Med. 78:* 18-24.
Robinson, D.S., Nies, A., Davis, J.N., Bunney, W.E., Davis, J.M., Colburn, R.W. Bourne, H.R., Shaw, D.M., and Coppen, A.J. (1972): Agine monoamines, and monoamine oxidase levels. *Lancet 1:* 290-291.
Robson, J.G., Burns, B.D., and Welt, P.J.L. (1960): The effect of inhaling dilute nitrous oxide upon recent memory and time estimation. *Canad. Anesth. Soc. J. 7:* 399-410.
Robustelli, F. (1966): Azione della nicotina sul condizionamento di salvaguardia di ratti di un mese. *Rend. Classe. Sci. Fisiche, Matemat e Naturali 40:* 490-497.
Rosen, H.J. (1975): Mental discipline in the elderly: pharmacotherapy (ergot alkaloids versus papaverine). *J. Amer. Geriatr. Soc. 23:* 169-174.
Roth, J.A., and Gillis, C.N. (1974): Inhibition of lung, liver and brain monoamine oxidase by imipramine and desipramine. *Biochem. Pharmacol. 23:* 1138-1140.
Ryback, R. (1969): The use of goldfish as a model for alcohol amnesia in man. *Quart. J. Stud. Alcohol. 30:* 877-882.
Ryback, R. (1969): State-dependent or "dissociated" learning with alcohol in the goldfish. *Quart. J. Stud. Alcohol. 30:* 598-608.
Ryback, R.S. (1970): Alcohol amnesia. *J.A.M.A. 212:* 1524.
Safer, D.J., and Allen, R.P. (1971): The central effects of scoploamine in man. *Biol. Psychiat. 3:* 347-355.
Sakalis, G., Oh, D., Gershon, S., and Shopsin, B. (1974): A trial of Gerovital H-3 in depression during senility. *Curr. Ther. Res. 16:* 59-63.
Samanin, R., Gumulka, W., and Valzelli, L. (1970): Reduced effect of morphine in midbrain raphe lesioned rats. *Europ. J. Pharmacol. 10:* 339-343.

Sandman, C.A., George, J.M., Nolan, J.D., Van Riezen, H., and Kastin, A.J. (1975): Enhancement of attention in man with ACTH/MSH 4-10. *Physiol. Behav. 15:* 427-431.
Schaaf, M., and Payne, C.A. (1966): Dystonic reactions to prochlorperazine in hypoparathyroidism. *New Engl. J. Med. 275:* 991-995.
Schaefer, G.J., Buchanan, D.C., and Ray, O.S. (1974): Effects of neonatal strychnine administration on active avoidance in rats. *Behav. Biol. 10:* 253-258.
Schenker, S., Breen, K.J., and Hoyumpa, A.M. (1974): Hepatic encephalopathy: current status. *Gastroenterology 66:* 121-151.
Schmidt, M.J., and Davenport, J.W. (1967): TZAP: Facilitation of learning in hypothyroid rats. *Psychonom. Sci. 7:* 185-186.
Sellers, E.M., and Koch-Weser, J. (1970): Potentiation of warfarin induced hypoprothrombinemia by chloral hydrate. *New Engl. J. Med. 283:* 827-831.
Sherlock, S. (1968): *Diseases of the Liver and Biliary System.* Blackwell, Oxford. 117.
Shin, K.C.L., and Sheon, Y.S. (1973): Influences of reserpine and chlorpromazine on the analgesic and metabolic effects of morphine. *Korean U. Med. J.* (Seoul) *10:* 653-661.
Signoret, J.L., Whiteley, A., and Lhermitte, F. (1978): Influence of choline on amnesia in early Alzheimer's disease. *Lancet 2:* 837.
Sitaran, H., Weingartner, H., Caine, E.D., and Gellin, J.C. (1978): Choline: selective enhancement of serial learning and encoding of low imagery. *Life Sci. 22:* 1555-1560.
Small, I.F., Sharpley, P., and Small, J.G. (1968): Influence of cylert upon memory changes with ECT. *Amer. J. Psychiat. 125:* 837-840.
Small, J.G., and Small, I.F. (1967): EEG spikes in non-epileptic psychiatric patients. *Dis. Nerv. Syst. 28:* 523-525.
Small, J.G., Small, I.F., Milstein, V., and Dian, D.A. (1977): Effects of ACTH 4-10 on ECT-induced memory dysfunctions. *Acta Psychiat. Scand. 55:* 241-250.
Smigel, J.O., Piller, J., Murphy, C., Lowe, D., and Gibson, J. (1960): H-3 procaine hydrochloride therapy in aging institutionalized patients. *J. Amer. Gerontol. Soc. 8:* 785-794.
Smith, R.G. (1967): Magnesium pemoline: Lack of facilitation in human learning and memory and performance tests. *Science 155:* 603-605.
Smith, W.L., Philippus, M.J., and Lowrey, J.B. (1968): A comparison of psychological and psychophysical test patterns before and after receiving papaverine HCl. *Curr. Therap. Res. 10:* 428-431.
Smith, C.M., Swash, M., Exton-Smith, A.N., Phillips, M.J., Overstall, P.W., Piper, M.E., and Bailey, M.R. (1978): Choline therapy in Alzheimer's disease. *Lancet 2:* 318.
Solyom, L., and Gallay, H.M. (1966): Effect of malononitrile dimer on operant and classical conditioning of aged white rats. *Int. J. Neuropsychiat. 2:* 577-584.
Soubrie, P., Simon, P., and Boissier, J.R. (1976): An amnesic effect of benzodiazepines in rats. *Experientia 32:* 359-360.
Stein, L. (1956): Reserpine and the learning of fear. *Science 124:* 1082-1083.
Stein, D.G. (1974): The effects of early saline injections and pentylenetetrazol on Hebb-Williams maze performance in the adult rat. *Behav. Biol. 1:* 415-422.
Stein, D.G., and Brink, J.J. (1969): Prevention of retrograde amnesia by injection of magnesium pemoline in dimethysulfoxide. *Psychopharmacologia 14:* 240-247.
Stein, H.H., and Yellin, T.O. (1967): Pemoline and magnesium hydroxide: lack of effect of RNA and protein synthesis. *Science 157:* 96-97.
Steinberg, H., and Summerfield, A. (1957): Influence of a depressant drug on acquisition in rote learning. *Quart. J. Exp. Psychol. 9:* 138-145.
Stetten, D., and Heron, S.Z. (1959): Intellectual level measured by Army classification battery and uric acid concentration. *Science 129:* 1737.

Stern, F.H. (1970): Management of chronic brain syndrome secondary to cerebral arteriosclerosis with special reference to papaverine hydrochloride. *J. Amer. Geriatr. Soc. 18:* 507-512.

Stern, W.C., and Heise, G.A. (1970): Failure of TCAP to facilitate acquisition of double alternation in rats. *Physiol. Behav. 5:* 449-452.

Stolerman, I.P., Fink, R., and Jarvik, M.E. (1973): Acute and chronic tolerance to nicotine measured by activity in rats. *Psychopharmacologia* (Berlin) *30:* 329-342.

Storm, T., and Caird, W.K. (1967): The effects of alcohol on serial verbal learning in chronic alcoholics. *Psychonom. Sci. 9:* 43-44.

Stratton, L.O., and Kastin, A.J. (1974): Avoidance learning at two levels of shock in rats receiving NSH. *Horm. Behav. 5:* 149-155.

Stratton, L.O., and Kastin. A.J. (1975): Increased acquisition of a complex appetitive task after MSH and MIF. *Pharmacol. Biochem. Behav. 3:* 901-904.

Stripling, J.S., and Alpern, H.P. (1974): Nicotine and caffeine disruption of the long-term store memory and proactive facilitation of learning in mice. *Psychopharmacologia* (Berline) *38:* 187-200.

Talland, G.A., Mendleson, J.W., Koz, G., and Aaron, R. (1965): Experimental studies of the effects of tricyano-aminopropene on the memory and learning capacities of geriatric patients. *J. Psychiat. Res. 3:* 171-179.

Talland, G.A., and Quarton, G.C. (1965): The effects of methamphetamine and pentobarbital on the running memory span. *Psychopharamacologia 7:* 379-382.

Tannen, R.L., Regal, E.M., Dunn, M.J., and Schrier, R.W. (1969): Vasopressin-resistant hyposthenuria in advanced chronic renal disease. *New Engl. J. Med. 280:* 1135-1141.

Teitelbaum, H.A., Newton, J.E.O., Gliedman, L.H., and Gantt, W.H. (1961): Conditioned reflex formation under pentobarbital. *Psychosom. Med. 23:* 446.

Teoh, P.C., and Cheah, J.S. (1973): Electrocardiographic changes in hyperthyroidism after adrenergic blockade with reserpine and propranalol. *Med. J. Australia* (Sydney) *2:* 116-118.

Thomson, H.T., and Cotterill, D. (1909): Note on the use of the scopolamine-morphine combination as an anaesthetic adjunct. *Edinb. Med. J. NS3:* 548.

Tissari, A.H., and Suurhasko, B.V.A. (1972): Effect of imipramine on the turnover of brain 5-HT in post-natal rats. *Acta. Pharmacol. Toxicol.* (Kobenhavn) *31:* (Suppl. 1), 29.

Tolman, E.C. (1917): Retroactive inhibition as affected by conditions of learning. *Psychol. Monogr. 18:* No. 107.

Turner, D.J., and Wilson, J. (1969): Effect of diazepam on awareness during caesarean section under general anaesthesia. *Brit. Med. J. 2:* 736-737.

Van Praag, H.M., and Leijnse, B. (1963): The influence of some antidepressives of the hydrazine type on the glucose metabolism in depressed patients. *Clin. Chim. Acta 8:* 466-475.

Veronin, L.G., and Napalkov, A.V. (1963): Complex systems of conditioned reflexes in the analysis of drug effects. In: Z. Votava, M. Horvath, and O. Vinar (Eds.), *Psychopharmacological Methods.* MacMillan, New York, p. 182.

Waldram, R.P.H., Davis, M., Nunnerley, H., and Williams, R. (1974): Emergency endoscopy after gastrointestinal haemorrhage in 50 patients with portal hypertension. *Brit. Med. J. 4:* 94-96.

Walk, R.D., Owens, J.W.M., and Davidson, B.S. (1961): Influence of reserpine on avoidance conditioning, exploratory behavior, and discrimination learning in the rat. *Psychol. Rep. 8:* 251-258.

Walsh, F.B. (1947): *Clinical Neuro-Ophthalmology.* Williams & Wilkins, Baltimore.

Weckowicz, T.E., Nutter, R., and Gibbs, J.T. (1974): The effect of tranylcypromine (Parnate) on eyelid conditioning and paired associate learning in depressed patients. *Pavlovian J. Biol. Sci. 9:* 122-123.

Weiss, B., and Laties, V.G. (1962): Enhancement of human performance by caffeine and the amphetamines. *Pharmacol. Rev. 14:* 1-36.

Weiss, B., and Laties, V.G. (1969): Behaviorial pharmacology and toxicology. *Ann. Rev. Pharmacol. 9:* 297-326.

Weissman, A. (1961): Interaction effects of imipramine and d-amphetamine on non-discriminated avoidance. *Pharmacologia 3:* 60.

Wenzel, D.C., and Davis, P.W. (1961): The effect of caffeine and nicotine as tension-inducing agents and the ability of meprobamate to counteract such effects upon performance. *Tech. Rep. Off. Nav. Res. Svc. Tech. Inf. Agency:* 1-11.

Wiechert, P., and Golinitz, G. (1969a): Stoffwechseluntersuchungen des cerebralen Anfallsgeschehens. Die Beteilung der Transaminasen und der Glutamat dehydrogenase am Krampfgeschehen. *J. Neurochem. 16:* 689-693.

Wiechert, P., and Gollnitz, G. (1969b): Staffwechseluntersuchungen des cerebralen Anfallsgeschehens. Die Konzentration des freien aminosauren in Anfalle. *J. Neurochem. 16:* 1007-1016.

Wilson, J., and Turner, D.J. (1969): Awareness during caesarean section under general anaesthesia. *Brit. Med. J. 1:* 280-283.

Wilson, W.A., and Escueta, A.V. (1974): Common synaptic effects of pentylenetetrazol and penicillin. *Brain Res.* (Amsterdam) *72:* 168-171.

Wolff, H.C., and Gantt, W.H. (1935): Sodium isoamylethyl-barbiturate, sodium functions. *Arch. Neurol. Psychiat. 33:* 1030-1057, Chicago.

Zieve, L. (1966): Pathogenesis of hepatic coma. *Arch. Int. Med. 118:* 211-223.

6

Neuropharmacological Perspectives in the Amnestic and Dysmnestic Syndromes

Walter B. Essman
Edward Sodaro

There are two major brain regions that have been generally implicated in human memory dysfunction: these include the diencephalon and the hippocampi. The dysmnestic syndromes which involve these structures include impairment of long-term data storage, disruption of the encoding of short-term into long-term storage, or a loss of decoding or access to the long-term data storage. This concerns the latter two problems. "Dysmnesia" is the preferred term describing a partial memory loss, in contrast to the term "amnesia" which implies a total memory loss. Amnesia may be viewed as an extreme on a broad continuum of dysmnestic syndromes, wherein mild dysmnestic illnesses occur more commonly than total amnesia.

There are several complex biochemical systems, involving several putative neurotransmitters, which subserve human information storage; these are apparently arranged in both parallel and serial processing frameworks which make research difficult because of several confounding experimental factors. Organic dysmnesia and amnesia can present either acutely or chronically as a result of lesions of a degenerative, space-occupying, traumatic, vascular, infectious, anoxic, metabolic, epileptic, nutritionally-induced, endocrinological, or other nature, with varying degrees of reversibility. Diffuse C.N.S. damage is associated with widespread cognitive impairment. In contrast, focal damage to some of the discrete regions considered in this chapter can produce a very specific type of memory loss with maintenance of other intellectual functions.

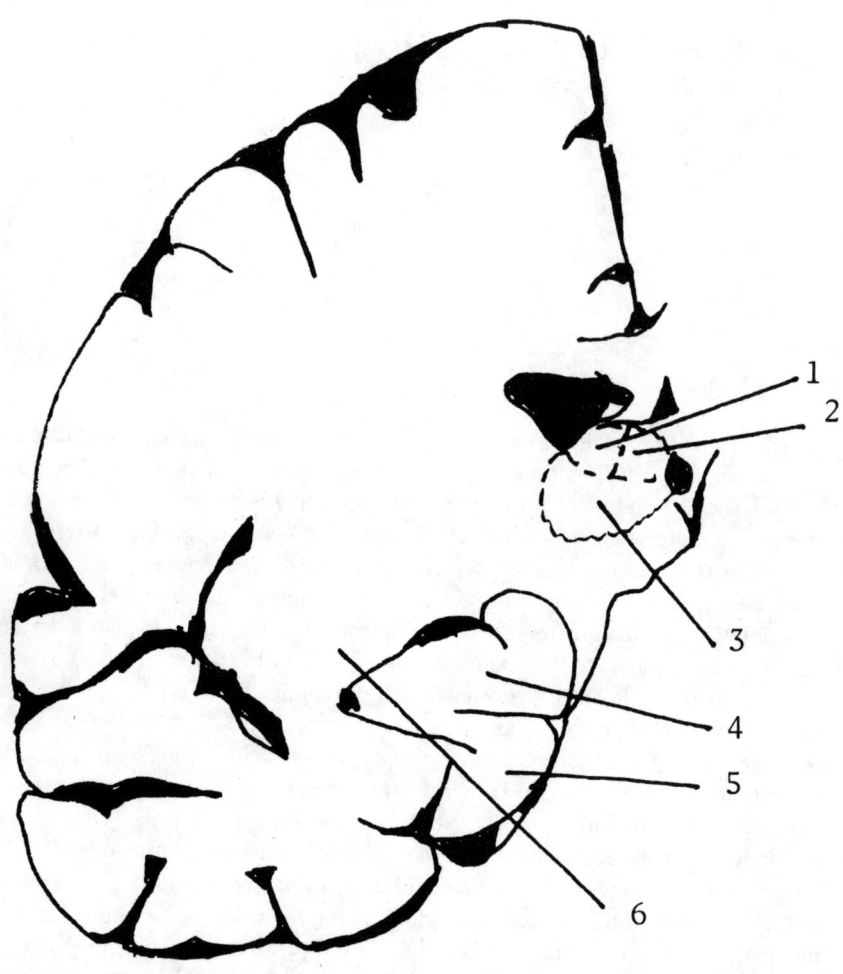

FIGURE 1. Schematic representation of the relationship between structures involved in memory and memory dysfunction. The frontal lobe shown anteriorly and the temporal lobe superiorly enclose, respectively, radiations to the frontal thalamus, which in turn provide mammillary body and sensory afferents; the latter encloses the uncus, amygdala, hippocampus, and dentate. The fornix anteriorly joins the mammillary body and posteriorly adjoins the dentate.

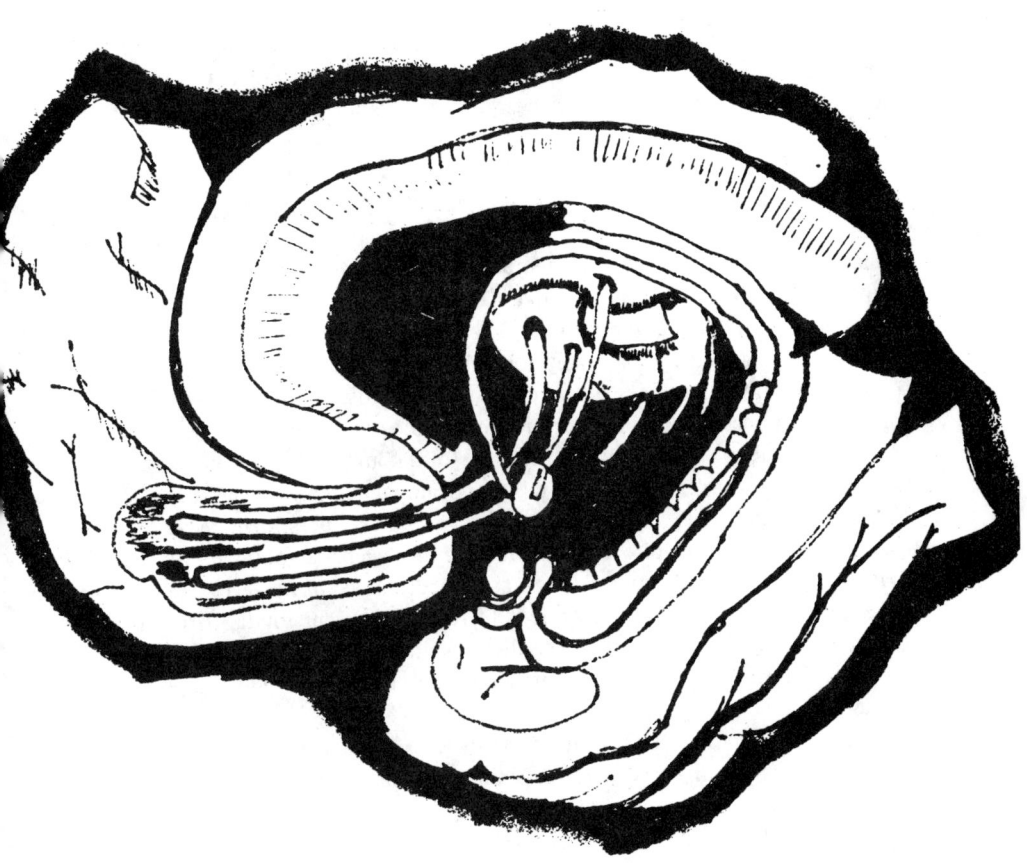

FIGURE 2. Frontal section through the right cerebral hemisphere with structures involved in the possible etiology of bitemporal amnesia, resulting from damage to the temporal stem (6); this band of white matter overlying the hippocampus (4) forms a connection between temporal neocortex and amygdala to the dorsomedial thalamic nucleus (2). The lateral thalamus (3) and anterior thalamic nucleus (1) as well as the hippocampal gyrus (5) remain distinctly separate particularly since these are almost always involved with unilateral lesions.

BEHAVIORAL MANIFESTATIONS OF THE DYSMNESTIC SYNDROMES

The dysmnesias found in both Korsakoff's and bilateral hippocampal syndromes have general similarities. Memory for any new data inputs is absent or deficient. Immediate memory, also termed ultra-short-term memory, is unimpaired so that the patient is able to recall brief series of digits within the limits of focused attention due to constant verbal rehearsal. Data storage is absent and memory is lost after several minutes due to an attention decrement. Preception, alertness, mood, social appropriateness, and affect may all appear to be perfectly normal.

The most prominent deficit in the dysmnestic syndromes is anterograde dysmnesia; this is characterized by severe impairment of new learning with its onset at the time of the original attack of illness, such as an episode of hypothiaminemia (Korsakoff's) or bilateral temporal herpes simplex encephalitis (hippocampal). The ability to place new data into information storage from the time of this illness is severely compromised. One result is the production of severe disturbances in orientation, especially for time.

It is important to distinguish recent memory loss from immediate memory preservation because the identification of dysmnesia could otherwise be missed. An alert, affable, friendly patient may perform completely normally on a standard digit span task. With bilateral hippocampal damage it has been shown (Drachman and Arbit, 1966) that verbal rehearsal may permit the recall of memory task material for quite a few minutes, and longer than observed for patients with Korsakoff's syndrome. As soon as distraction occurs however, the memory trace is lost. Also, severe impairment of recall can occur for tasks that require the learning of lists longer than the digit span. Some degree of recall recovery is possible for Korsakoff patients, but is less likely to be observed for hippocampal patients.

Memory loss for events prior to the onset of illness, termed retrograde dysmnesia, exists to varying degrees of severity for all patients. The severity of the retrograde memory problem decreases as a function of the time since the onset of physical illness. The most severe degree of dysmnesia occurs for those events within the limits of the retrograde dysfunction, with a disorganization in the recall sequence for those events which may be recalled (Lishman, 1978).

Anterograde time sense is also distorted particularly for Korsakoff patients. Long periods of time may be subjectively experienced as condensed. Events that occur over short time periods may be recalled as having occurred over many years. Sequence of events is also disturbed. Events occurring at different times may be recalled as a single episode. The dysmnestic or amnestic patient may then be described as being, in effect, lost in time. It has been suggested (Sanders and Warrington, 1971) that when time-related stimuli are of equal difficulty, the temporal gradient for retention loss disappears. The temporal gradient of retrograde amnesia was studied in alcoholic Korsakoff's patients to indicate a steep gradient; this was independent of task difficulty and memory impairment occurred for all time sequences tested (Albert et al., 1979).

Coherent, orderly but entirely falsified or confabulated histories can occasionally be obtained from non-malingering Korsakoff patients, but not from hippocampal patients. This symptom appears to be a function of a number of factors including loss of time sense and premorbid alcoholic personality disorder.

STRUCTURAL CORRELATES OF KORSAKOFF'S SYNDROME

The mammillary bodies of the hypothalamus, nucleus medialis dorsalis of the thalamus, and other gray matter surrounding the third ventricle appear to be critical sites of the lesions which produce the Korsakoff syndrome; such lesions are symmetrical. Other regions may also be involved, but to a lesser degree; these include the terminal portions of the fornices (near the mammillary bodies) and gray matter surrounding the aqueduct and fourth ventricle. Lesions of the ventricular surface portion of the nucleus medialis dorsalis invariably occur in Korsakoff's syndrome. Korsakoff's syndrome often involves other thalamic regions, especially the pulvinar and nucleus anteromedealis. Damage only rarely occurs in the cerebral cortex, cingulate gyri, hippocampi, and other regions (Victor et al., 1971).

Korsakoff's syndrome often follows an attack of Wernicke's encephalopathy and several investigators view the disorders as a unitary Wernicke-Korsakoff syndrome. Careful neuropathological studies have correlated the Wernicke symptoms of ophthalmoplegia with lesions of the third and sixth cranial nerve nuclei, ataxia from cerebellar lesions, and nystagmus from lesions of the medial vestibular nuclei.

Alcoholics in general are at risk for cerebellar degeneration, central pontine myelinosis, and lesions of the corpus callosum (the latter in Marchiafava-Bignami syndrome). These disorders and Korsakoff's amnestic syndrome relate to nutritional factors, notably a reduced blood level of thiamine (hypothiaminemia). Thiamine or its phosphorylated form are requisites for the coenzyme for pyruvate decarboxylation and also for the enzymes, α-ketoglutarate decarboxylase and transketolase. Thiamine deficiency, therefore, leads to increased blood and tissue levels of pyruvate and decreased activity of enzymes, reflecting an impairment in both the tricarboxylic acid cycle and the pentose phosphate pathway (Brin et al., 1960; Dreyfus, 1962). Neural tissue surrounding the third and fourth ventricles and aqueduct are particularly prone to lesions in thiamine depletion states, possibly as a result of a transketolase deficiency. Blass and Gibson (1977) have reported a transketolase defect (a thiamine dependent enzyme) in fibroblasts from skin biopsy cultured from patients with Korsakoff's syndrome. These investigators suggested that those individuals who develop

Korsakoff's syndrome possess an abnormality in the kinetics of the enzyme. Since the alteration in the fibroblasts persisted for more than 20 generations of culture, the authors suggested a genetic factor and a genetic variation in the susceptibility to thiamine deficiency.

Conditions other than alcoholism can also produce dysmnesia as a result of lesions from hypothiaminemia. These include debilitated infectious states, intestinal obstruction, pernicious anemia, starvation, and other forms of malnutrition. Deficiencies of the other B vitamins may also contribute to the state. Some authors have reserved the term "Korsakoff's" to refer only to the dysmnestic syndrome found in chronic alcoholics, although most workers use the term for any nutritionally derived illness with the characteristic memory disturbance.

There is some controversy as to the precise site of hypothiaminemia-induced lesions. Classically most reports have documented characteristic bilateral lesions of the mammillary bodies. In one series Victor and colleagues (1971) noted that symmetrical mammillary damage was localized to the medial and central regions. While these authors confirmed the well known invariable appearance of mammillary lesions in Korsakoff patients, they also reported data from five patients with bilateral mammillary lesions and no memory disturbance. Their neuropathological data were highly consistent for a relationship between amnesia and lesions of the magnocellular part of the nucleus medialis dorsalis of the thalamus. A good, but not perfectly consistent relationship was found between memory disruption and lesions of the mammillary bodies and pulvinar.

The nucleus medialis dorsalis and the mammillary bodies constitute portions of the diencephalon in which the latter consist mainly of the spherical medial mammillary nuclei which form the characteristic two bulges at the base of the brain posterior to the pituitary body. These medial nuclei consist of small cells surrounded by a capsule of myelinated fibers. A rather small intermediate (also termed intercalated) mammillary nucleus is encountered upon outward extension. Some histologists have described the cells as larger in the intermediate than in the medial nucleus, while others have described completely the opposite. More laterally a larger lateral mammillary nucleus occurs, which in spite of its size, does not significantly contribute to the bulge of the mammillary body. The large cells of the lateral nucleus are identical with and merge with the structure of the posterior hypothalamic region, the latter being associated with sympathetic nervous system control.

Intraconnnections within the mammillary bodies and between them and nearby other hypothalamic regions may exist but have not been clearly defined. Fibers of the medial forebrain bundle pass in closs proximity with the mammillary bodies and may provide bidirectional interconnections with diverse regions extending from the forebrain through the preoptic and hypothalamic regions and into the midbrain. An important point to be given later consideration concerns possible connections between the mammillary bodies and the supraoptic nuclei.

The hippocampus and mammillary area are uniquely interconnected by hippocampohypothalamic fibers which mainly travel through the fornix. A flow of information is probably unidirectional and terminates in the mammillary region (the interconnections through the fornix, on the other hand, are largely bidirectional). This specific pathway is also a portion of Papez' limbic system circuit, the proposed physiological substrate for emotional behavior.

The fibers of the fornix are separated into pre- and post-commissural divisions depending upon their relationship to the anterior commissure. The fornix will be discussed in greater depth later, but the post-commissural portion is of particular relevance for the present issue. The greatest number of afferent fibers to the medial mammillary nucleus drive from the post-commissural fornix. Lesions of this nucleus occur most frequently in Korsakoff's syndrome, although five cases of severe destruction in the absence of memory disturbance were reported, as noted previously. Lesions of the terminal portions of the postcommissural fornix have also often been observed in the spectrum of Korsakoff pathology. Fibers from the post-commissural fornix are also distributed to the thalamus, mainly to the anterior and intralaminar nuclei. The anterior nuclei receive as many direct fibers from the fornix as from the mammillothalamic tract (Powell et al., 1957). Post-commissural fibers also descend adjacent to the mammillary bodies and then join nearby fiber bundles which enter the midbrain (Nauta, 1958).

Amygdalohypothalamic fibers travel to the hypothalamus via the stria terminalis and the ventral amygdalofugal pathway. While clearly distributing to other regions of the hypothalamus, it is not known if these fibers provide any mammillary afferents.

Afferents from the brain stem and the reticular activating system are also relevant. The mammillary peduncles provide for fibers from the dorsal and ventral tegmental nuclei of the midbrain that terminate mainly in the lateral mammillary nucleus.

Fibers within the dorsal longitudinal fasciculus extend from the central gray of the midbrain to the periventricular gray matter near the mammillary complex. This fiber bundle relays impulses both rostrally and caudally; those regions served by this fiber bundle are all highly sensitive to thiamine and may be involved in the lesions of the Korsakoff syndrome. In addition, there is evidence that the gray matter surrounding the third ventricle, where the fasciculus terminates, contains vasopressin receptors; this finding bears upon another aspect of memory functions that will be considered in this chapter.

Mammillary efferent fibers arise mainly from the medial mammillary nucleus, but there are some efferents that derive from the intermediate and lateral nuclei. The efferents briefly travel together dorsally as the fasciculusmammillaris princeps and then divide into the mammillothalamic and mammillotegmental tracts.

The mammillothalamic tract, another element of the Papez circuit, provides fibers from the medial mammillary nucleus which extend to the ipsilateral anteroventral and anteromedial thalamic nuclei. The mammillothalamic tract also provides fibers bilaterally from the lateral mammillary nucleus to both anterodorsal thalamic nuclei (Frid et al., 1963). Hippocampal fibers from the fornix join the mammillothalamic tract and project directly to the thalamus (Valenstein and Nauta, 1959).

As noted earlier, recent import has been given to the nucleus medialis dorsalis of the thalamus, particularly the magnocellular portion, as the critical site for the memory-disruptive lesions of the Korsakoff syndrome. The magnocellular portion of this thalamic nucleus lies most medially along the surface of the third ventricle, a region of interest for the possible locus of receptor sites for vasopressin, a functionally relevant neuropeptide with a role in memory processes to be discussed later.

The nucleus medialis dorsalis (NMD) occupies much of the region between the internal medullary laminar and the periventricular gray matter just discussed. The magnocellular portion contains fairly large, deeply-staining polygonal cells, and lies dorsomedially and rostrally. The larger parvocellular region contains clusters of small pale-staining cells. The medialis dorsalis has connections with the centromedianus, other intralaminar nuclei, and the lateral nuclei. The nucleus medialis dorsalis is thought to be involved in the integration of complex somatic and viseral inputs, aside from its role in memory. This region also represents a site where psychosurgery is believed to alter effective states through interruption of diverse projections to the frontal lobes. The parvocellular portion of the NMD projects in an organized distribution to the entire frontal cortex rostral to Brodman areas 6 and 32. The magnocellular portion of the NMD receives inputs, via the inferior thalamic peduncle, from the amygdala, temporal neocortex, orbital frontal cortex, and possibly from the substantia innominata. The inferior thalamic peduncle with fibers interconnecting the amygdala and preoptic regions constitutes the ansa peduncularis (Carpenter, 1976). There are presumably interconnections between the magnocellular and parvocellular portions of the NMD with considerable transmission of impulses likely from the magnocellular into the parvocellular regions.

It is relevant that vasopressin is capable of exerting trophic effects other than its more familiar properties as a neurohormone with antidiuretic and pressor activities. Data suggests that vasopressin has a role in memory processes through secretion into the third ventricle with receptors in the periventricular gray matter (the same highly thiamine-dependent tissue that is damaged in Korsakoff's syndrome). Exogenous vasopressin and its analogues, when injected intraventricularly, facilitate the consolidation of learned responses. Vasopressing antibodies, which biologically inactivate vasopressin, block memory consolidation when injected into the third ventricle, thus approximating a memory defect resembling that of the Korsakoff syndrome. The memory consolidation process usually refers to the transfer of information from short-term rehearsal (a period during which the as-yet unstable memory trace is vulnerable to the disruptive effects of several agents or events) into long-term storage.

Vasopressin has been used in a number of animal studies in which it presumably facilitates the consolidation of the memory trace for simple avoidance tests in rats (deWied et al., 1975). The application of vasopressin to studies of memory function in man, without clinical or measured biochemical changes, has suggested that intranasal installation of 16 i.u. of lysine-8-vasopressin significantly improved performance of 12 patients on attention tasks, motor performance, and visual retention, recognition, and recall (Legros et al., 1978). Vasopressin has also been used with some success in the treatment of alcoholic as well as post-traumatic amnesias (Oliveros et al., 1978).

Vasopressin has been used with reported success in the treatment of Korsakoff's syndrome (Le Bouef et al., 1978). The treatment involves nasal spray administration of the vasopressin three times a day. Replication of these reports would be extremely important. In animal studies vasopressin has been shown to facilitate memory consolidation, presumably through its selective action upon the hippocampus (Wimersma-Greidanus and deWeid, 1977) and the suggestion for its application as a therapeutic medium in memory dysfunction in humans has been made (Legros et al., 1978; Oliverso et al., 1978). This line of research has lead to a "vasopressin theory" of Korsakoff syndrome wherein the dysmnesia results from levels of exogenous vasopressin due to periventricular tissue damage. Both effector as well as some receptor gray matter are destroyed to varying degrees, by the characteristic lesions of Korsakoff's syndrome thereby influencing the potential responsivity of such sites to therapeutic vasopressin. Sysmnestic syndromes, so common in older adults, seem correlated with lowered blood levels of vasopressin in men and women over 50 years of age.

In addition to the studies with vasopressin, a "noradrenergic theory" of the Korsakoff syndrome has been proposed. It has been noted that the Korsakoff lesions lie along monoaminergic pathways that have been carefully delineated in histofluorescence studies. In one systematic study (McEntee and Mair, 1978) CSF metabolites of serotonin, dopamine, and norepinephrine were measured in Korsakoff patients. The concentration of MHPG, the primary metabolite of norepinephrine, was decreased in Korsakoff patients as compared with controls. The concentration of MHPG in the CSF was also correlated with psychometric measures of memory impairment, such that individuals with the lowest concentration of the norepinephrine metabolite showed the greatest degree of memory impairment. More recent data favoring a noradrenergic deficit in Korsakoff syndrome has emerged in a study of eight patients in which significant improvement on memory tests occurred after two weeks of treatment with the a-noradrenergic agonist, clonidine (McEntee and Mair, 1980). These findings have been viewed as a Korsakoff-selective diminished pre-synaptic effect of clondine (favoring enhanced learning and memory), providing for unopposed post-synaptic a-adrenergic receptor effect.

Animal experiments support this relationship between the noradrenergic system and memory functions. Lesions of the locus coeruleus in rats is associated with impairment of subsequent learning and decreased cortical levels of norepinephrine (Anzelark et al., 1973). Agents that decrease brain norepinephrine level produce amnesia for well learned tasks; such impairment is reversible by the administration of drugs which elevate norepinephrine levels (Roberts et al., 1970). One cannot ignore several complex interactions between the noradrenergic and vasopressin systems.

THE HIPPOCAMPAL SYNDROME

Bilateral lesions of the hippocampus produce a dysmnestic syndrome symptomatologically quite similar to Korsakoff's syndrome. Unilateral hippocampal lesions do not produce such cognitive changes. Even though this structure-function relationship exists, the hippocampus is only rarely affected in the Korsakoff syndrome. The production of dysmnesia by bilateral hippocampal lesions was initially observed as an iatrogenic effect of surgical ablation of the temporal lobe for intractable epilepsy (Scovell and Milner, 1957). The critical lesions are those which bilaterally affect the hippocampi, on the medial surfaces of the temporal lobes. Damage to the temporal neocortex, amygdala, and uncus have no effect upon memory. Other causes of such bilateral hippocampal damage include cerebrovascular accidents and encephalitis, expecially herpes simplex. The proportion of hippocampal tissue damage is roughly proportional to the severity of the dysmnestic syndrome produced (Milner, 1966). Hippocampal damage also produces a deficit in spatial orientation.

The hippocampal formation (also called Ammon's Horn) includes the hippocampus proper, the dentate gyrus, and according to many authors, the subiculum. The lips of the hippocampal fissure are formed respectively by the dentate gyrus and hippocampus. The ventricular (lateral) surface of the hippocampus is covered by the alveus which is white matter composed of axons from the hippocampus. These fibers eventually enter the fiber bundle of the fornix.

The parahippocampal gyrus is demarcated by the hippocampal fissure and the collateral sulcus. The sequence of transition between the six-layered parahippocampal cortex and the three layered hippocampus is: parahippocampal cortex, presubiculum, subiculum, prosubiculum, and hippocampus. The pre- and prosubiculum areas represent zones of transition.

The anterior portion of the parahippocampal gyrus, the uncus, and the lateral olfactory atria form the pyrifrom lobe. The rhinal sulcus, a rostral continuation of the collateral sulcus, separates the parahippocampal gyrus from the more lateral neocortex. The pyriform cortex can be divided into the prepyriform, periamygdaloid, and entorhinal regions. The prepyriform cortex (also called the lateral olfactory gyrus) can be viewed as an extension of the lateral olfactory stria, and is regarded as an olfactory relay center. The periamygdaloid region is a small dorsal region rostrally overlying the amygdala, and has many connections with the prepyriform zone. All of these regions are anterior to the hippocampus. The most posterior portion of the pyriform lobe is the entorhinal lobe which corresponds histologically to Bradmann area 28. The entorhinal cortex does not receive fibers from the olfactory bulb. The prepyriform cortex projects to the entorhinal region as well as to the nucleus medialis dorsalis of the thalamus. The entorhinal cortex, but not the periamygdaloid and prepyriform zones, projects to the hippocampus. The more intrinsic features of the hippocampus consist of three fundamental layers: the polymorphic, pyramidal, and molecular (the latter has also been termed the external plexiform layer). A second nomenclature is based upon the arrangements of neurons and their processes; from the superficial to the deep layers, these include (1) stratum moleculare, (2) stratum lacunosum (which both contain afferent fibers from the entorhinal area and terminal branches of pyramidal apical dendrites), (3) the stratum radiatum, (4) stratum pyramidale, and (5) stratum oriens.

The stratum radiatum contains afferent fibers (including commissural fibers from the other hippocampus) and shafts of pyramidal apical dendrites. The prominent stratum pyramidale contains Golgi type II cells (short axon) as well as large and small pyramidal cells. Some of the pyramidal cells are termed double pyramids because of dense dendritic plexuses arising from both poles. Basket cells are found near the border between the stratus oriens but still within the stratum pyrimidale. Their axons loop back through the stratum radiatum to form a basket plexus around pyramidal cells. The stratus oriens contains polymorphic cells and pyramidal cell dendrites and afferent fibers which enter from the entorhinal cortex or from the fornix.

On the basis of intrinsic structural differences, the hippocampus is divided into several subzones: CA 1, CA 2, CA 3, and CA 4. The CA subdivisions are along the 'surface' of the hippocampus and can be viewed as analogous to Brodmann areas. CA 4 lies within the hilus of the dentate gyrus, while at the other end of the hippocampus, CA 1 is continuous with the subiculum region. The smallest pyramidal cells are found in CA 1, while the largest are in CA 4.

The dentate gyrus also consists of three layers: molecular, granular, and polymorphic. The molecular layer of the dentate is continuous with the hippocampal molecular layer, i.e., continuous with the strata radiatum, lacunosum, and moleculare. The granular layer consists of small round cells which give rise to axons which pass through the polymorphic layer to terminate in CA 3 near the roots of pyramidal cell apical dendrites. These granule cell derived processes are termed mossy fibers, which are part of a recurrent excitation network. The endings of such mossy fibers are mainly cholinergic.

The major inputs into the dentate and hippocampus derive from the lateral entorhinal area (Brodmann area 28) through the perforant or direct temporo-ammonic path. Perforant path fibers traverse the subiculum, then traverse the lower lip of the hippocampal fissure and terminate in the stratum moleculare of CA 1, CA 2, CA 3, and the dentate. Synapses are made with apical dendrites of the pyramidal cells and dendrites of granule cells.

The medial entorhinal area serves as the origin of the alvear (or temporo-alvear) path. These fibers pass through and distribute themselves in the deep layers of the subiculum. The remnant fibers then pass along the ventricular or alvear surface of the hippocampus, sending fibers along the way deeply to terminate in CA 1.

A crossed temporoammonic path from the contralateral entorhinal area terminates in the subiculum after travelling through the fornix and its commissure, the psalterium. The hippocampal commissure tends to be less distinct and less developed in man than in many lower species. The medial forebrain bundle and septal area send fibers to the hippocampal formation through the fornix. The medial septal nucleus projects to the dentate, CA 3, and CA 4. The majority of fibers passing through the psalterium terminate in all regions of the contralateral hippocampus and dentate. Some commissural fibers, after decussating, eventually enter the perforant path to terminate in apical dendrites of the pyramidal cells. Commissural fibers to the dentate end on the inner portion of the granule cell dendritic tree, in contrast to the perforant path terminations which occur on the outer portion of the dendrites.

Other inputs into the hippocampal region come from the cingulum, a large fiber bundle which travels through the core of the cingulate gyrus. The temporal continuations of the cingulum terminate in the presubiculum and entorhinal areas to form a key link in the Papez circuit. The supracallosal gyrus (or induseum griseum) is embryologically related to and sends fibers to the hippocampus. The axons of CA 3 pyramidal cells project to CA 2 and especially CA 1 pyramidal all apical dendrites through what are termed Shaeffer collaterals, an important functional arrangement system with the mossy fibers for recurrent excitation. System complexity is enhanced by other pyramidal cell collaterals which synapse with basket cells to recurrently inhibit other pyramidal cells.

Efferent fibers from pyramidal cell neurons exit chiefly through the fornix. As the fornix passes under the splenium and body of the corpus callosum, the hippocampal commissure occurs. Further forward the body of the anterior commissure passes orthogonally through the now descending fornix, with approximately half of all fibers going into each division. The anterior commissure is a structure largely unrelated to the fornix with importance for olfactory and cortical interconnections. Precommissural fibers distribute to the septal nuclei, the lateral portion of the preoptic region, anterior hypothalamus, and nucleus of the diagonal band of Broca. The remaining fibers are joined by septal efferents to form Zuckerkandl's bundle, a major component of the medial forebrain bundle, to distribute to central gray matter in the brain stem. It is relevant that regions associated with production of vasopressin (the anterior hypothalamus) and norepinephrine (the locus cocruleus) appear to receive precommissural fibers from the hippocampus. The anterior commissure interconnects the anygdala and entorhinal and pyriform corteces but not the hippocampi.

Approximately one-third to one-half of the post commissural output projects to the mammillary bodies, chiefly to the medial mammillary nuclei. Many, if not the majority, of post-commissural fibers project to the thalamus, chiefly to the anterior group, intralaminar nuclei, and lateralis dorsalis. An interesting modification of the Papez circuit theory lies in the observation that as many fibers from the hippocampi may project directly to the anterior thalamic nuclei as come from the mammillary bodies. Post-commissural fibers also join the medial forebrain bundle to descend and distribute widely.

Recent work by Raisman and colleagues (1965, 1966) has clarified the relation of the hippocampus to other regions. Post commissural efferents arise from CA 1 (anterior part) and CA 2 to terminate in thalamic and mammillary regions. Pre-commissural fibers arise from CA 1 (posterior part), CA 3, and CA 4 to terminate bilaterally to the diagonal band and lateral septum, and unilaterally to the medial septum. Further complex interrelationships have been observed; the dentate projects via mossy fibers to CA 3 pyramidal cells which, in turn, project to the septum and diagonal band, and then project back to CA 3. Shaeffer collaterals from CA 3 excite CA 1, and connect to the prosubiculum, which in turn projects to the supachiasmatic and arcuate nuclei of the hypothalamus.

Through these complex efferent systems the hippocampus can influence cortical activity and sensation. For example, hippocampal stimulation can inhibit cortical evoked responses from sensory inputs. Electrical stimulation of the hippocampus in man is capable of evoking autonomic functions, such as salivation, pupillary dilation, and the release of TSH and ACTH. Increased voltage and reduced frequency in the ipsilateral frontal cortex is produced by electrical stimulation of the hippocampus.

The theta wave of the EEG is hippocampal in origin and is produced by visual, auditory, comatosensory, or olfactory stimulation. This 4 to 7 Hertz wave can also be elicited by stimulation of the medial septal region, lateral hypothalamus (sites of norepinephrine fiber tracts), anterior hypothalamus (site of vasopressin productions) and reticular activating system. When the theta wave is recorded from hippocampus, the neocortex shows fast low voltage arousal activity. The inverse relationship between theta wave hippocampal activity and alpha wave neocortical activity may be due to inhibitory control of the hippocampus by periaqueductal and medial tegmental gray matter (Peele, 1977). These latter regions are affected in Korsakoff's disease. Further data are necessary to define the inhibitory functions of norepinephrine pathways to the hippocampus; this would provide a critical link in a more unified concept of memory mechanisms.

Loss of hippocampal theta wave rhythm through medial septal lesions in rats produced dysmnestic syndromes with prominent spatial memory deficits (Winson, 1978). In rabbits, hippocampal EEG data taken before the onset of training predicts subsequent learning rate even over a period of several days. The higher the proportion of pretraining theta wave activity, the better the memory for a learned task. Conversely, the greater the proportion of high frequency (8-22 Hertz) activity, the slower the rate of learning. The amount of theta activity determines the capacity for memory consolidation (Berry and Thompson, 1978).

Injection of moderate doses of eserine produces enhanced theta activity, which is dependent upon the septohippocampal fornix pathway with the pacemaker in the septal region. Both acetylcholine transferase and choline acetylase activity are dramatically reduced in the hippocampus following section of the septohippocampal pathways. Acetylcholinesterase accumulates on the septal side of this lesion (Shute and Lewis, 1963). In the hippocampus, there is a laminar distribution pattern of acetylcholinesterase. The septum appears to regulate theta activity through a cholinergic septohippocampal excitatory pathway.

Glutamic acid is the most significant and powerful hippocampal excitatory putative neurotransmitter having its effect on the dendritic tree, but not the cell bodies of pyramidal cells on proximal dendritic regions (Schwartzkrain and Anderson, 1975). The most significant inhibitory hippocampal neurotransmitter is gamma-aminobutyric acid (GABA), which acts upon pyramidal cell soma receptors to inhibit both induced and spontaneous hippocampal pyramidal activity. Recurrent excitatory mechanisms previously discussed, such as mossy fiber and Shaeffer collateral systems appear to utilize glutamic acid, while recurrent inhibition mechanisms, such as the basket cell system, appear to involve GABA. Complex interaction between septal pacemaker, recurrent inhibition, and recurrent excitation are probably responsible for spontaneous hippocampal electrical activity.

Other neurotransmitters found in high concentration in the hippocampus include serotonin, norepinephrine, and epinephrine. Unlike the other putative neurotransmitters mentioned, these substances do not show characteristic patterns of structural neuropharmacology and are found diffusely in high concentration throughout the hippocampus (Anderson, 1975). Norepinephrine probably has an important function in the memory functions of the hippocampus due to its concentration and wide distribution. The neuropharmacology and neurophysiology of norepinephine-dependent limbic systems may be the key to a unified theory of memory consolidation.

One of the dysmnestic syndromes involving the hippocampi, but sparing the mammillary complex or nucleus medialis dorsalis is Alzheimer's disease. Aside from the well-documented clinical picture of this disorder, the major gross pathological characteristic is atrophy, although this finding is a normal accompaniment of aging. The dysmnestic disorder is more directly associated with the development of neurofibrillary tangles; these are paired helically arranged filamentous structures (Kidd, 1963; Wiśnewski, et al., 1976) that are believed to result from modified protein synthesis (Iqbal et al., 1975) or as a reaction from neuronal cell body injury (Torack, 1979). Neurons of the hippocampus containing neurofibrillary tangles from patients with Alzheimer's dementia have been shown to contain high aluminum content in the nuclear region (Perl and Brody, 1980). In the cytoplasm of neurofibrillary tangle containing neurons from demented patients there was almost a 30 percent incidence of aluminum presence, as compared with only 11 percent in non-demented elderly patients. Other pathological findings in Alzheimer's disease include senile plaques and granulovaculor degeneration. Plaques identical with those found in Alzheimer's disease have been studies in senile monkeys (Wiśnewski et al., 1973). Several abnormalities were noted, including scattered neurites, fibrillar material, vascular amyloidosis, lipofuscin accumulation, dark neurons undergoing phagocytosis, enlarged mitochondria, myelin remodeling, virus-like particles, electron-dense croplets, and paracrystalline mitochondrial inclusions. In patients with Alzheimer's disease, electron microscopic examination of biopsy material has revealed enlarged axons, presynaptic axon terminals, and probably dendrites, containing fibrils, branching vesicular profiles, and multilaminar bodies (Gonatas et al., 1967). The enlarged axon terminals seen in Alzheimer's disease resemble those seen in some retardation syndromes. A reduction in the number of presynaptic terminal vesicles very likely is a reflection of an altered disposition for neurotransmitters, which undoubtedly function to mediate memory functions.

Biochemical changes associated with dementia have been documented for the frontal gray matter (Bowen et al., 1973); these include a pronounced decrease in a neuronal-type protein, neuronin S-6, and a slightly increased concentration of the glia-associated protein, S-100. These changes may reflect neuronal loss and glial hypertrophy, as observed in the Alzheimer type of dementia. Related enzymatic findings in senile dementia (Bowen et al., 1974; Bowen and Davison, 1975) have documented a pronounced depletion of glutamic acid decarboxylase (GAD) in the frontal and temporal cortex. Lower activity of choline acetyltransferase were also observed in the cerebral cortex and caudate of patients with senile dementia (Bowen et al., 1976). The activity of choline acetyltransferase, was reduced in several brain regions of patients with dementia (Perry et al., 1977), and for several of such areas, enzyme activity was significantly lower in the Alzheimer-type of dementia as compared with multi-infarct dementia; these areas included the temporal cortex, parietal cortex, and hippocampus—all interestingly bearing upon the general issue of memory function and amnesia. Because of the obvious role of neurotransmitter synthesizing enzymes in determining the disposition of specific amines and the suggested relationship of some of these substances to memory functions, there have been several bases for a neurotransmitter role in memory dysfunction.

A summary of the putative neurotransmitter changes that have been measured in Alzheimer's disease and in animal models is given in Tables 1 and 2. Several of these changes may have a bearing upon suggested aminergic substrates for memory consolidation—the stage of the memory process that appears to be principally impaired in the amnesic component of Alzheimer's dementia. A potential role for catecholamines (Kety, 1967), serotonin (Essman, 1978), and acetylcholine (Drachman, 1977) in memory functions has been suggested and simple neurotransmitter concentration status changes, *per se,* may not be adequate to describe the mechanism by which memory dysfunction in aging or dementia occurs. For example, changes in concentration, turnover, or effects at specific receptor sites may depend upon specific triggering events, an interaction with nutritional factors. Preliminary reports of the potential application of dietary cholinergic replacement regimens (Lecithin, choline) for the treatment of memory dysfunction associated with Alzheimer's and other dementias have appeared (Wurtman, 1980). Certainly this approach appears somewhat promising in view of animal studies showing increased brain acetylcholine content in animals treated with dietary lecithin (Hirsch and Wurtman, 1978; Wurtman et al., 1977) or choline (Cohen and Wurtman, 1976). Dietary choline may also act to stimulate cholinergic receptors (Karczmar, 1979; Karczmar and Dun, 1978). In several studies with oral choline therapy for memory dysfunction in presenile dementia, variable results have emerged. Some reduced confusional behavior in approximately one-third of patients receiving choline (9g/day x 2 wks.) was observed but no change in memory tests was noted (Smith et al., 1978). Little cognitive benefit was observed from oral choline (5g/day x 2 wks. + 10g/day x 2 wks.) in elderly patients (Boyd et al., 1977), but some improvement in younger patients with a shorter history of Alzheimer's disease was noted after 3 weeks of choline treatment (9g/day), when memory tests were given (Signoret et al., 1978). Although no memory testing changes were noted in patients with Alzheimer's disease treated with lecithin (25g/day + additional 25g/wk. for 4 wks.), learning scores and visual retention scores did improve (Etienne et al., 1978). Choline chloride (2g, q.i.d.) given to elderly subjects for 21 days had no effect upon performance on memory storage tasks, retrieval tasks or digit-symbol substitution (Mohs et al., 1980). The failure of choline to consistently improve memory functions in elderly subjects in patients with memory dysfunction of Alzheimer's disease may reside in the weak cholinergic agonist activity of this agent, or in the failure of choline, *per se,* to effect nerve ending acetylcholine release. Finally, choline as an acetylcholine precursor, does not provide for increased hippocampal acetylcholine (Jenden, 1979)—a site-specific referent to the memory dysfunction to which a cholinergic hypothesis has been applied.

A possible parallel to the effects of oral cholinergic precursors or receptor agonists in memory functions may reside in clinical studies utilizing cholinergic drugs to study a variety of memory deficits. A summary of such studies may be found in Table 3.

TABLE 1. Putative Neurotransmitter and Related Metabolic Changes in Patients with Alzheimer's Disease or Senile Dementias

Acetylcholine
Reduced cholinergic neurons in temporal lobe
(35%) — Bowen et al., 1979
Reduced choline acetyltransferase
    frontal cortex — Bowen et al., 1976
    hippocampus — Perry et al., 1977
Reduced acetylcholinesterase activity — Davies and Maloney, 1976; Davies, 1979

Hippocampal muscarinic cholinergic receptors
    - decreased — Reisine et al., 1978
    - no change — White et al., 1977; Davies and Verth, 1978

Dopamine
Reduced dopamine
    striatum — Finch, 1972
    Median eminence
    posterior pituitary — Finch, 1978
    Thalamus
    Pons — Adolfson et al., 1978
Reduced dopaminergic cells
Reduced homovanillic acid
    corpus striatum — Gottfries et al., 1969, 1970

Norepinephrine
Reduced norepinephrine — Winblad et al., 1978
    Putamen
    frontal cortex
    hypothalamus — Finch, 1972

Serotonin
Reduced serotonin
    brain stem
    cortex
    hippocampus — Meek et al., 1977
Reduced serotonin receptor activity
    temporal lobe — Bowen et al., 1979
    no change in neocortex — Reisine et al., 1978

GABA
Reduced Glutamate decarboxylase activity
    neocortex — Bowen et al., 1976
Reduced GABA receptors — Perry et al., 1977; Reisine et al., 1978

References cited in this table agree with text citations or are referred to in appropriate text citations.

TABLE 2. Neurotransmitter and Enzyme Changes in the Aging Brain and Dementia

Tyrosine hydroxylase	↓	McGeer and McGeer, 1976
DOPA decarboxylase	↓	McGeer and McGeer, 1976
Catechol-O-methyl transferase (hippocampus)	↓	Roginson, et al., 1977
Monoamine oxidase	↑	Cote and Kremzner, 1974; Grote et al., 1974; Robinson et al., 1972
MAO-B	↑	Gottfries et al., 1975
Dopamine	↓	Carlsson and Winblad, 1976
Norepinephrine	↓	Robinson et al., 1972, 1977
HVA (CSF)	↓	Gottfries et al., 1969, 1970, 1974
5-HIAA (CSF)	↓	Gottfries et al., 1969, 1970
Glutamic acid cecarboxylase	↓	Bowen et al., 1974
choline acetyltransferase	↓	McGeer and McGeer, 1976; Perry et al., 1977; Spillane et al., 1977

References cited in this table agree with text citations or are referred to in appropriate text citations.

TABLE 3. Cholinergic Agents and Memory Effects in Man

Physostigmine

Improvement of memory in normal volunteers	Davis et al., 1978
Reversal of anticholinergic-induced memory impairment	Choneim and Mewaldt, 1977
Antagonism of scopolamine-induced memory dysfunction	Drachman, 1978

Scopolamine

Memory impairment in normal subjects	Drachman and Leavitt, 1974; Drachman, 1978

References cited in this table agree with text citations or are referred to in appropriate text citations.

DISCUSSION

The similar clinical manifestations of the Korsakoff and hippocampal syndrome have complex underlying structural and neuropharmacological substrates. The fornix is the fiber bundle that interconnects the two regions that are neuropathologically correlated with these dysmnestic syndromes. One would expect, on theoretical grounds, that lesions of the fornix would produce a dysmnestic syndrome. However the evidence has been inconsistent (Brierly, 1977; Hacaen and Albert, 1978; Lishman, 1978, and Peele, 1977). While there are cases where discrete fornical damage is indeed associated with amnesia, there are also patients with total fornical section who show no associated memory deficit. These latter cases represent an extremely puzzling neurophyschological finding. One conclusion that might be drawn is that there are at least two separate subsystems essential for memory consolidation.

Pribram (1971) has proposed a provocative holographic theory of human memory which deserves discussion. Holography, although popularized as three-dimensional photography, is actually a much more general process which can be applied in any media, including biological systems. The critical feature of holography is the ability to utilize Fourier mathematical spatial transformations as stored representations of information. Pribram presents a variety of neuropsysiological data to support his contention that the human C.N.S. does indeed operate using a Fourier transform mode to store memory. The hologram produced would be the broad expanse of neocortical tissue. The hippocampal and diencephalic systems discussed earlier would function in encoding and might also have a role in the decoding of holographically stored data. Holograms have the property of equipotentiality. In the case of the cerebral cortex, data is stored throughout all constituent gray matter and all portions of cortex have an equal capacity to store information. Long-term memories are therefore never destroyed completely by focal lesions, but only more diffuse. The law of mass action is also obeyed by holograms with the clarity of stored information directly proportional to the amount (mass) of the hologram available for decoding from Fourier transform mode. RNA dependent conformational changes in protein molecules of the cerebral cortex would play a role in information storage analogous to the photographic silver nitrate emulsion crystals in optic holograms.

Anterograde dysmnesia is represented by a loss of encoding capacity while dysfunctional decoding is retrograde dysmnesia. The loss of cerebral cortical tissue is associated with a reduction in the clarity of long-term memory storage. Lashley's laws of mass action and equipotentiality as well as clinical features of Korsakoff's and the hippocampal syndromes can be explained in terms of the holographic theory.

Research on the neuropharmacology of dysmnesia must take structural considerations such as holographic theory into account. Studies of noradrenergic, cholinergic, glutaminergic, GABA-eric, serotonergic, dopaminergic, and vasopressin-dependent limbic neurotransmitter systems should help clarify encoding and decoding mechanisms of human memory. In another respect, research concerned with RNA-dependent protein synthesis and conformational changes, could probably be useful as a basis for understanding the nature of long-term storage. The complex interactions between these subsystems remains to be further clarified to provide structural neuropharmacology research with methods of clarifying the unknowns and complexities of the human dysmnesia syndromes.

REFERENCES

Adolfsson, R., Gottfries, C.G., Oreland, L., Roos, B.E., and Winblad, B. (1978): Reduced levels of catecholamines in the brain and increased activity of monoamine oxidase in platelets in Alzheimer's disease. Therapeutic implications. In: R. Katzman, R.D. Terry and K.L. Bick (Eds.), *Alzheimer's Disease and Related Dementias.* Raven Press, New York, pp. 441-451.
Albert, M.S., Butters, N., and Levin, J. (1979): Temporal gradients in the retrograde amnesia of patients with alcoholic Korsakoff's disease. *Arch. Neurol. 36;* 211-216.
Anderson, P. (1975): Organization of hippocampal neurons and their interconnections. In: R. Issacson, and K. Pribam, Eds., *The Hippocampus.* Plenum Press, London.
Anzelark, G., Crow, T., and Greenberg, T. (1973): Impaired learning and decreased cortical norepinephrine after bilateral locus coeruleus lesions. *Science 191:* 682-684.
Berry, S. and Thompson, T. (1978): Prediction of learning rate from hippocampal electroencephalogram. *Science 200:* 1298-1300.
Blass, J.P. and Gibson, G.E. (1977): Abnormality of a thiamine-requiring enzyme in patients with Wernicke-Korsakoff syndrome. *N. Eng. J. Med. 297:* 1367-1370.
Bowen, D.M. and Davison, A.N. (1975): Extrapyramidal diseases and dementia. *Lancet 1:* 1199-1200.
Bowen, D.M., Smith, C.B., and Davison, A.N. (1973): Molecular changes in senile dementia. *Brain 96:* 849-856.
Bowen, D.M., Smith, C.B., White, P., and Davison, A.N. (1976): Neurotransmitter-related enzymes and indices of hypoxia in senile dementia and other abiotropies. *Brain 99:* 459-496.
Bowen, D.M., White, P., Flack, R.H.A., Smith, C.B., and Davison, A.N. (1974): Brain-decarboxylase activities as indices of pathological change in senile dementia. *Lancet 1:* 1247-1249.
Bowen, D.M., White, P., Spillane, J.A., Goodhart, M.J., Curzon, G., Iwangoff, P., Meier-Ruge, W., and Davison, A.N. (1979): Accelerated aging or selective neuronal loss as an important cause of dementia? *Lancet 1:* 11-14.
Boyd, W., Graham-White, I., and Blackwood, G. (1977): Clinical effects of choline in Alzheimer senile dementia. *Lancet 2:* 711.
Brierly, J. (1977): The neuropathology of amnestic states. In: C. Whitty and O. Zangwill, *Amnesia, 2nd ed.* Butterworths, London.
Brin, M., Tal, M., Ostashever, A.S., and Kalinsky, H. (1960): Effect of thiamine deficiency on activity of erythrocyte hemolysate transketolase. *J. Nutr. 71:* 273-280.
Carpenter, M. (1976): *Human Neuroanatomy.* Williams and Wilkins, Baltimore.
Cohen, E.L. and Wurtman, R.J. (1976): Brain acetylcholine: control by dietary choline. *Science 191:* 561-562.
Cote, L.J., and Kremzner, L.T. (1974): Changes in neurotransmitter systems with increasing age in human brain. *Trans. Am. Soc. Neurochem. 5:* 83.

Davies, P. and Maloney, A.J.F. (1976): Selective loss of cholinergic neurons in Alzheimer's disease. *Lancet 2:* 1403.
Davies, P. (1979): Neurotransmitter-related enzymes in senile dementia of the Alzheimer type. *Brain Res. 171:* 319-327.
Davies, P., and Verth, A.H. (1978): Regional distribution of muscarinic acetylcholine receptor in normal and Alzheimer's-type dementia brains. *Brain Res. 138:* 385-392.
Davis, K.L., Mohs, R.C., Tinklenberg, J.R., Hollister, L.E., Pfefferbaum, A., and Kopell, B.S. (1978): Physostigmine: Enhancement of long-term memory functions on normal subject. *Science 201:* 274-276.
De Weid, D., Witter, A., and Greven. H.M. (1975): Behaviourally active ACTH analogues. *Biochem. Pharmacol. 24:* 1463-1468.
Drachman, D.A. (1977): Memory and cognitive function in man: Does the cholinergic system have a specific role? *Neurology 27:* 283-290.
Drachman, D.A. (1978): Memory, dementia, and the cholinergic system. In: R. Katzman, R.D. Terry, and K.L. Bick, Eds., *Alzheimer's Disease: Senile Dementia and Related Disorders (Aging, Vol. 7).* Raven Press, New York, 141-148.
Drachman, D.A. and Arbit, J. (1966): Memory and the hippocampal complex. *Arch. Neurol. 5:* 15-61.
Drachman, D.A. and Leavitt, J. (1974): Human memory and the cholinergic system: A relationship to aging. *Arch. Neurol. 30:* 113-121.
Dreyfus, P.M. (1962): Clinical application of blood transketolase determinations. *N. Eng. J. Med. 267:* 496-598.
Essman, W.B. (1978): Serotonin in learning and memory. In: W.B. Essman, Ed., *Serotonin in Health and Disease: Vol. III.* Spectrum, New York, 69-143.
Etienne, P., Gauthier, S., and Dastoor, D. (1978): Lecithin in Alzheimer's disease. *Lancet 2:* 1206.
Finch, C.E. (1972): Cellular pacemakers of aging in mammals. In: R. Harris and D. Viza (Eds.), *Proc. 1st European Conference on Cell Differentiation.* Munkesgaard, Copenhagen. pp. 123-126.
Finch, C.E. (1978): Neurochemical and neuroendocrine changes during aging in rodent models. In: R. Katzman, D. Terry and K.L. Bick (Eds.), *Alzheimer's Disease: Senile Dementia and Related Disorders.* Raven Press, New York. pp. 461-468.
Fry, W., Krumins, R., Fry, F., Thomas, G., Borbely, S., and Ades, H. (1963): Origins and distribution of some efferent pathways from the mammillary nuclei of the cat. *J. Comp. Neurol. 120:* 195-258.
Ghoneim, M.M. and Mewaldt, S.P. (1977): Studies on human memory. The interactions of diazepam, scopolamine and physostigmine. *Psychopharmacology 52:* 1-6.
Gonatas, N.K., Anderson, W., and Evangelista, I. (1967): The contribution of altered synapses in the senile plaque: An electron microscopic study in Alzheimer's dementia. *J. Neuropathol. Exp. Neurol. 26:* 25-39.
Gottfries, C.G., Gottfries, I., and Roos, B.E. (1969): The investigation of homovanillic acid in the human brain and its correlation to senile dementia. *Brit. J. Psychiat. 115:* 563-574.
Gottfries, C.G., Gottfries, I., and Roos, B.E. (1970): Homovanillic acid and 5-hydroxyindole acetic acid in cerebrospinal fluid related to mental and motor impairment in semile and presenile dementia. *Acta Psychiatr. Neurol. Scand. 46:* 99-103.
Gottfries, C.G., Kjallquist, A., Ponten, U., Roos, B.E., and Sundbarg, G. (1974): Cerebrospinal fluid pH and monoamine and glucolytic metabolites in Alzheimer's disease. *Brit. J. Psychiat. 124:* 280-287.
Gottfries, C.G., Oreland, L., Wiberg, A., and Winblad, B. (1975): Lowered monoamine oxidase activity in brains from alcoholic suicides. *J. Neurochem. 25:* 667-673.

Grote, S.S., Moses, S.G., Robins, E., Hudgens, R.W., and Croninger, A.B. (1974): A study of selected catecholamine metabolizing enzymes: A comparison of depressive suicides and alcoholic suicides with controls. *J. Neurochem. 23:* 791-802.

Hacaen, H. and Albert, M. (1978): *Human Neuropsychology.* Wiley, New York.

Hirsch, M.J. and Wurtman, R.J. (1978): Lecithin consumption elevates acetylcholine concentrations in rat brain and adrenal gland. *Science 202:* 223-225.

Iqbal, K., Wisniewski, H.M., Grundke-Iqbal, I., Korthals, J.K., and Terry, R.D. (1975): Chemical pathology of neurofibrils: Neurofibrillary tangles of Alzheimer's presenile-senile dementia. *J. Histochem. Cytodhem. 23:* 563-569.

Jenden, D.J. (1979): The neurochemical basis of acetylcholine precursor loading as a therapeutic strategy. In: K.L. Davies and P.A. Berger, Eds., *Brain Acetylcholine and Neuropsychiatric Disease.* Plenum Press, New York. 483-514.

Karczmar, A. (1979): Overview: Cholinergic drugs and behaviour—what effects may be expected from a "cholinergic diet?" In: J. Growdon, R.J. Wurtman, and A. Barbeau, Eds., *Uses of Choline and Lecithin in Neurological and Psychiatric Disorders.* Raven Press, New York.

Karczmar, A. and Dun, N. (1978): Cholinergic synapses: Physiological, pharmacological and behavioral correlates. In: M. Lipton, A. DiMascio, and K. Killam, Eds., *Psychopharmacology: A Generation of Progress.* Raven Press, New York. 293-305.

Kety, S.S. (1967): The central physiological and pharmacological effects of the biogenic amines and their correlations with behavior. In: G.C. Quinton, T. Melneckich, and F. Schmidt, Eds., *The Neurosciences.* Rockefeller University Press, New York. 444-452.

Kidd, M. (1963): Paired helical filaments in electron microscopy of Alzheimer's disease. *Nature* (Lond.) *197:* 192-193.

LeBoeuf, A., Lodge, J., and Eames, P.G. (1978): Vasopressin and memory in Korsakoff syndrome. *Lancet 2:* 1370.

Legros, J.J., Gilot, P., Seron, X., Claessens, J., Adam, A., Moeglen, J.M., Audibert, A., and Berchier, P. (1978): Influence of vasopressin on learning and memory. *Lancet 1:* 41-42.

Lishman, W. (1978): *Organic Psychiatry: The Psychological Consequences of Cerebral Disorder.* Blackwell, Oxford.

McEntee, W.J. and Mair, R.G. (1978): Memory Impairment in Korsakoff's psychosis: A correlation with brain nonadrenergic activity. *Science 202:* 905-907.

McEntee, W.J. and Mair, R.G. (1980): Memory enhancement in Korsakoff's psychosis by clonidine: Further evidence for a noradrenergic deficit. *Ann. Neurol. 7:* 466-470.

McGeer, E.G., and McGeer, P.L. (1976): Neurotransmitter metabolism in the aging brain. In: R.D. Terry and S. Gershon (Eds.) *Aging. Vol. 3.* Raven Press, New York. pp. 389-403.

Meek, E.G., and Bertilsson, L., Cheney, D.L., Zsilla, G., and Costa, E. (1977): Aging-induced changes in acetylcholine and serotonin content of discrete brain nuclei. *J. Gerontol. 32:* 129-131.

Milner, G. (1966): Amnesia following operation on the temporal lobes. In: C. Whitty and O. Zangwill, Eds., *Amnesia* (1st ed.) Butterworths, London.

Mohs, R.C., Davis, K.L., Tinklenberg, J.R., and Hollister, L.E. (1980): Choline chlordie effects on memory in the elderly. *Neurobiology of Aging 1:* 21-25.

Nauta, J. (1958): Hippocampal projections and related neural pathways in the midbrain of the cat. *Brain 81:* 319-340.

Oliveros, J.C., Jandali, M.K., Timsit Berthier, M., Remy, R., Benghezal, A., Audibert, A., and Moeglen, J.M. (1978): Vasopressin in amnesia. *Lancet 1:* 42.

Peele, T. (1977): *The Neuroanatomical Basis for Clinical Neurology.* McGraw-Hill, New York.

Perl, D.P. and Brody, A.R. (1980): Alzheimer's Disease: X-ray spectrometric evidence of aluminum accumulation in neurofibrillary tangle-bearing neurons. *Science 208:* 297-299.

Perry, E.K., Perry, R.H., Blessed, G., and Tomlinson, B.E. (1977): Neurotransmitter enzyme abnormalities in senile dementia—choline acetyltransferase and glutamic acid decarboxylase in necropsy brain tissue. *J. Neurol. Sci. 34:* 247-265.

Perry, E.K., Perry, R.H., Gibson, P.H., Blessed, G., and Tomlinson, B.E. (1977): A cholinergic connection between normal aging and senile dementia in the human hippocampus. *Neurosci. Lett. 6:* 85-89.

Powell, T., Bullery, R., and Loman, W. (1957): A quantitative study of the fornix-mammillothalamic system. *J. Anat. 91:* 419-432.

Pribam, K. (1971): *Languages of the Brain.* Prentice Hall, Englewood Cliffs, N.J.

Raisman, G., Cowen, W., and Powell, T. (1965): The extrinsic afferent, commissural, and association fibers of the hippocampus. *Brain 88:* 963-996.

Raisman, G., Cowen, W., and Powell, T. (1966): An experimental analysis of the efferent connections of the hippocampus. *Brain 89:* 83-108.

Reisine, T.D., Bird, E.D., Spokes, E., Enna, S.J., and Yamamura, H.I. (1978): Pre and postsynaptic neurochemical alterations in Alzheimer's disease. *Trans. Am. Soc. Neurochem. 9:* 203.

Roberts, R.B., Flexner, J.B., and Flexner, L.B. (1970): Some evidence for the involvement of adrenergic sites in the memory trace. *Proc. Nat. Acad. Scie. 66:* 310-313.

Robinson, D.S. Davies, J.M., and Nies, A. (1972): Aging, monoamines, and monoamine oxidase level. *Lancet 1:* 290-291.

Robinson, D.S., Sourkes, T.L., Nies, A., Harris, L.S., Spector, S., Barlett, D.L., and Kaye, L.S. (1977): Monoamine metabolism in human brain. *Arch. Gen. Psychiatry 34:* 89-92.

Sanders, H.L. and Warrington, E.K. (1971): Memory for remote events in amnesic patients. *Brain 94:* 661-668.

Schwartzdrain, P. and Anderson, P. (1957): Glutamic acid sensitivity of dendrites in hippocampal slices in vitro. In: G. Dreuzberg, Ed., *Properties of Dendrites.* Raven Press, New York.

Scovell, W.B. and Milner, B. (1957): Loss of recent memory after bilateral hippocampal lesions. *J. Neurol. Neurosurg. Psychiat. 20:* 11-25.

Shute, C. and Lewis, P. (1963): Cholinesterase containing systems of the brain of the rat. *Nature 199:* 1160-1164.

Signoret, J., Whiteley, A., and Lhermitte, F. (1978): Influence of choline on amnesia in early Alzheimer's disease. *Lancet 2:* 837.

Smith, C.M., Swash, M., Exton-Smith, A.N., Phillips, M.J., Overstall, P.W., Piper, M.E., and Bailey, M.R. (1978): Choline in Alzheimer's disease. *Lancet 2:* 318.

Spillane, J.A., White, P., Goodhardt, M.J., Flack, R.H.A., Bowen, D.M., and Davison, A.N. (1977): Selective vulnerability of neurons in organic dementia. *Nature* (Lond.) *266:* 558-559.

Torack, R.M. (1979): Adult dementia: history, biopsy, pathology. *Neurosurg. 4:* 434-442.

Valenstein, F. and Nauta, W. (1959): A comparison of the distribution of the fornix system in the rat, guinea pig, and monkey. *J. Comp. Neurol. 113:* 337-363.

Van Wimersma Greidanus, T. B. and De Weid, D. (1977): The physiology of the neurophypophyseal system and its relation to memory processes. In: A.N. Davidson, Ed., *Biochemical Correlates of Brain Function.* Academic Press, London. 284-289.

Victor, M., Adams, R., and Collins, G. (1971): *The Wernicke-Korsakoff Syndrome.* Blackwell, Oxford.

White, P., Goodhardt, M.J., Keet, J.P., Hiley, C.R., Carrasco, L.H., Williams, I.E.I., and Bowen, D.M. (1977): Neocortical cholinergic neurones in elderly people. *Lancet 1:* 668-670.

Winblad, B., Adolfsson, R., Gottfries, C.G., Oreland, L., and Roos, B.E. (1978): Brain monoamines, monoamine metabolites and enzymes in physiological aging and senile dementia. In: A. Grigerio, Ed., *Recent Developments in Mass Spectrometry in Biochemistry and Medicine*, 1. Plenum, New York. 253-267.

Winson, J. (1978): Loss of hippocampal theta activity results in spatial memory deficit in rats. *Science 201:* 160-163.

Wiśniewski, H.M., Ghetti, B., and Terry, T.D. (1973): Neuritic (senile) plaques and filamentous changes in aged rhesus monkeys. *J. Neuropathol. Exp. Neurol. 32:* 566-584.

Wiśniewski, H.M., Narang, H.K., and Terry, R.D. (1976): Neurofibrillary tangles of paired helical filaments. *J. Neurol. Sci. 27:* 173-181.

Wurtman, R. (1980): Memory disorders. *Trends in Neurosciences,* VII-X.

Wurtman, R.J., Hirsch, M.I., and Grodon, J.H. (1977): Lecithin consumption raises serum-tree-choline levels. *Lancet 1:* 68-69.

7

Localization of Substance P and Enkephalin in the Spinal Cord: Relationship to Pain Pathways

N. Eric Naftchi
Susan Abrahams
Henry St. Paul
Linda Vacca

It has long been known that the perception of pain in the central nervous system is first integrated in the spinal cord, in the narrow band of gray matter at the apex of the dorsal horns known as the substantia gelatinosa. Primary afferent neurons terminate in the substantia gelatinosa, and interact with many small inter-neurons found in this region. High concentrations of the peptides substance P, leucine-enkephalin and methionine-enkephalin have been found in the substantia gelatinosa comprising Rexed's lamina II and II and Rexed's lamina I (Abrahams et al., 1978; Brownstein et al., 1976; Elde et al., 1976; Hökfelt et al., 1975a, 1975b, 1977; Kanazawa and Jessel, 1976; Naftchi et al., 1978). Additionally, a dense population of opiate receptors have been demonstrated in the substantia gelatinosa (Atweh and Kuhar, 1977). These three neuropeptides, thus have been implicated in the mediation of pain and analgesia.

Substance P was extracted in 1931 from equine brain and intestine by Von Euler and Gaddum (1931). It was found to possess a vasodilatory effect and stimulate smooth muscle. It was not until 1970, however, that Chang and Leeman (1970) isolated a sialogogic peptide from bovine hypothalamus which was purified, characterized as substance P, and synthesized. It was found to be an undecapeptide (Chang et al., 1971). Subsequently, antibodies to substance P were prepared and using radioimmunoassay, it was found that substance P had an uneven distribution in the central nervous system (Powell et al., 1973). Its highest concentrations occurred in the substantia nigra, hypothalamus, pineal gland and the dorsal gray matter of the spinal cord (Brownstein et al., 1976). These results have been confirmed by immunofluorescence and immunoperoxidase methods in a variety of animals; human, cat, rat, and monkey (Hökfelt et al., 1975a, 1975b, Naftchi et al., 1978; Cuello et al., 1976). In the substantia gelatinosa, the immunoreactivity seems to occur within thin unmyelinated fibers classically known to carry thermal and pain stimuli. This finding suggests that substance P is the first chemical signal of exteroceptive perception in the spinal cord (Cuello et al., 1976). Physiological evidence indicates that substance P can produce slow, long-lasting excitation in spinal neurons when applied iontophoretically. These neurons include motoneurons, Renshaw cells, and dorsal horn inter-neurons in the substantia gelatinosa and Rexed's lamina V (Henry, 1976; Henry et al., 1975). The data support the view that substance P may be a transmitter or modulator involved in the perception of pain.

In 1973, binding of radioactive opiates, including morphine, to brain synaptosomal membranes was independently reported by three groups (Pert and Snyder, 1973; Simon et al., 1973; Terenius, 1973). The binding could be blocked stereospecifically by the opiate antagonists naloxone and naltrexone. It was postulated, therefore, that opiates must bind to selective sites, or receptors, located on the surface of nerve cells in the CNS, before they can produce their characteristic pharmacological responses; analgesia, euphoria, sleep, and relaxation. The antagonists, which may also possess some agonist effect, would then bind to these specific sites first, and thereby prevent opiate (agonist) binding (Simon, 1976).

Accordingly, opiate receptors have been reported in various regions of the brain, in especially high amounts in the limbic system (except the hippocampus), in the spinal cord, especially the dorsal gray matter, and in the intestine (Simon, 1976; Kuhar, 1975). Additionally, opiate receptor binding sites have been demonstrated by radiobinding assay and by autoradiography in brain and spinal cord (Atweh and Kuhar, 1977; Pert et al., 1976; Hiller et al., 1973).

The presence of the opiate receptors in the CNS led to the thinking that a biological ligand(s) for opiate receptors might exist in the CNS and might be a naturally occurring endogenous morphine-like substance(s). Several studies reported that electrical stimulation of certain parts of the brain could cause analgesia which was prevented by injections of naloxone (Liebeskind et al., 1974; Mayer and Hayes, 1975; Mayer and Liebeskind, 1974). These studies suggested a release of an endogenous opiate-like substance. In a search for a substance with morphine-like effects on smooth muscle that could be blocked by naloxone, Hughes and Kosterlitz (Hughes, 1975; Hughes et al., 1975) screened pig brain extracts. After extensive purification, two such morphine-like substances were characterized as pentapeptides and were called "enkephalins." These compounds were also isolated by Simantov and Snyder (1976) from calf brain. One of the enkephalins was found to have the amino acid sequence (Tyr-Gly-Gly-Phe-Met) and was called methionine-enkephalin. The other had the amino acid sequence (Tyr-Gly-Gly-Phe-Leu) and was named leucine-enkephalin. β-Endorphin, a fragment of β-lipoprotein, which is a pituitary peptide, also has a very potent opiate-like effect. The name endorphins was proposed by Simon to denote endogenous morphine-like substances.

The roles of endorphin, leu- and met-enkephalin have not yet been elucidated. At present they are thought to be neurotransmitters or neuromodulators probably involved in pain pathways as well as pathways involving higher mental processes.

These peptides have been demonstrated in rat central nervous system by immunofluorescence (Elde et al., 1976; Hökfelt et al., 1975b; Simantov et al., 1077). In the brain, fluorescence was confined to neurons, as opposed to glia, and was found most intensely in nerve endings where it would be expected to be concentrated if the peptides were acting as neurotransmitters. In our laboratory, we have investigated the changes in substance P and leu-enkephalin in spinal cord transected rats, cats, and monkeys using a sensitive and specific peroxidase-antiperoxidase immunocytochemical method (Abrahams et al., 1978; Naftchi et al., 1978). At varying intervals of time after transection, the distribution and changes of substance P and leu-enkephalin were studied in the spinal cord both above and below the lesion.

In order to assess further the roles of the opiate receptor, substance P, and the enkephalins in spinal pain pathways, we have studied the effects of chronic morphine treatment *in vivo*. Stereospecific opiate receptor binding is reduced in the substantia gelatinosa after dorsal rhizotomy (LaMotte et al., 1976). Conceivably the opiate receptors are associated presynaptically with substance P-containing primary afferent fibers in the substantia gelatinosa. There is further evidence that opiate receptor sites interact with the enkephalins in this region (LaMotte et al., 1976). We have been exploring the neural circuits between these substances to elucidate the interaction between these peptides and their involvement in pre- and post-synaptic and inter-neuronal events.

TRANSECTION OF THE SPINAL CORD

Rats, cats or monkeys were anesthetized with Ketamine or Nembutal. A dorsal laminectomy was performed and the spinal cord was exposed and transected at mid to low thoracic levels. Small pieces of sterile gelfoam were placed between the cut ends of the cord which immediately stopped any bleeding that had occurred. The gelfoam was left in place and the animals were sutured. Animals were not fed or watered for one day following surgery but were allowed to eat and drink ad libitum. Thereafter, their bladders were expressed three times daily.

TISSUE PREPARATION

At varying time intervals after transection, tissue from paraplegic and normal control animals was processed for immunocytochemistry. The animals were anesthetized with Nembutal and sacrificed by perfusion through the ascending aorta with 4 percent paraformaldehyde in 0.1 M phosphate buffer, pH 7.2 for ten minutes. Sections of spinal cord were removed from above and below the lesion and were immediately immersed in picric acid-formaldehyde fixative for about six hours after which time they were cut into smaller pieces. The tissues were then rinsed in phosphate buffered saline for two hours to overnight, dehydrated through a graded series of ethanol solutions, put through several changes of xylene and paraffin and finally embedded in paraffin. Sections were cut at a thickness of 4-5 μm and affixed to albumin-coated glass slides. Once prepared, these slides could be incubated for immunoreactivity at any future time.

ANTISERA

Rabbit antiserum to substance P was generously supplied by Dr. Susan Leeman. Prior to incubation of the tissue, the antiserum was diluted 1:100 with 0.5 M Tris-Saline (pH 7.6) and incubated for two hours at 37°C with rat liver acetone powder (20 mg liver powder per milliliter of diluted serum). This was stored overnight at 4°C and filtered the next morning through a 0.2 μm millipore filter. It was then further diluted with 0.5 M Tris-Saline. Final dilutions used in this series of experiments ranged from 1:400 to 1:1000. Antiserum to leu-enkephalin was prepared by the method of Moore et al. (1977). This was diluted with 0.5 Tris-Saline and used in the dilution range of 1:200 to 1:500.

IMMUNOHISTOCHEMICAL STAINING

The peroxidase-anti-peroxidase immunohistochemical method as first described by Sternberger (1974) and modified by Pickel et al., (1977) was performed on 5 μm tissue sections for localization of substance P and leu-enkephalin in tissues (Naftchi et al., 1978). In some cases, a "double bridge" modification was used which amplified staining (Vacca et al., 1975, 1979).

Nonspecific protein binding was reduced by incubating the sections with 3 percent goat serum in Tris-Saline before they were incubated with anti-substance P or anti-leu-enkephalin antisera for one hour or overnight. Goat anti-rabbit immunoglobulin (Miles Labs) was applied for 30 minutes after two brief rinses with Tris-Saline. Following two more rinses, the PAP reagent (Dako Accurate Chemicals) was applied in 1:25 to 1:50 dilution for 30 minutes. The slides were then incubated for 15-30 minutes with 0.05 percent 3,3'-diaminobenzidine (Sigma) and 0.01 percent hydrogen peroxide solution in Tris buffer (pH 7.6). A brown precipitate was formed characteristic of polymerized diaminobenzidine. The reaction involves the donation of electrons by peroxidase to hydrogen peroxide. The oxidized enzyme is then reduced by diaminobenzidine and, thus, converted to the active form. The oxidative intermediate of diaminobenzidine is polymerized to an insoluble brown precipitate. After several washes in distilled water, the slides were dehydrated and mounted with coverslips.

Sham-operated animals served as controls for paraplegic animals. Tissues from these animals were processed in the same manner as above.

MORPHINE-TREATED ANIMALS

Rats were chronically exposed to morphine sulfate (10 mg/kg, i.p.) for 10 days, and sacrificed by perfusion. Their spinal cords were removed and the tissues were processed as above. Saline-injected animals served as controls.

IMMUNOHISTOCHEMICAL CONTROLS

In order to control for immunohistochemical specificity, normal rabbit serum was routinely substituted for specific rabbit antibody to substance P or leu-enkephalin in all experiments.

The degree of cross-reactivity between the peptide, methionine-enkephalin with antibody to leucine-enkephalin, was assessed by first incubating leu-enkephalin antibody with serial dilutions of either leu- or met-enkephalin antigen prior to application to the slides. It was possible to totally erase the immunoreactive staining when leu-enkephalin was added to the antibody. In the same dilution range, however, negligible staining persisted when met-enkephalin was added to the antibody indicating the presence of slight cross reactivity.

All the sections were examined with a Jena light microscope at magnifications of 25X to 630X.

SUBSTANCE P

Tissue from normal and sham-operated cats and rats (Figures 1a and 1b) displayed peroxide-positive staining which appeared as a band of nerve terminals in the dorsal horn at the junction between the white and gray matters, the substantia gelatinosa which corresponds to laminae II and III of Rexed (1954). Substance P specific staining was also found in Rexed's lamina I.

Two and five days after transection of the spinal cord of the rats and cats, respectively, there was a sharp increase in the amount of substance P below the lesion which had outlined both dorsal horns and bridged the two together. Above the lesion, in the region of the substantia gelatinosa, the number of punctate bodies was fewer and the intensity of staining around the dorsal horn was less than that in sections obtained from below the lesion. This pattern was repeated in sections from chronic cats sacrificed one to 12 weeks and chronic rats one to three weeks following spinal cord transection. Substance P specific immunoreactive staining in sections cut from above the lesion (Figures 2a and 3a) was little compared with the great amount of staining found in sections cut from below the lesion (Figures 2b and 3b). In addition to punctate bodies, long

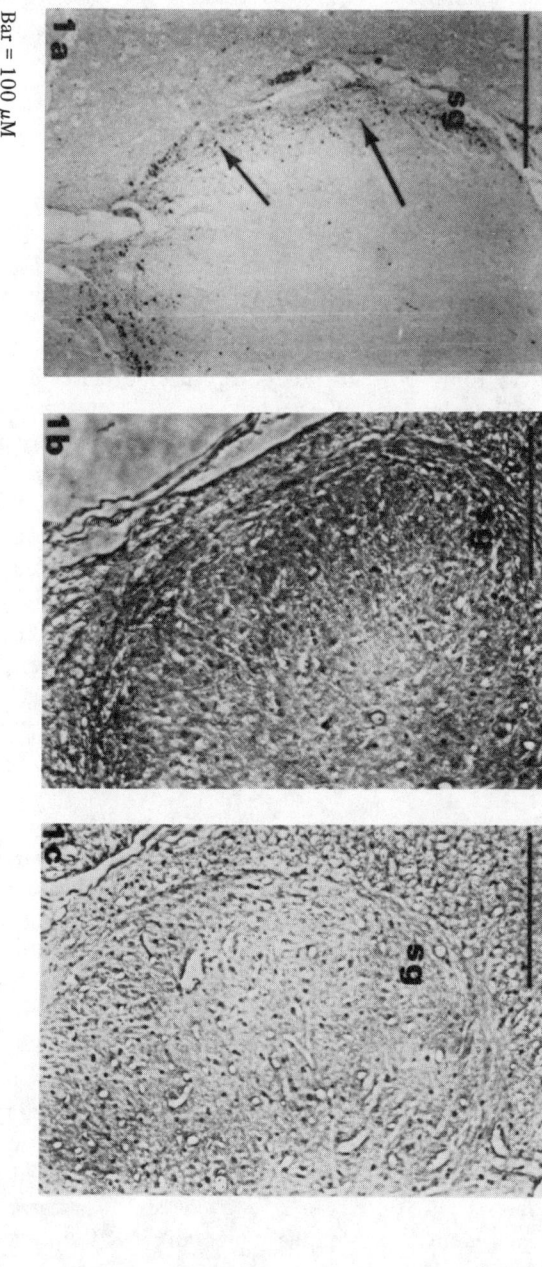

Bar = 100 μM

FIGURE 1a. Section from T 11-12 region of the spinal cord of a sham-operated cat. Arrow points to immunoreactive substance P (SP) specific bodies in dorsal horn (area of substantia gelatinosa, SG). X 200

FIGURE 1b. Phase contrast micrograph of the same dorsal horn region seen in a. The section was incubated for SP immunoreactivity. Note the presence of a dark ring in the SG region, indicating the area of immunoreactivity. X 200

FIGURE 1c. Phase contrast micrograph of the same dorsal horn region seen in a. The section was incubated with normal rabbit serum. Compared with b, the absence of any SP-specific staining is evident. X 200

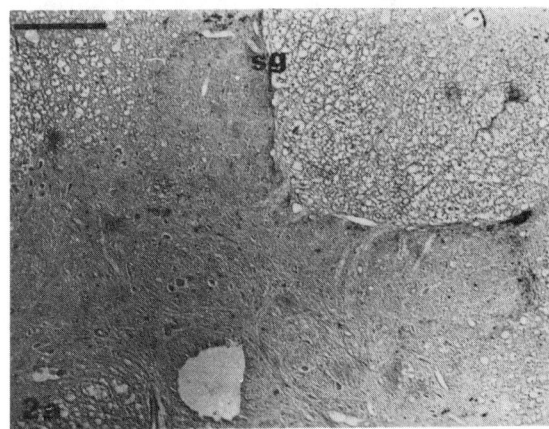

Bar = 100 μM
NOTE: all photographs on this page have been reduced 5% from authors' originals.

FIGURE 2a. Field showing dorsal horns *above* the lesion from a cat transected 5 weeks before perfusion. SG shows slight staining. X 125

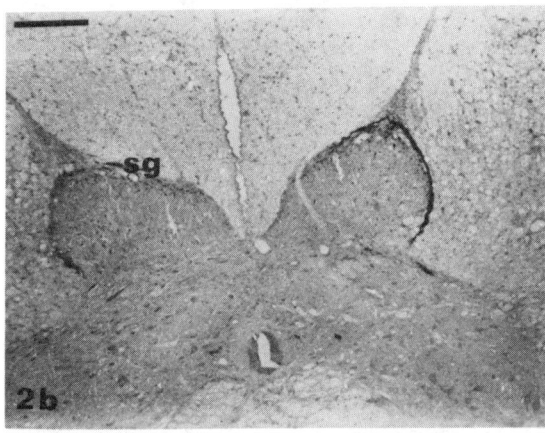

FIGURE 2b. Tissue from the same cat as in Figure 2a sectioned *below* the lesion. Note the intense reaction product delineating both dorsal horns. X 100

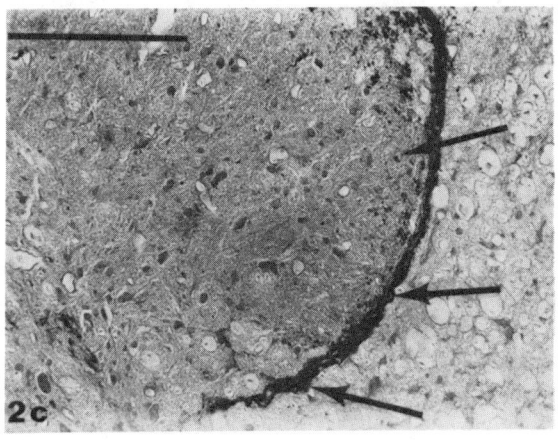

FIGURE 2c. The detail of the SG seen in Figure 2b. Arrows point to darkly stained SP-immunoreactive punctate bodies and an intense band of bead-like varicosities delineating the entire SG. X 250

Bar = 100 μM
NOTE: all photographs on this page have been reduced 48% from authors' originals.

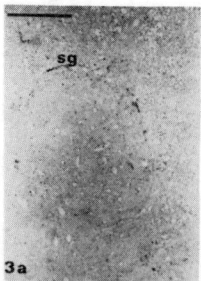
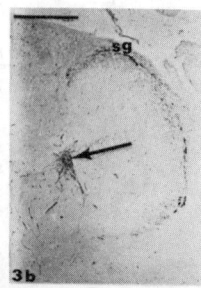

FIGURE 3a. Section from *above* the lesion of a cat transected 12 weeks before sacrifice. Note sparse staining surrounding the dorsal horn in the SG. X 160

FIGURE 3b. Tissue from the same cat as in Figure 3a, sectioned *below* the lesion. The staining of the bank of nerve terminals in the SG is much more intense in this section than that in the section *above* the lesion. Note the appearance of the nerve plexus (arrow) near the center (Lamina V) of the dorsal horn. X 160

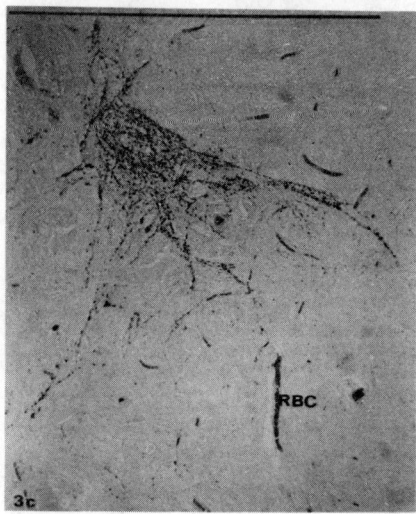

FIGURE 3c. A detail of the nerve plexus from Figure 3b. Immunoreactive substance P appears bead-like, fibrillar varicosities which may be nerve terminals originating from dorsal roots and entering the spinal cord. RBC = red blood cells present in small capillaries. X 960

fibers and varicosities were present in sections taken from below the lesion (figure 2c). A network of fibers located centrally within each dorsal horn (Rexed laminae IV and V) from rats and cats sacrificed three and 12 weeks, respectively, after transection were found to be immunoreactive for substance P (Figures 3b and 3c). Some staining was often seen in the ventral horn in the form of small, dense punctate bodies scattered randomly throughout the horn (Figure 4a). It was difficult to assess whether the amount of staining in the ventral horn changed with time either above or below the lesion. In chronically lesioned monkeys (six months or longer after spinal cord transection) ventral horn and central canal region staining was more prominent compared with cats and rats (Figure 4b). Using a modified PAP method which amplifies immunological staining, especially in sparsely innervated regions (Vacca et al., 1979), ventral horn staining became more prominent in the rat around the motoneurons and other ventral horn cells and along the ventrolateral fringe of the ventral horn (Figure 4c). Additionally, using this modified technique, punctate bodies and subependymal processes were sometimes seen in the central canal region (Figure 4d). In normal rat tissue, sometimes laminae IV and V gave positive staining when the double bridge amplification method was used (Figure 4e).

Substitution of normal serum for immune serum as a control showed no staining in the gray matter of the spinal cord with the exception of red blood cells which contain endogenous peroxidase (Figure 1c). In some specimens, immunoreactive staining did appear in the white matter which could be attributed, in part, to nonspecific affinity of the rabbit serum for the membranes in the regions where the myelin had leached out since the same type of light-brown background staining appeared in control sections where normal rabbit serum was substituted for the specific antiserum. There were, however, some small, immunoreactive, substance P specific, dark punctate bodies present in the myelinated axons of the white matter in the ventrolateral and dorsolateral parts of the spinal cord. This may suggest rostral axonal flow of substance P within myelinated fibers possibly belonging to lateral spinothalamic tracts or to shorter tracts concerned with segmental transmission. In monkey tissue additional white matter staining appeared to be selective for substance P; ventral white matter was bilaterally stained in a uniform, symmetrical pattern which extended to the ventrolateral white region (Figure 4f).

EFFECT OF MORPHINE ON SUBSTANCE P IMMUNOREACTIVITY

Immunocytochemical examination of the rats treated chronically (10 days) with morphine sulfate revealed a non-uniform increase in substance P in certain regions of the spinal cord compared with tissue from saline-treated rats (Figure 5). Substance P was increased in the substantia gelatinosa, Rexed's laminae I, IV and V, and the ventral horn around the medial and lateral groups of moto-

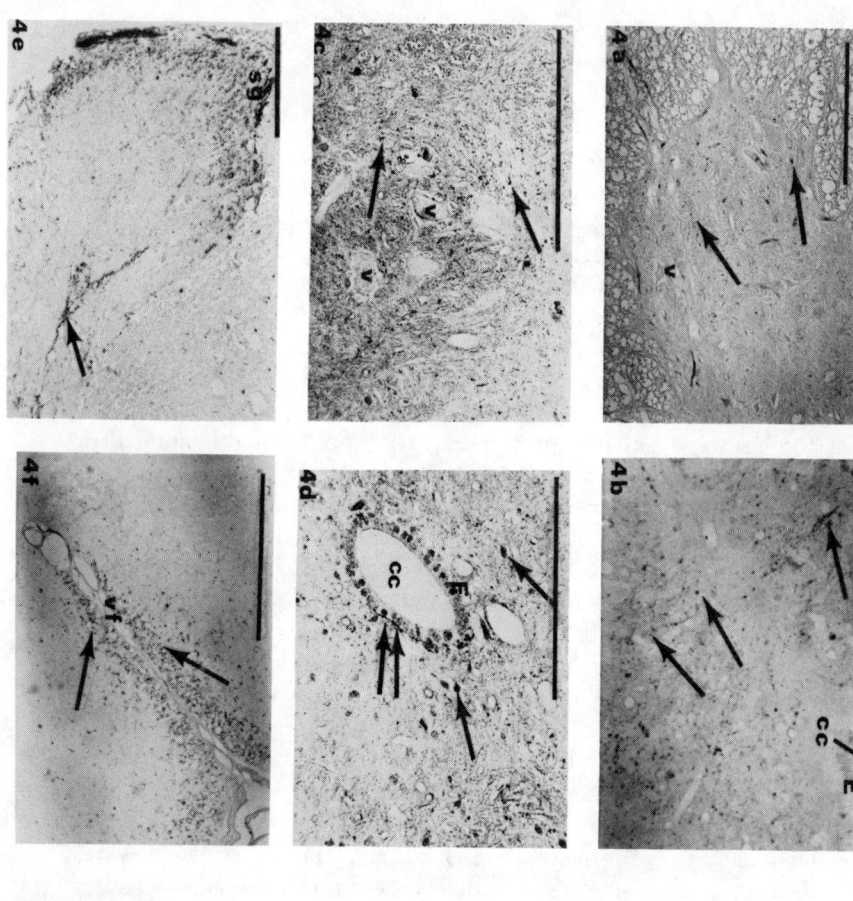

Bar = 100 μM
NOTE: all photographs on this page have been reduced 28% from authors' originals.

FIGURE 4a. Section of the ventral horn from below the lesion of a cat transected 5 weeks before sacrifice. Ventral horn cells (V) are present. Arrows point to immunopositive bodies that are scattered throughout. X 250

FIGURE 4b. Section of the area lateral and ventral to the central canal (CC) of a sham-operated monkey. Arrows point to a few of the large number of immunopositive bodies present. Endothelial cells (E) surround the CC. X 300

FIGURE 4c. Section of normal rat ventral horn to which the double bridge PAP method was applied. Arrows point to immunopositive punctate bodies. Ventral horn cells (V) are present. X 400

FIGURE 4d. Section of normal rat central canal area to which the double bridge PAP method was applied. A fiber (double arrow) which abuts on the ependymal cells (E) appears positively stained. Many stained punctate bodies are present (arrows). X 400

FIGURE 4e. Section from a normal rat dorsal horn area stained by the double bridge PAP method showing SP localization in lamina V (arrow) as well as in the SG. X 200

FIGURE 4f. Area showing the ventral fissure (VF) of the spinal cord of a 4 week transected monkey. Small bodies (arrows) which appear positively stained for SP bilaterally ring the fissure in the ventral white matter. X 300

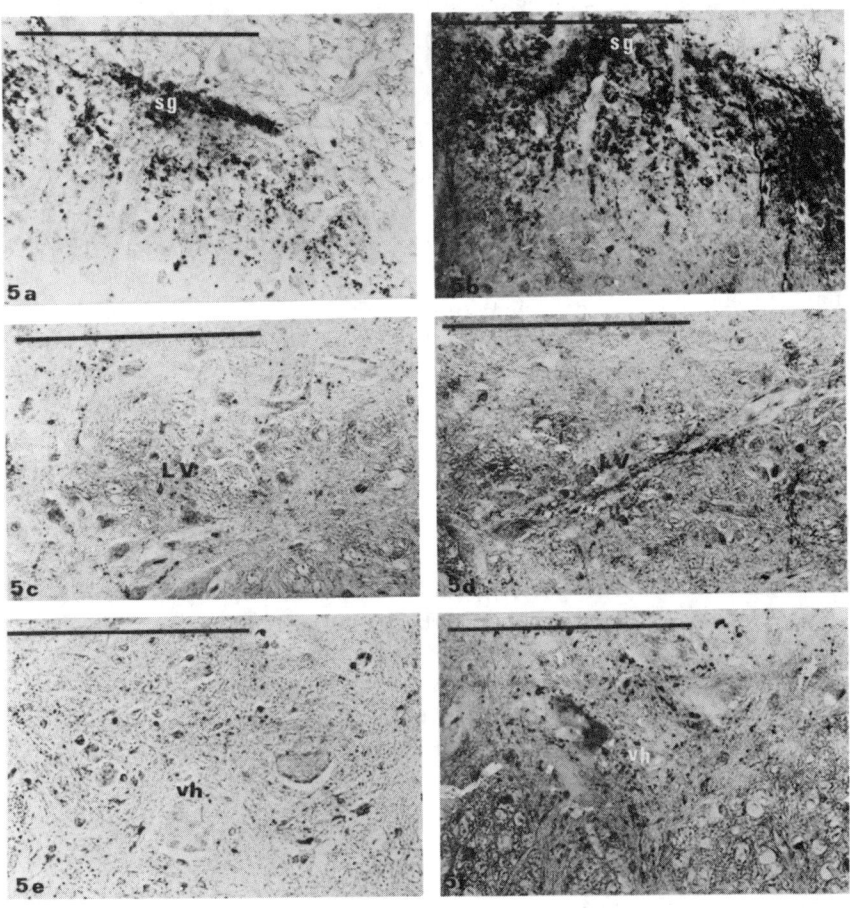

Bar = 100 μM
NOTE: all photographs on this page have been reduced 35% from authors' originals.

FIGURE 5. Tissue from rats chronically injected with morphine, 10 mg/kg for 10 days, compared with saline-injected controls. The double bridge PAP method was used.
FIGURE 5a is a section of the SG region of the dorsal horn of a saline control.
FIGURE 5b is a comparable section from a morphine-treated animal.
FIGURE 5c is a section through lamina V (LV) of the dorsal horn of a saline control.
FIGURE 5d is a comparable section from a morphine-treated animal.
FIGURE 5e is a section of the ventral horn (VH) from a saline control.
FIGURE 5f is a comparable section from a morphine-treated animal.
At each of these levels (Dorsal horn, lamina V, ventral horn) there is more immunoreactivity in the morphine-treated animals than in the saline control. X 500

neurons and traveling along the ventral roots. Substance P, however, did not increase within processes found around the central canal.

LEUCINE-ENKEPHALIN

Spinal cord sections from sham-operated cats taken from the T5 region displayed a pattern of immunoreactive bodies in the substantia gelatinosa (Figure 6a), a fairly dense region lateral and dorsal to the central canal (Figure 6c), and a substantial scattering of immunoreactive bodies throughout the entire ventral horn (Figure 7a). In the substantia gelatinosa of the cat spinal cord, specific leu-enkephalin immunoreactivity in the sections from below the level of the lesion was never as great as that found in comparable tissue sections reacted for substance P.

In contrast to substance P, there was no apparent difference in the amount or distribution of staining with time after spinal cord transection, nor was there any difference in immunoreactivity above or below the level of the lesion (Figure 6b).

The immunoreactive substance was mostly in the shape of punctate bodies, many of which were present in the substantia gelatinosa. Stained varicosities were often seen extending for short distances into the dorsal white matter (Figure 6b). In the ventral horn, long fibrous elements were present which seemed to extend to the ventral horn cells after stretching a distance within the gray matter (Figure 7a). Some long bead-like fibrillar processes were also seen extending a long distance from gray to white matters (Figure 7b). In some instances immunoreactive fibers appeared to run for some distance along the ventral root fibers into the white matter (Figure 7c). A great deal of immunoreactivity was visualized both dorsal and lateral to the central canal region, mostly in the form of varicosities (Figures 6c and 6d).

No specific immunoreactivity was present when normal serum was substituted for immunoserum or when leu-enkephalin antiserum was preincubated with the peptide leu-enkephalin.

The abundance of substance P immunoreactive nerve terminals in the substantia gelatinosa suggests that substance P is contained in the primary afferent fibers which penetrate the substantia gelatinosa and dorsolateral funiculus radially and terminate in the dorsal horn. These regions are classically associated with pain transmission. Additionally, some SP-containing processes penetrated the intermediate gray regions and extended to the heavily innervated lamina V region and the ventral horn.

Otsuka et al., (1975) ligated the dorsal roots of the cat and found that substance P concentration increased on the ganglion side of the ligature and decreased centrally. The findings suggested that substance P was synthesized in dorsal root ganglia and its presence in afferent fibers suggested a role in neuro-

Bar = 100 µM
NOTE: *all photographs on this page have been reduced 26% from authors' originals.*

FIGURE 6a. Section showing part of the dorsal horn region of the spinal cord at T 11-12 of a sham-operated cat. Immunoreactive leucine-enkephalin (LE) specific bodies outline the SG. X 200

FIGURE 6b. Section showing the SG from *below* the lesion of a cat transected 2 weeks before sacrifice. The amount of immunoreactive LE-specific bodies is comparable to Figure 3a. Immunoreactivity is also present in fibers (arrows) extending into the white matter. X 200

FIGURE 6c. Region around the central canal (CC) area of a sham-operated cat. Many immunoreactive bodies (arrows) are seen in the region. X 200

FIGURE 6d. Region lateral to the central canal in a sham-operated cat. LE positive punctate bodies as well as a beaded fiber (arrow) are seen. Red blood cells (RBC) in a small vessel are present. X 500

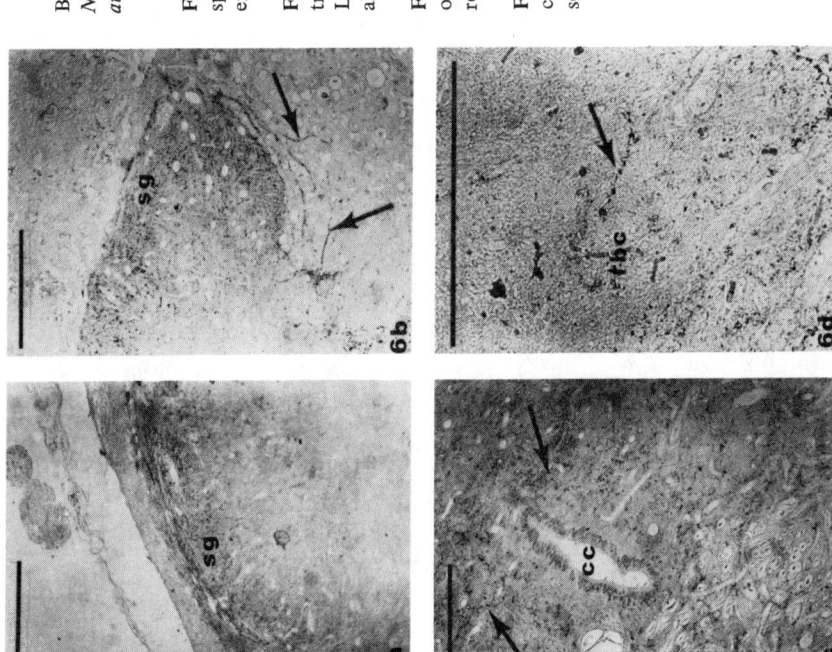

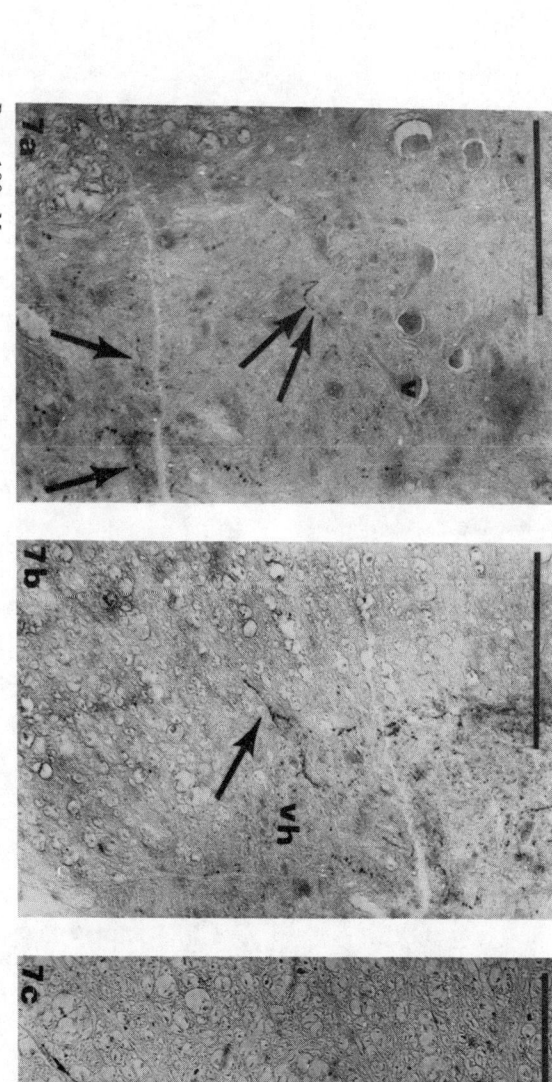

Bar = 100 μM

FIGURE 7a. Field from the ventral horn of a sham-operated cat. Ventral horn cells (V) are present. LE positive fibers (arrows) can be noted and at one point (double arrow) seem to surround one of the ventral horn cells. X 250

FIGURE 7b. Field showing LE immunopositive bodies at the edge of the ventral horn (VH) in a sham-operated cat. Arrow points to a stained branching fiber extending into the white matter. X 250

FIGURE 7c. Long, distinct LE immunopositive fibers (arrows), extending well into the white matter, appear to travel along with the ventral root fibers that exit from the ventral horn (VH) in this section taken from a sham-operated cat. X 250 transmission. Iontophoretic application of substance P to spinal neurons by Henry (Henry, 1976; Henry et al., 1975) produced a strong but slow and prolonged excitatory action on nearly half the neurons tested in the lumbar spinal cord of the cat. It is noteworthy that all units excited by substance P were also excited by noxious thermal stimulation of the skin. The highest number of units excited by substance P was found in lamina VI and the lowest in lamina IV. In two cases, treatment with substance P led to a response to noxious heat by units which had previously been unresponsive to thermal stimulation. Henry suggested, therefore, that substance P may be involved specifically in afferent units associated with pain sensation. Hökfelt also observed that substance P-containing fibers in peripheral afferent nerves are unmyelinated and that in the skin these fibers terminate in free nerve endings usually associated with pain transmission (Hökfelt et al., 1975a, 1975b).

Using immunohistochemical techniques for localization of substance P, our finding of extensive staining of the nerve plexus in lamina V below the lesion (Figures 3b and 3c) shows the presence of a network of varicosities in the nerve endings in the area classically known to be concerned with noxious transmission. Lamina V networks were never observed in the sections above the lesion. The results demonstrate accumulation of substance P below the lesion and suggest its rostral direction by axoplasmic flow in the spinal cord.

The slow time course of substance P action by Henry et al., (1975) was incompatible with a role as the main excitatory transmitter of primary afferent terminals, but its strong excitatory action might have functional significance as sensitizer or modulator over a long period. Recently, Pickel et al., (1977) using immunocytochemical techniques, reported that within axon terminals substance P appeared to be associated with one type of organelle, a large, round vesicle 60-80 nm in diameter. In addition, in the same axon terminal, small, unlabeled vesicles were also present. It is generally accepted that such small vesicles serve as storage sites for most neurotransmitters. This finding further supports the suggestion that substance P may act as a modulator rather than the neurotransmitter initiating synaptic events.

Konishi and Otsuka (1974) showed that on the isolated frog spinal cord preparation, substance P was about 200 times more active on a molar basis than L-Glutamate in depolarizing spinal motoneurons. The depolarizing action persisted after synaptic transmission was blocked by Ca++ deficient Ringer's solution or by tetrodotoxin. They concluded, therefore, that substance P exerted a transsynaptic action on motoneurons and was probably a candidate for the excitatory transmitter of primary sensory neurons. In our work, immunoreactive susbstance P endings could often be seen in close association with motoneurons.

Our data concur with those of other investigators, suggesting a pathway for substance P starting from the dorsal root ganglion via primary afferent fibers toward their terminals in the dorsal horn of the spinal cord. It further extends the work by demonstrating that substance P accumulates in the dorsolateral part of the dorsal horn below the level of the lesion indicating an upward flow of this peptide in the spinal cord in contrast to the downward movement from the brain stem of monoamine transmitters by axoplasmic flow (Dahlstrom, 1971; Naftchi et al., 1974). Although our data indicate an anterograde direction of substance P in the spinal cord it does not elucidate whether it arises in the collaterals of primary afferent fibers or in second order fibers.

It was of interest to note the presence of some fibers stained for substance P in the ventral horn. The amount of immunoreactive product appeared to remain constant above and below transection suggesting that the substance P fibers in the ventral horn are involved in spinal segmental transmission. The cellular origin of these fibers is not known at present, nor is the relationship between these processes in the ventral gray matter and those which appear more dorsally understood. However, there are indications that they may derive from the processes which enter the intermediate gray regions (Vacca et al., 1979). Such considerations, while speculative, may implicate substance P in mechanisms of visceral pain. The fact that other substance P fibers cross in the dorsal gray commissure, a region which also contains sympathetic innervation, lends credence to this idea.

The immunocytochemical findings from morphine-treated rats demonstrate that the concentration of intraneuronal substance P increased in three regions of the spinal cord: the substantia gelatinosa plus Rexed's lamina I, Rexed's lamina IV and V, and the ventral horn. The data suggest that morphine analgesia inhibits the release of intra-neuronal substance P. Inhibition of substance P release has been demonstrated in slices of trigeminal nucleus *in vitro* (Jessel and Iverson, 1977). Furthermore, by immunocytochemistry, we have shown that morphine blocks the release of substance P in certain regions of the spinal cord which are specifically associated with pain transmission: the substantia gelatinosa and lamina V. Similarly, these regions accumulate substance P below the level of spinal cord transection. Yaksh (1978) has shown that lamina V neurons in the dorsal horn are discharged by the application of noxious stimuli to their receptive fields and by $A\delta$ and C fiber activation. Administration of narcotics in doses sufficient to produce analgesia will depress these discharges. Previously, LaMotte et al., (1976) demonstrated that opiate binding, which is high in the substantia gelatinosa, was reduced when the dorsal roots were cut. This finding implies that opiate receptors which bind morphine occur on primary afferent fibers (from the dorsal root ganglion), some of which contain substance P. They thus hypothesized that their data indicated that the opiate receptors are presynaptic, and can thereby block the release of a pain transmitter such as substance P.

In addition to causing an accumulation of substance P in the substantia gelatinosa and in lamina V, morphine treatment also resulted in a buildup of substance P in the ventral horn. This phenomenon raises questions concerning the relationship of the ventral horn fibers with pain transmission. After morphine

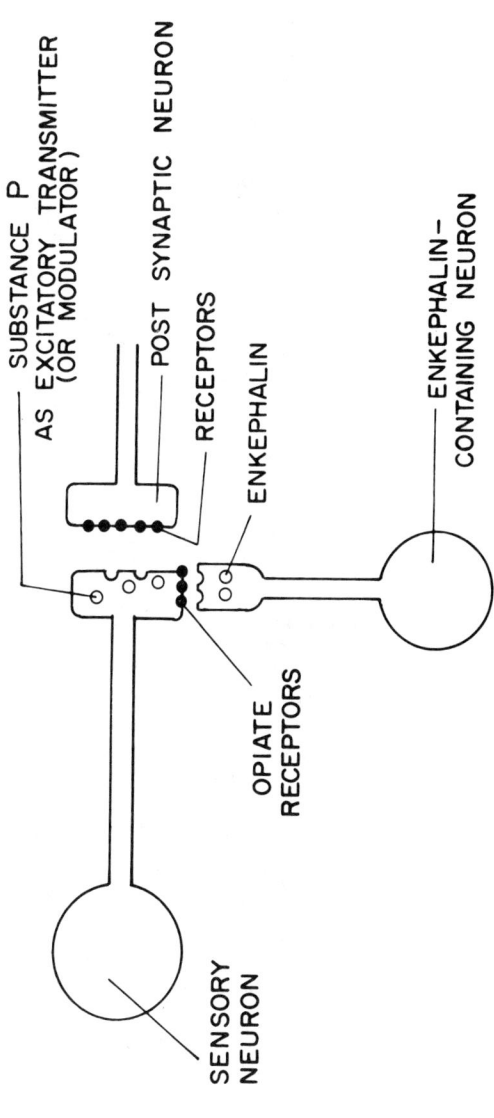

Bar = 100 μM

FIGURE 8. A hypothetical model of presynaptic inhibition of substance P action by enkephalinergic inhibitory interneurons. Enkephalin released from an interneuron would bind to opiate receptors present on the terminal of a sensory neuron, preventing its release of substance P and thereby disrupting the transmission of pain.

treatment, however, certain other substance P containing processes which appeared around the central canal, crossing in the dorsal gray commissure, and subependymally did not differ from those in the controls.

Such differential effects may reflect regional differences in numbers and types of opiate receptors, or in their pre- and post-synaptic locations. More detailed dose response and opiate binding studies are in progress.

Work by Hökfelt et al., (1977) has correlated enkephalin-positive nerve terminals in areas where morphine is known to produce behaviorial analgesia. In the spinal cord, these regions also contain high concentrations of substance P. In our studies, spinal cord transection did not produce any changes in the concentration of leu-enkephalin-positive nerve terminals. These findings confirm Hökfelt's results which have demonstrated that enkephalin-containing cells are probably interneurons within the spinal cord.

These data implicate the mutual involvement of substance P, a probable pain transmitter, and leu-enkephalin, an endogenous opiate, in the transmission of pain and control of pain and analgesia, as illustrated in the following neural circuit (Figure 8). The scheme depicts enkephalin-containing interneurons impinging upon primary afferent neurons which contain substance P. Enkephalin, like morphine, binds to the pre-synaptic opiate receptors, thereby preventing the release of the pain transmitter. This mechanism provides a working hypothesis for the control of pain by natural physiological substances.

REFERENCES

Abrahams, S.J., Naftchi, N.E., St. Paul, H.M., Lowman, E.W., and Schlosser, W. (1978): Localization and changes in substance P and leu-enkephalin in spinal cord of paraplegic cats. *Fed. Proc. 37:* 439.
Atweh, S.F. and Kuhar, M.J. (1977): Autoradiographic localization of opiate receptors in rat brain. I. Spinal cord and lower medulla. *Brain Res. 124:* 53-67.
Brownstein, M.J., Mroz, E.A., Kizer, J.S., Palkovits, M., and Leeman, S.E. (1976): Regional distribution of substance P in the brain of the rat. *Brain Res. 116:* 229-305.
Chang, M.M. and Leeman, S.E. (1970): Isolation of a sialogogic peptide from bovine hypothalamic tissue and its characterization as substance P. *J. Biol. Chem. 245:* 4787-4790.
Chang, M.M., Leeman, S.E., and Niall, H.D. (1971): Amino acid sequence of substance P. *Nature New Biol. 232:* 86-87.
Cuello, A.C., Polak, J.M., and Pearse, A.G.E. (1976): Substance P: a naturally occurring transmitter in human spinal cord. *Lancet:* 1054-1056, Nov. 13.
Dahlstrom, A. (1971): Axoplasmic transport. *Phil. Trans. B. 261:* 325-358.
Elde, R., Hökfelt, T., Johansson, O., and Terenius, L. (1976): Immunohistochemical studies using antibodies to leucine-enkephalin: initial observations on the nervous system of the rat. *Neuroscience 1:* 349-351.
Henry, J.L. (1976): Effects of substance P on functionally identified units in cat spinal cord. *Brain Res. 114:* 439-451.
Henry, J.L., Krnjević, K., and Morris, M.E. (1975): Substance P and spinal neurones. *Canad. J. Physiol. Pharmacol. 53:* 423-432.

Hiller, J.M., Pearson, J., and Simon, E.J. (1973): Distribution of stereospecific binding of the potent narcotic analgesic etorphine in the human brain; predominance in the limbic system. *Res. Commun. in Chem. Pathol. and Pharm. 6:* 1052-1062.

Hökfelt, T., Kellerth, J.O., Nillson, G., and Pernow, B. (1975): Substance P: localization in the central nervous system and some primary sensory neurons. *Science 190:* 889-890.

Hökfelt, T., Kellerth, J.O., Nillson, G., and Pernow, B. (1975): Experimental immunohistochemical studies on the localization and distribution of substance P in cat primary sensory neurons. *Brain. Res. 100:* 235-252.

Hökfelt, T., Ljungdahl, A., Terenius, L., Elde, R., and Nillson, G. (1977): Immunohistochemical analysis of peptide pathways possibly related to pain and analgesia: enkephalin and substance P. *Proc. Nat. Acad. Sci. 74:* 3081-3085.

Hughes, J. (1975): Isolation of an endogenous compound from the brain with properties similar to morphine. *Brain Res. 88:* 295-308.

Hughes, J., Smith, T., Kosterlitz, H.W., Fothergill, L.A., Morgan, B., and Morris, H.R. (1975): Identification of two related pentapeptides from the brain with potent opiate agonist activity. *Nature 258:* 577-579.

Jessel, J.M. and Iverson, L. (1977): Opiate analgesics inhibit substance P release from rat trigeminal nucleus. *Nature 268:* 549-551.

Kanazawa, I. and Jessel, I (1976): Post mortem changes and regional distribution of substance P in the rat and mouse nervous system. *Brain Res. 117:* 362-367.

Konishi, S. and Otsuka, M. (1974): The effects of substance P and other peptides on spinal neurons of the frog. *Brain Res. 65:* 397-410.

Kuhar, M.J., Pert, C.B., and Snyder, S.H. (1975): Regional distribution of opiate receptor in rat brain. *Life Sci. 16:* 1849-1854.

LaMotte, C., Pert, C.B., and Snyder, S.H. (1976): Opiate receptor binding in primate spinal cord: distribution and changes after dorsal root section. *Brain Res. 112:* 407-412.

Liebeskind, J.C., Mayer, D.J., and Akil, H. (1974): Central mechanisms of pain inhibition: studies of analgesia from focal brain stimulation. In: J.J. Bonica (Ed.), *Advances in Neurology,* Vol. 4. International Symposium on Pain, Raven Press, New York. p. 261-268.

Mayer, D.J. and Hayes, R. (1975): Stimulation-produced analgesia: development of tolerance and cross-tolerance to morphine. *Science 188:* 941-943.

Mayer, D.J. and Liebeskind, J.C. (1975): Pain reduction by focal electrical stimulation of the brain: an anatomical and behavioral analysis. *Brain Res. 68:* 73-93.

Moore, G., Lutterodt, A., Burford, G., and Lederis, K. (1977): A highly specific antiserum for arginine vasopressin. *Endocrinology 101:* 1421-1435.

Naftchi, N.E., Demeny, M., Kertesz, A., Viau, A.T., and Lowman, E.W. (1974): Effect of spinal cord transection on mammalian biogenic amines, c-AMP, and tyrosine hydroxylase activity in CNS, adrenals and heart. *Trans. Amer. Soc. Neurochem 5:* 80.

Naftchi, N.E., Abrahams, S.J., St. Paul, H., Lowman, E.W., and Schlosser, W. (1978): Localization and changes of substance P in spinal cord of paraplegic cats. *Brain Res. 153:* 507-513.

Otsuka, M., Konishi, S. and Takahashi, T. (1975): Hypothalamic substance P as a candidate for transmitter of primary afferent neurons. *Fed. Proc. 34:* 1922-1928.

Pert, C.B. and Snyder, S.H. (1973): Opiate receptor: demonstration in nervous tissue. *Science 179:* 1011-1014.

Pert, C.B., Kuhar, M.J., and Snyder, S.H. (1976): Opiate receptor: autoradiographic localization in rat brain. *Proc. Nat. Acad. Sci. 73:* 3729-3733.

Pickel, V.M., Reis, D.J., and Leeman, S.E. (1977): Ultrastructural localization of substance P in neurons of rat spinal cord. *Brain Res. 122:* 534-540.

Powell, D., Leeman, S., Tregear, G.W., Niall, H.D., and Potts, J.T. (1973): Radioimmunoassay for substance P. *Nature New Biol. 241:* 252-254.

Rexed, B. (1954): A cytoarchitectonic atlas of the spinal cord in the cat. *J. Comp. Neurol. 100:* 297-379.

Simantov, R. and Snyder, S.H. (1976): Morphine-like peptides in mammalian brain: isolation, structure, elucidation and interaction with the opiate receptor. *Proc. Nat. Acad. Sci. 73:* 2515-2519.

Simantov, R., Kuhar, M.J., Uhl, G.R., and Snyder, S.H. (1977): Opioid peptide enkephalin: immunohistochemical mapping in the rat central nervous system. *Proc. Nat. Acad. Sci. 74:* 2167-2171.

Simon, E.J. (1976): The opiate receptors. *Neurochem. Res. 1:* 3-28.

Simon, E.J., Hiller, J.M., and Edelman, I. (1973): Stereospecific binding of the potent narcotic analgesic ^{3}H-etorphine to rat brain homogenate. *Proc. Nat. Acad. Sci. 70:* 1947-1949.

Sternberger, L. (1974): *Immunocytochemistry*. Prentice-Hall, Englewood Cliffs, New Jersey.

Terenius, L. (1973): Stereospecific interaction between narcotic analgesics and a synaptic plasma membrane fraction of rat cerebral cortex. *Acta Pharmacol. Toxicol. 32:* 317-320.

Vacca, L.L., Rosario, S., Zimmerman, E.A., Tomachefsky, P., Ng, P.-Y., and Hsu, K.G. (1975): Application of immunoperoxidase techniques to localize horseradish peroxidase tracer in the central nervous system. *J. Histochem. Cytochem. 23:* 208.

Vacca, L.L., Abrahams, S.J. and Naftchi, N.E. (1979): A modified peroxidase anti-peroxidase procedure for improved localization of tissue antigens: localization of substance P in rat spinal cord. *J. Histochem. Cytochem.* (Submitted).

Von Euler, U.S. and Gaddum, J.H. (1931): An unidentified depressor substance in certain tissue extracts. *J. Physiol. 72:* 74-87.

Yaksh, T.L. (1978): Opiate receptors for behavioral analgesia resemble those related to the depression of spinal nociceptive neurons. *Science 199:* 1231-1232.

8

Gilles De La Tourette's Syndrome: An Overview

L. Valzelli

INTRODUCTION

Our knowledge of neuropsychiatric diseases is still unsatisfactory, despite the considerable technological advances made in the field of medical science. This situation occurs mainly as a result of the obvious impossibility of directly examining the human nervous system; this results in a recurrent controversy between psychological and organic approaches to the study of neuropsychiatric disorders. The situation is illustrated by the explanation of the origin of tics. Tics are brief, involuntary, and purposeless movements of a body part, occurring at random intervals and continuing for varying lengths of time. They were believed to be psychogenic in origin by Wilson (1927), while others have suggested developmental (Balthasar, 1957) or inflammatory disorders (Creak and Gurrman, 1935) of the basal ganglia as possible causes.

There has been considerable interest of late in re-examination of some clinical entities whose psychological and organic components have not been clearly established. One such example, in the field of tics, is the Gilles De la Tourette's syndrome. A review of the pertinent literature indicates that, because of the protean characteristics, this disease being intermittently shifted between the disciplines of psychology and medicine (Abuzzahab and Anderson, 1973; Alliez and Audon, 1977). Gilles De la Tourette's syndrome was initially believed to be and was described as a rare, sporadic condition but its incidence is now rapidly increasing, so that its rarity today can be questioned. In this framework, clinical interest in Tourette's syndrome now also lies in the fact that an early and correct diagnosis will minimize the harmful effects imposed by a delay in the administration of available pharmacotherapy.

SYMPTOMATOLOGICAL PROFILE

Gilles De la Tourette's syndrome is classically listed among the atypical psychoses as an idiopathic syndrome of rare occurrence (Lehmann, 1975). It was sometimes referred to as *tic convulsif* by French clinicians and in the German literature as *mimische Krampfneurose*. This uncommon disorder was described in detail in 1825 by Itard, who reported the very first case. Sixty years later, however, De la Tourette (1885) gave a further account of nine cases and established the configuration of the disease syndromes in the form known at the present.

The characteristic features of the syndrome are:
(a) the onset of symptoms in childhood, usually in children between the ages of 2 and 14 years, and generally not beyond the 18th year of age, with males outnumbering females in a ratio of three or four to one (Shapiro et al., 1972).
(b) multiple motor tics, and sudden involuntary and purposeless movements, which may include vulgar gestures *(copropraxia)* and compulsive touching;
(c) vocal tics, consisting in explosive, involuntary and repetitive utterances, including both inarticulate noises (barks, yelps, grunts, coughs) and articulated obscenities *(coprolalia)*; and
(d) imitative phenomena, either verbal *(echolalia)* or behavioral *(echopraxia)* (Fernando, 1967, 1976; Goforth, 1974; Perera, 1975; Pollack et al., 1977; Sarteschi, 1956; Sweet et al., 1973; Woodrow, 1974).

Diagnosis is commomly based on the presence of items (b) and (c), since almost all patients present both motor and verbal tics. Coprolalia develops in about half the patients, while echopraxia and echolalia are present in approximately 20 percent of cases. Copropraxia remains confined to a minority of subjects.

In more than one-third up to half of the patients, either compulsive or phobic-obsessive, components are clearly present (Abuzzahab and Anderson, 1976; Charcot, 1899; De la Tourette, 1899; Penna and Lion, 1975; Walsh, 1962; Yaryura-Tobias, 1975, 1979; Yaryura-Tobias and Neziroglu, 1977). Further, overtly hostile and violent behavior has been recently reported in more than half of the case studies (Moldofsky et al., 1974; Yaryura-Tobias and Neziroglu, 1977), including self-destructive and auto-mutilative behavior (Van Woert et al., 1976). Finally, left-handedness has been found in some 35 percent of patients (Shapiro et al., 1972), whereas left-handed individuals are calculated as normally representing from 5 to 10 percent of the general population (Hecaen and de Ajuriaguerra, 1964).

EPIDEMIOLOGY

Estimates of the occurrence and frequency of Tourette's syndrome vary enormously. This variability very likely depends either on the still limited number of cases reported in the world literature or on the large number of undiagnosed cases. Accordingly, estimates vary from 0.25 to 4 cases per 100,000 population (Woodrow, 1974). Patients with Tourette's syndrome have been reported in England, France, Italy, Germany, Finland, Ireland, Japan, Australia and other countries, but sixty-seven percent of the patients studied by Shapiro et al., (1972) had an East European Jewish ethnic background.

As already stated, the disorder is recognized as occurring more frequently in males than in females, with a ratio of approximately 3.5 to 1 (Challas et al., 1967; Corbett et al., 1969; Fernando, 1968; Lucas, 1970; Lucas et al., 1967; Shapiro et al., 1972).

DIFFERENTIAL DIAGNOSIS

Frequent reference has been made to some similarities between Tourette's disease and analogous cross-cultural syndromes such as "latah" (Malaysia), "myriachit," "the jumpers of Maine" (United States), "Saint Vito's dance" (Italy), "imubacco" (Japan), "piblokto" (Arctic hysteria, Eskimos), and possibly others (Aberle, 1952; Beard, 1880; Chapel, 1970; De la Tourette, 1884, 1885; Hammond, 1884, 1892; Lehmann, 1975; Mazur, 1953). These syndromes have in common a startle response, with echolalia, echopraxia, automatic obedience and sometimes coprolalia, but unlike Tourette's syndrome, they are induced by an external startling stimulus, none has motor or verbal tics, and their onset is after adolescence.

Disorders of infancy and childhood like Huntington's chorea, Sydenham's chorea, Pelizaeus-Merzbacher disease, tics of childhood, and others, are easily differentiated, mostly on the basis of the characteristics of the movement disorder and the absence of vocal tics (Bruun and Shapiro, 1972). Consequently, the consensus is that Gilles De la Tourette's syndrome evidently comprises a separate entity (Chapel, 1970; Eisemberg et al., 1959).

COURSE

The syndrome has a notably consistent course, with onset at a mean age of seven, with 85 percent of cases beginning before ten years of age (Corbett et al., 1969; Fernando, 1968; Moldofsky, 1971; Shapiro et al., 1972).

Although exceptions can obviously be found, the progression of symptoms tends to be cephalocaudal. Nevertheless, since in the course of time the symptoms may change insidiously, initial symptoms being retained or gradually lost and substituted by new ones, the patent or his family often report an inaccurate account of symptom progression.

The first symptoms are usually simple movements most frequently involving the face, nose, head, and shoulders. Then eyelid blinking, facial twitching, grimaces, and purposeless neck movements become evident. Later, movements of the shoulders, in form of sudden shoulder raising or rapid "shrugging" movements, sudden movement of upper extremities and chest appear, with the lower extremities last to be involved, if at all (Bruun and Shapiro, 1972; Fernando, 1968, 1976; Shapiro et al., 1972; Sweet et al., 1973). The movements, usually brief and explosive (Stevens, 1964), may sometimes be more complex and may include slapping the face, wringing the hands, jumping, squatting, kicking, hitting, repetitively touching various objects, touching or kissing people, and many others (Bruun and Shapiro, 1972; Corbett et al., 1969; Fernando, 1968; Eisenberg et al., 1959).

Vocal tics, sounds or words, eventually appear in all patients from months to years after the earliest symptoms. Generally they first become evident as inarticulate sounds, varying from explosive noises, throat clearing, snorting, to barking, grunting and yelping, and superficially resemble animal noises or nonsense sounds. The last verbal symptom that appears in only slightly more than 50 percent of patients, is the explosive utterance of obscenities (Bruun and Shapiro, 1972; Chapel, 1966; Fernando, 1976). Such forced shouting of obscenities, or coprolalia, not a necessary component of the syndrome, may last for only brief periods of the illness, one third of patients also showing spontaneous remission of this symptom. It may be of interest to observe that mental coprolalia, or compulsive thoughts of obscene terms, can occur in absence of verbal coprolalia (Bruun and Shapiro, 1972), and that verbal coprolalia has been observed in patients as young as four years old (Shapiro et al., 1973 a). Vocal tics or even coprolalia may sometimes be the starting symptoms of the syndrome. Imitative speech (echolalia) and movements (echopraxia) may occasionally occur.

Motor and vocal tics may be minimally influenced by voluntary efforts at inhibition. The entire symtomatology is characteristically reduced under circumstances of fairly relaxed emotional conditions, and is entirely absent during sleep (Sarteschi, 1956). The symptoms commonly increase in frequency and intensity with anxiety states, anger, fear, or prolonged periods of emotional stress, while voluntarily inhibiting them frequently causes the explosion of other symptoms (Ascher, 1948; Bruun and Shapiro, 1972; Challas et al., 1967; Field et al., 1966). Compulsive, phobic, and obsessive components, especially in the form of dwelling on intrusive thoughts, doubting, double-checking, rituals, repetitive touching of objects or persons have been reported as always associated with the syndrome, even when not overt (Ascher, 1948; Corbett, 1971; Eldridge et al., 1977; Milman, 1975; Penna and Lion, 1975; Walsh, 1962; Yaryura-Tobias, 1975, 1979). Furthermore in from 40 to 65 percent of the cases, hostile-violent and/or self-destructive behavior has been observed (Modolfsky et al., 1974; Van Woert et al., 1976; Yaryura-Tobias and Neziroglu, 1977).

The entire syndrome is characterized by alternating waxing and waning, and although its course is usually progressive, it has been said that it may stop at any stage (Mazur, 1953), and spontaneous complete remissions have been reported (Challas et al., 1967; Fernando, 1968; Mazur, 1953). It has also been reported that patients may show intellectual impairment (Moldolfsky et al., 1974), though others maintain that mental and neurologic deterioration does not occur, nor is the outcome psychosis (Bruun and Shapiro, 1972; De la Tourette, 1885; Lucas, 1970; Shapiro et al., 1972).

ETIOLOGY

The prime cause of Tourette's syndrome is still unknown, and there has been widespread speculation about possible precipitating factors. Nevertheless, a certain number of features are known to be common to most of the patients of Tourette's syndrome, and can be identified.

Personality Characteristics

The most diffuse personality characteristics of these patients are extroversion and compulsivity. Extroversion gives a "friendly" and "gregarious" mark to the patient (Eisenberg et al., 1959), who however is more commonly described as an obsessive-compulsive individual. He is usually obedient, well-mannered, perfectionistic, and anxious (Corbett et al., 1969), and has visible difficulty in overtly expressing his anger (Ascher, 1948; Chapel, 1966).

In this framework, motor and verbal tics are interpreted as possible symbolic expressions of unacceptable hostile impulses (Moldofsky, 1971), and coprolalia in particular has been seen as a compulsive expression of verbal aggression (Yaryura-Tobias, 1979). The shifting of personal feelings of hostility to more generalized hostile expressions through coprolalia, represents the defense mechanism most directly involved in these patients (Ascher, 1948; Moldofsky, 1971).

Parental Components

As for other neuropsychiatric conditions, hereditary factors have been implicated in Tourette's syndrome (Field et al., 1966; Golden, 1978) and denied (Corbin, 1970; Stevens, 1964). Recent analyses of 60 families of children with Tourette's disease revealed either the presence of the syndrome or of chronic motor tics in a large percentage of the familial milieu of the patients (Eldridge et al., 1977; Golden, 1978), such to suggest an autosomal dominal mode of inheritance (Golden, 1977, 1978). Similar conclusions have also been reached by others

(Eldridge et al., 1977; Fernando, 1967; Friel, 1973; Moldofsky et al., 1974; Sanders, 1973), and in this respect, Tourette's syndrome and chronic motor tics are proposed as conditions along a continuum with a hereditary basis (Golden, 1978).

Family psychopathology indicates that at least one of the patient's parents is often rigid, demanding, controlling, punitive, and dominant (Chapel, 1966; Lucas, 1970). Other studies show that in 60 percent of the cases one of the parents has overtly paranoid or strongly dominant characteristics, greater than might be expected (Challas et al., 1967; Shapiro et al., 1972). The presence of depressive disorders and schizophrenia in the family of some patients has also been reported (Corbett et al., 1969; Fernando, 1967; Shapiro et al., 1972). It must be strongly emphasized that there is no clinical evidence that Tourette's syndrome is in any way related to schizophrenia (Shapiro et al., 1972; Woodrow, 1974).

Other Concomitants

Factors related to birth history, such as toxemia, prematurity, prolonged labor, neonatal pneumonitis, and other birth abnormalities are not significantly different for Tourette patients than for the general population (Corbett et al., 1969; Mahler et al., 1945; Shapiro et al., 1972). Psychogenic precipitants of the syndrome have been said to include episodes of fearfulness, starting school, separation from a sibling, birth of a sibling, parental illness, parental separation and other emergent stressful events (Corbett et al., 1969; Fernando, 1967). Unimpressive, non-specific neurological abnormalities, not indicative of focal pathology, have been observed in about 50 percent of cases (Lucas, 1970; Shapiro et al., 1973 a; Sweet et al., 1973).

NEUROCHEMICAL CORRELATES

A relatively recent trend, started some 15 years ago by Schildkraut (1965), is to search for the neurochemical correlates of various neuropsychiatric disorders (Berger, 1976; Randrup et al., 1975; Valzelli and Sarteschi, 1977), in the more extended framework of the neurochemical correlates of behavior (Valzelli, 1978 a). From this standpoint, the theoretical significance of Tourette's syndrome lies in its repetitive and purposeless repetitive behavior induced by amphetamine intoxication. The neurochemical change responsible for the stereotyped movements induced in experimental animals by amphetamine is increased dopaminergic activity in the brain (Snyder, 1972; Snyder et al., 1970). This fact is observable in the brain of experimental animals, but obviously cannot be matched by any correspondingly direct evidence in humans, in whom only indirect approaches and interpretations are possible.

Haloperidol is an almost selective blocking agent of brain dopaminergic receptors (Nyback et al., 1968), and is also considered the best drug for treating Tourette's syndrome (Shapiro et al., 1973 b; Van Woert et al., 1976). Consequently, patients have been considered as having dopaminergic hyperactivity or hypersensitivity of brain dopamine receptors to the mediator. Interestingly, in a somewhat opposite situation, represented by Parkinsonism, tic-like movements of the mouth and limbs are often seen in patients following an overloading treatment with 1-Dopa (Saks et al., 1970) and, accordingly, 1-Dopa treatment accentuates the symptoms of Tourette's syndrome (Messiha and Knopp, 1976). In addition, Tourette's patients have an increased urinary excretion of dopamine and of its metabolite, 3-methoxytyramine (Knopp et al., 1973; Messiha and Knopp, 1976), and high concentrations of another dopamine metabolite, homovanillic acid, in the cerebrospinal fluid (Van Woert et al., 1976). Cerebrospinal fluid levels of brain biogenic amine metabolites have been used as indicators of changes in the brain metabolism of these amines (Moir et al., 1970), and probenecid loading with analysis of acidic-amine metabolite variations in cerebrospinal fluid provides a means of assessing brain dopamine and serotonin turnover (Neff and Tozer, 1968). This method thus makes it possible to detect alterations of neurotransmitter metabolism in the human brain, not easily discovered through analysis of their metabolites under steady-state conditions.

When the probenecid technique is applied to Tourette patients, low dopamine turnover is revealed (Butler et al., 1979), a fact that may depend on either increased production of brain dopamine or increased sensitivity at dopamine receptors, both resulting in a negative feedback response in the presynaptic dopamine neurons (Friednoff, 1977). These data clearly support the already formulated hypothesis of hyperactivity of the dopaminergic system in Tourette's syndrome (Moldofsky et al., 1974). The alternative hypothesis of specific involvement of norepinephrine as the crucial mediator of the syndrome (Meyerhoff and Snyder, 1973) has not been further confirmed (Lake et al., 1977).

There is in fact indirect evidence of reduced activity of brain serotonergic neurons in Tourette's syndrome, as suggested by positive results in patients given chlorimipramine, a tricyclic antidepressant that blocks serotonin reuptake (Yaryura-Tobias, 1979; Yaryura-Tobias and Neziroglu, 1977), or clonazepam, a benzodiazpine that has been reported to increase brain serotonin content (Chadwick et al., 1975; Gonce and Barbeau, 1977; Jenner et al., 1975). Others have used the serotonin precursor, 5-hydroxy-trytophan, to increase brain serotonin production in their patients (Van Woert et al., 1977). Recently, measurements of the main serotonin metabolite, 5-hydroxy-indoleacetic acid, in the cerebrospinal fluid of patients have shown no significant differences from control values, whereas the probenecid technique indicates there is reduced serotonergic activity (Butler et al., 1979).

The neurochemical profile of Gilles De la Tourette's syndrome seems to be characterized by increased dopaminergic activity in the presence of reduced serotonergic control in the brain. This feature could also represent a neurochemical defect in the make-up of the brain, a hereditary or familial feature that, depending on the magnitude of the imbalance, may underlie other similar neuropsychiatric disorders. Lastly, with regard to the hostile manifestations of the syndrome, it may be of interest to note that the same type of neurochemical imbalance is either typically seen in some experimental models of abnormal aggression induced in laboratory animals, or reasonably deducible in several examples of human violent behavior (Valzelli, 1980).

NEUROANATOMY

The neurochemical changes described are currently believed to take place in the corpora striata (Moldofsky et al., 1974) and especially in the striatal-pallidal connections (Lucas, 1964; Snyder et al., 1970) and nigro-striatal system (Moldofsky et al., 1974; Randrup and Munkvad, 1976). It is also of interest to note that corpora striata send projections to the amygdala and that repeated chemical or electrical stimulation of this structure, or amygdaloid kindling, induces a long-term alternation of behavior in laboratory animals characterized by facial twitching, masticatory convulsions, head jerks, and rapid clonic movements of the limbs (Goddard, 1969; Goddard et al., 1960; Racine, 1972 a, b). In addition, with regard to the hostile and destructive components of the syndrome, the amygdala is known to play a very important role in the regulation of aggressive behavior (Valzelli, 1978 b).

TREATMENT

Modern pharmacotherapy provides for suitable management of Tourette's syndrome. Most clinicians consider haloperidol the treatment of choice, resulting in marked improvement in about 90 percent of treated patients (Bruun and Shapiro, 1972; Challas et al., 1967; Craven, 1976; Fernando, 1976; Izmeth, 1979; Moldofsky et al., 1974; Perera, 1975; Seignot, 1961; Shapiro et al., 1972, 1973 b; Woodrow, 1974). The side effects most often encountered are dyskinesia, akathisia, akynesia, and parkinsonism, and almost all patients on daily doses above 2 mg of this drug require antiparkinsonian medication. The therapeutic range varies from 6 to 180 mg per day, and it must be noted that haloperidol's efficacy is greatly affected by social and familial situations, so that stressful events and stimulation may even abolish its effect (Surwillo et al., 1978).

Then too, a variety of biological, psychosocial, emotional and developmental issues bear upon the individual response to haloperidol treatment. In addition, side effects of the drug, especially hypokynesia, can be troublesome, and the experience of loss of vivacity or spontaneity may prove intolerable to many patients (Moldofsky et al., 1974). Haloperidol has also been reported to cause a significant deficit of temporal information processing by patients (Goldstone and Lhamon, 1976), and may occasionally lead to psychotic symptoms (Caine et al., 1978).

Pimozide, a relatively new neuroleptic drug with more specific antidopaminergic activity than haloperidol (Seeman and Lee, 1975) and fewer adverse effects (Ayd, 1971), has been recently proved superior to haloperidol in the clinical management of Tourette's syndrome, and was associated with significantly fewer complaints of lethargy (Ross and Moldofsky, 1977, 1978).

With regard to the serotonergic implications already discussed, partial relief of symptoms has been described following treatment with the benzodiazepine derivative clonazepam (Gonce and Barbeau, 1977), while the use of chlorimipramine is proposed as an alternative to haloperidol therapy because of the high efficacy, lack of toxicity and mild side effects of this antidepressant derivative (Yaryura-Tobias, 1979; Yaryura-Tobias and Neziroglu, 1977). Along the same lines, 1-trytophan has been suggested as helpful (Yaryura-Tobias, 1979), and the association of a dopaminergic blocker with a serotonergic stimulant may provide a very effective combination in treating the syndrome.

Careful attention must be paid to avoid confusion between Tourette's syndrome and hyperactive manifestations of minimal brain dysfunction, since administration of methylphenidate or dexamphetamine, the drugs of choice for treating hyperactive children, will precipitate, exacerbate, or even occasionally induce Tourette's syndrome (Bremness and Sverd, 1979; Fras and Karlavage, 1977; Pollack et al., 1977). This is obviously due to the intense brain catecholaminergic stimulation induced by these drugs, and physicians prescribing them should carefully inquire about the presence of tics in patients and their families.

REFERENCES

Aberle, D.F. (1952): "Arctic hysteria" and latah in Mongolia. *Transactions of the New York Academy of Sciences, 14*: 291-297.
Abuzzahab, F.S., Sr. and Anderson, F.O. (1973): Gilles De la Tourette's syndrome; international registry. *Minnesota Medicine 56*: 492-496.
Abuzzahab, F.S., Sr. and Anderson, F.O. (1976): Gilles De la Tourette syndrome. In: *International Registry* Vol. 1, Mason Publ., Saint Paul, MN.
Alliez, J. and Audon, S. (1977): La maladie des tics de Gilles De la Tourette. *Annales Medico-Psychologiques 135*: 489-522.
Ascher, E. (1948): Psychodynamic considerations in Gilles De la Tourette's disease (maladie des tics). *American Journal of Psychiatry 105*: 267-276.
Ayd, F.J. (1971): Pimozide: a promising neuroleptic. *International Drug Therapy Newsletter 6*: 17-20.

Balthasar, K. (1957): Uber das anatomische Substrat der generalisierten Tic-krankheit (maladie des tics, Gilles De la Tourette): Entwicklungshemmung des corpus striatum. *Archiv für Psychiatrie und Nervenkrankheiten 195*: 531-549.

Beard, G.M. (1880): Experiments with the "jumpers" or "jumping Frenchmen of Maine." *Journal of Nervous and Mental Diseases 7*: 487-490.

Berger, F.M. (1976): Aminergic factors in mental illness. *Current Developments in Psychopharmacology 3*: 125-153.

Bremness, A.B. and Sverd, J. (1979): Methylphenidate-induced Tourette syndrome: Case report. *American Journal of Psychiatry 136*: 1334-1335.

Bruun, R.D. and Shapiro, A.K. (1972): Differential diagnosis of Gilles De la Tourette syndrome. *Journal of Nervous and Mental Disease 155*: 328-334.

Butler, I.J., Koslow, S.H., Seifert, W.E., Caprioli, R.M., and Singer, H.S. (1979): Biogenic amine metabolism in Tourette syndrome. *Annals of Neurology 6*: 37-39.

Caine, E.D., Margolin, D.I., Brown, G.L., and Ebert, M.H. (1978): Gilles De la Tourette's syndrome, tardive dyskenesia, and psychosis in an adolescent. *American Journal of Psychiatry 135*: 241-243.

Chadwick, D., Harris, R., Jenner, P., Reynolds, E.H., and Marsden, C.D. (1975): Manipulation of brain serotonin in the treatment of myoclonus. *Lancet 2*: 434-435.

Challas, G., Chapel, J.L. and Jenkins, R.L. (1967): Tourette's disease: Control of symptoms and its clinical course. *International Journal of Neuropsychiatry 3*: suppl. 1, 96-104.

Chapel, J.L. (1966): Gilles De la Tourette's disease: The past and the present. *Canadian Psychiatric Association Journal 11*: 324-329.

Chapel, J.L. (1970): Gilles De la Tourette syndrome: Latah, myriachit and jumpers revisited. *New York State Journal of Medicine 70*: 2201-2204.

Charcot, P. (1899): Des tics des ticqueurs. *Annales Medico-Chirurgicals 5*: 1-5.

Corbett, J.A. (1971): The nature of tics and Gilles De la Tourette's syndrome. *Journal of Psychosomatic Medicine 15*: 403-409.

Corbett, J.A., Mathews, A.M., Connell, P.H., and Shapiro, D.A. (1969): Tics and Gilles De la Tourette's syndrome: A follow-up study and critical review. *British Journal of Psychiatry 115*: 1229-1241.

Corbin, K.B. (1970): Gilles De la Tourette's syndrome: Common neurophysiological factors reported in literature. *New York State Journal of Medicine 70*: 2193-2197.

Craven, E.M. (1969): Gilles De la Tourette syndrome treated with haloperidol. *Journal of American Medical Association 210*: 134.

Creak, M. and Guttmann, E. (1935): Chorea, tics and compulsive utterances. *Journal of Mental Sciences 81*: 834-839.

De la Tourette, G.G. (1884): Jumping, latah, myriachit. *Archives de Neurologie 8*: 68-74.

De la Tourette, G.G. (1885): Etude sur une affection nerveuse caractérisée par l'incoordination motrice accompagnée d'écholalie de coprolalie (jumping, latah, myriachit). *Archieves de Neurologie 9*: 19-42 and 158-200.

De la Tourette, G.G. (1899): La maladie des tics convulsifs. *La Semaine Medicale 19*: 153-157.

Eisenberg, L., Ascher, E., and Kanner, L. (1959): A clinical study of Gilles De la Tourette's disease (maladie des tics) in children. *American Journal of Psychiatry 115*: 715-723.

Eldridge, R., Sweet, R., Lake, C.R., Ziegler, M., and Shapiro, A.K. (1977): Gilles De la Tourette's syndrome: Clinical, genetic, psychologic, and biochemical aspects in 21 selected families. *Neurology 27*: 115-124.

Fernando, S.J.M. (1967): Gilles De la Tourette's syndrome: A report on four cases and a review of published case reports. *British Journal of Psychiatry 113*: 607-617.

Fernando, S.J.M. (1968): Gilles De la Tourette's syndrome. *British Journal of Psychiatry 114*: 123-125.

Fernando, S.J.M. (1976): Six cases of Gilles De la Tourette's syndrome. *British Journal of Psychiatry 128*: 436-441.
Field, J.R., Corbin, K.B., Goldstein, N.P., and Klaas, D.W. (1966): Gilles De la Tourette's syndrome. *Neurology 16*: 453-462.
Fras, I. and Karlavage, J. (1977): The use of methylphenidate and imipramine in Gilles De la Tourette's disease in children. *American Journal of Psychiatry 134*: 195-197.
Friedhoff, A.J. (1977): Receptor sensitivity modification (RSM)–a new paradigm for the potential treatment of some hormonal and transmitter disturbances. *Comprehensive Psychiatry 18*: 309-317.
Friel, P.B. (1973): Familial incidence of Gilles De la Tourette's disease, with observations on aetiology and treatment. *British Journal of Psychiatry 122*: 655-658.
Goddard, G.V. (1969): Analysis of avoidance conditioning following cholinergic stimulation of amygdala in rats. *Journal Comparative and Physiological Psychology 68*: monograph suppl. no. 2, pt. 2, 1-18.
Goddard, G.V., McIntyre, D.C., and Leech, C.K. (1969): A permanent change in brain function resulting from daily electrical stimulation. *Experimental Neurology 25*: 295-330.
Goforth, E.G. (1974): A single case study: Gilles De la Tourette's syndrome. *Journal of Nervous and Mental Diseases 158*: 306-309.
Golden, G.S. (1977): Tourette syndrome. The pediatric perspective. *American Journal of Disease of Children 131*: 531-534.
Golden, G.S. (1978): Tics and Tourette's: A continuum of symptoms? *Annals of Neurology 4*: 145-148.
Goldstone, S. and Lhamon, W.T. (1976): The effects of haloperidol upon temporal information processing by patients with Tourette's syndrome. *Psychopharmacology 50*: 7-10.
Gonce, M. and Barceau, A. (1977): Seven cases of Gilles De la Tourette syndrome: Partial relief with clonazepam: A pilot study. *Canadian Journal of Neurological Sciences 4*: 279-283.
Hammond, G.M. (1892): Convulsive tic, its nature and treatment. *Medical Records 41*: 236-239.
Hammond, W.A. (1884): Myriachit: A newly described disease of the nervous system and its analogues. *British Medical Journal 1*: 758-759.
Hecaen, H. and de Ajuriaguerra, J. (1964): *Left-handedness: Manual Superiority and Cerebral Dominance.* Grune and Stratton, New York.
Itard, J.M.G. (1925): Memoire sur quelques fonctions involuntaires des appareils de la locomotion, de la préhension et de la voix. *Archives Generales de Medecine 8*: 385-407.
Izmeth, A. (1979): Gilles De la Tourette syndrome. *Journal of Mental Deficiency Research 23*: 25-27.
Jenner, P., Chadwick, D., Reynolds, E.H., and Marsden, C.D. (1975): Altered 5-HT metabolism with clonazepam, diazepam and diphenyl-hydantoin. *Journal of Pharmacy and Pharmacology 27*: 707-710.
Knopp, W., Arnold, L.E., and Messiha, F.S. (1973): Gilles De la Tourette's disease; Implications for research in Huntington's chorea. *Advances in Neurology 1*: 135-145.
Lake, R.C., Ziegler, M.G., Eldridge, R., and Murphy, D.L. (1977): Catecholamine metabolism in Gilles De la Tourette's syndrome. *American Journal of Psychiatry 134*: 257-260.
Lehmann, H.E. (1975): Unusual psychiatric disorders and atypical psychoses. In: *Comprehensive Textbook of Psychiatry*, 2nd. ed. vol. 2, edited by A.J. Freedman, H.I. Kaplan, and B.J. Sadock, pp. 1724-1736, Williams & Wilkins, Baltimore.
Lucas, A.R. (1964): Gilles De la Tourette's disease in children: Treatment with phenothiazine drugs. *American Journal of Psychiatry 121*: 606-608.

Lucas, A.R. (1970): Gilles De la Tourette's disease. An overview. *New York State Journal of Medicine 70*: 2197-2200.
Lucas, A.R., Kauffman, P.E., and Morris, E.M. (1967): Gilles De la Tourette's disease. A clinical study of fifteen cases. *Journal of American Academy of Child Psychiatry 6*: 700-722.
Mahler, M.S., Luke, J.A., and Daltroff, W. (1945): Clinical and follow-up study of the tic syndrome in children. *American Journal of Orthopsychiatry 15*: 631-647.
Mazur, W.P. (1953): Gilles De la Tourette's syndrome. *Edinburgh Medical Journal 60*: 427-433.
Messiha, F.S. and Knopp, W. (1976): A study of endogenous dopamine metabolism in Gilles De la Tourette's disease. *Diseases of the Nervous System 37*: 470-473.
Meyerhoff, J. and Snyder, S.H. (1973): Catecholamines in Gilles De la Tourette's disease: A clinical study with amphetamine isomers. *Advances in Neurology 1*: 123-134.
Milman, D.H. (1975): Gilles De la Tourette syndrome; extended follow-up. *New York State Journal of Medicine 75*: 892-895.
Moir, A.T.B., Ashcroft, G.W., Crawford, T.B.B., Eccleston, D., and Gultberg, H.C. (1970): Cerebral metabolites in cerebrospinal fluid as a biochemical approach to the brain. *Brain 93*: 357-368.
Moldofsky, H. (1971): A psychophysiological study of multiple tics. *Archives of General Psychiatry 25*: 79-87.
Moldofsky, H., Tullis, C., and Lamon, R. (1974): Multiple tic syndrome (Gilles De la Tourette's syndrome). Clinical, biological, and psychosocial variables and their influence with haloperidol. *Journal of Nervous and Mental Disease 159*: 282-292.
Neff, N.H. and Tozer, T.N. (1968): "In vivo" measurement of brain serotonin turnover. *Advances of Pharmacology 6A*: 97-109.
Nybäck, H., Borzecki, A., and Sedvall, G. (1968): Accumulation and disappearance of catecholamines formed from tryosine-^{14}C in mouse brain; effect of some psychotropic drugs. *European Journal of Pharmacology 4*: 395-403.
Penna, M.W. and Lion, J.R. (1975): Gilles De la Tourette's syndrome and depression: A case report. *Diseases of the Nervous System 36*: 41-43.
Perera, H.V. (1975): Two cases of Gilles De la Tourette's syndrome treated with haloperidol. *British Journal of Psychiatry 127*: 324-326.
Pollack, M.A., Cohen, N.L., and Friedhoff, A.J. (1977): Gilles De la Tourette's syndrome. Familial occurrence and precipitation by methylphenidate therapy. *Archives of Neurology 34*: 630-632.
Racine, R.J. (1972a): Modification of seizure activity by electrical stimulation. I. Afterdischarge threshold. *Electroencephalography and Clinical Neurology 32*: 269-279.
Racine, R.J. (1972b): Modification of seizure activity by electrical stimulation. II. Motor seizure. *Electroencephalography and Clinical Neurophysiology 32*: 281-294.
Randrup, A. and Munkvad, I. (1967): Stereotyped activities produced by amphetamine in several animal species and man. *Psychopharmacologia 11*: 300-310.
Randrup, A., Munkvad, I., Fog, R., Gerlach, J., Molander, L., Kjellberg, B., and Scheel-Krüger, J. (1975): Mania, depression, and brain dopamine. *Current Developments in Psychopharmacology 2*: 205-248.
Ross, M.S. and Moldofsky, H. (1977): Comparison of pimozide with haloperidol in Gilles De la Tourette syndrome. *Lancet 1*: 103.
Ross, M.S. and Moldofsky, H. (1978): A comparison of pimozide and haloperidol in the treatment of Gilles De la Tourette's syndrome. *American Journal of Psychiatry 135*: 585-587.
Sacks, O.W., Ross, S.J., and De Paola, D.P. (1970): Abnormal mouth-movements and oral damage associated with L-dopa treatment. *Annals of Dentistry 29*: 130-144.

Sanders, D.G. (1973): Familial occurrence of Gilles De la Tourette syndrome. *Archives of General Psychiatry 28*: 326-328.
Sarteschi, P. (1956): Sulla delimitazione della malattia di Gilles De la Tourette. Presentazione di un caso di tics multipli. *Rassegna di Studi Psichiatrici 45*: 960-970.
Schildkraut, J.J. (1965): The catecholamine hypothesis of affective disorders: A review of supporting evidence. *American Journal of Psychiatry 122*: 509-522.
Seeman, P. and Lee, T. (1975): Antipsychotic drugs: Direct correlation between clinical potency and presynaptic action on dopamine neurons. *Science 188*: 1217-1219.
Seignot, J.N. (1961): Un cas de maladie des tics de Gilles De la Tourette gueri par le R-1625. *Annales Medico-Psychologiques 119*: 578-579.
Shapiro, A.K., Shapiro, E., and Wayne, H. (1972): Birth, developmental, and family histories and demographic information in Tourette's syndrome. *Journal of Nervous and Mental Disease 155*: 335-344.
Shapiro, A.K., Shapiro, E., and Wayne, H. (1973b): Treatment of Tourette's syndrome. With haloperidol, review of 34 cases. *Archives of General Psychiatry 28*: 92-97.
Shapiro, A.K., Shapiro, E., Wayne, H., and Brunn, R.D. (1973a): Tourette's syndrome: Summary of data on 34 patients. *Psychosomatic Medicine 35*: 419-435.
Snyder, S.J. (1972): Catecholamines in the brain as mediators of amphetamine psychosis. *Archives of General Psychiatry 27*: 169-179.
Snyder, S.J., Taylor, K.M. Coyle, J.T., and Meyerhoff, J.L. (1970): The role of brain dopamine in behavioral regulation and the actions of psychotropic drugs. *American Journal of Psychiatry 127*: 199-207.
Stevens, H. (1964): The syndrome of Gilles De la Tourette and its treatment. Report of a case. *Medical Annals of the District of Columbia 33*: 277-279.
Surwillo, W.W., Shafi, M., and Barrett, C.L. (1978): Single case study. Gilles De la Tourette syndrome. A 20 month study of the effect of stressful life events and haloperidol on symptom frequency. *Journal of Nervous and Mental Diseases 166*: 812-816.
Sweet, R.D., Solomon, G.E., Wayne, H., Shapiro, E., and Shapiro, A.K. (1973): Neurological features of Gilles De la Tourette's syndrome. *Journal of Neurology, Neurosurgery and Psychiatry 36*: 1-9.
Valzelli, L. (1978a): Affective behavior and serotonin. In: *Serotonin in Health and Disease*, vol. 3, *The Central Nervous System*, edited by W.B. Essman, pp. 145-201, Spectrum Publ., New York.
Valzelli, L. (1978b): Human and animal studies on the neurophysiology of aggression. *Progress in Neuro-Psychopharmacology 2*: 591-611.
Valzelli, L. (1980): *Psychobiology of aggression and violence*, Raven Press, New York, in press.
Valzelli, L. and Sarteschi, P. (1977): *Considerazioni in tema di schizofrenia*. Edizioni Medico Scientifiche, Torino.
Van Woert, M.H., Jutkowitz, R., Rosenbaum, D., and Bowers, M.B., Jr. (1976): Gilles De la Tourette's syndrome: Biochemical approaches. In: *The Basal Ganglia*, edited by M.D. Yahr, pp. 459-465, Raven Press, New York.
Van Woert, M.H., Rosenbaum, D., Howieson, J., and Bowers, M.B., Jr. (1977): Long-term therapy of myoclonus and other neurologic disorders with L-5-hydroxytryptophan and carbidopa. *New England Journal of Medicine 296*: 70-75.
Walsh, P.J.F. (1962): Compulsive shouting and Gilles De la Tourette's disease. *British Journal of Clinical Practice 16*: 651-655.
Wilson, S.A.K. (1927): The tics and allied conditions. *Journal of Neurology and Psychopathology 8*: 93-109.
Woodrow, K.M. (1974): Gilles De la Tourette's disease. A review. *American Journal of Psychiatry 131*: 1000-1003.

Yaryura-Tobias, J.A. (1975): Chlorimipramine in Gilles De la Tourette's disease. *American Journal of Psychiatry 132*: 1221.

Yaryura-Tobias, J.A. (1979): Gilles De la Tourette syndrome. Interactions with other neuropsychiatric disorders. *Acta Psychiatrica Scandinavica 59*: 9-16.

Yaryura-Tobias, J.A. and Neziroglu, F.A. (1977): Gilles De la Tourette syndrome: A new clinical approach. *Progress in Neuro-Psychopharmacology 1*: 335-338.

9

Psychopharmacology of Clonidine[1]

Gary T. Shearman
Harbans Lal

INTRODUCTION

There are thousands of chemical substances which show significant potential as pharmacological agents. However, only a handful of them ever become investigational tools of a kind that stimulates the type of research which is critical for the development of pharmacology itself. Clonidine is one such substance. Originally synthesized to relieve symptoms associated with the common cold and sinusitis, clonidine was subsequently found to offer a new approach to the control of hypertension.

The antihypertensive action of clonidine involves a unique mechanism. Hypertension was once thought to be caused primarily by the faulty functioning of peripheral blood vessels and has usually been treated by drugs acting at peripheral sites. Clonidine acts directly on the central nervous system. The finding that a centrally acting drug could control a peripheral malfunction aroused great interest among medical researchers throughout the world and led to investigation of clonidine not only as a tool of research in the hypertensive disease process but also as a means of developing new approaches to the treatment of several other disease states.

While the central sites of clonidine's action on hypertension are well recognized, possible psychopharmacological actions of this drug have not drawn appropriate attention. It may be noted that the early human volunteers taking clonidine nose drops experienced some drowsiness, and during this period, the

---

[1] Similar reviews were recently published elsewhere (Fielding and Lal, 1980; Lal and Shearman, 1981).

blood pressure-lowering effect of clonidine was first observed. This was the first evidence of possible psychopharmacological effects of clonidine. Since then, many other observations on the behavioral effects of clonidine have been reported. In order that proper perspectives may be developed regarding the potential usefulness of this drug in behavioral disorders, we undertook to review the available literature in this area and are describing below the known psychopharmacological actions of clonidine.

MOTOR BEHAVIOR

Locomotor Activity

It has been suggested that locomotor activity is mediated by both the dopaminergic and the noradrenergic systems within the brain (Anden et al., 1976). Locomotor activity in laboratory animals is often measured by the number of times the subject interrupts a light beam in a photocell chamber (Seiden and Dykstra, 1977). Each time the light beam is interrupted, a count is recorded, and thus the number of counts varies proportionately with the subject's locomotor activity.

Peripheral administration of clonidine (0.05-25.0 mg/kg) has been reported to cause a dose-dependent decrease in the locomotor activity of mice and rats measured in the above manner (Maj et al., 1972, 1975; Strombom, 1976; Tilson et al., 1977) and to antagonize the increase in locomotor activity induced by d-amphetamine (0.5 mg/kg) in rats in a dose-dependent manner (Skolnick et al., 1978).

Bilateral administration of dopamine (5-10 μg) or d-amphetamine into the nucleus accumbens stimulated locomotor activity, whereas norepinephrine (1–10 μg) or clonidine (1-10 μg) decreased locomotor activity (Pijneberg et al., 1976). Clonidine (5 μg) caused only a slight reduction in the locomotor activity induced by ergotamine when both drugs were injected into the nucleus accumbens, whereas the imidazoline derivative 3,4-dihydroxy-phenylamino-2-imidazoline (DPI) strongly inhibited this effect of ergotamine (Pijneberg et al., 1976a). Low doses of clonidine (0.025-0.05 mg/kg i.p.), which either did not affect or only slightly affected the motor activity of control mice, markedly suppressed ethanol-induced motor stimulation (Strombom et al., 1977).

While clonidine (1-25 mg/kg) potentiated the decrease in locomotor activity caused by pretreatment with the neuroleptic spiroperidol (Maj et al., 1972), it did not influence the depression of locomotor activity due to pretreatment with reserpine (Anden et al., 1970a, 1973, 1976; Maj et al., 1972; Menon et al., 1977), alpha-methyl-paratyrosine (Anden et al., 1972; Maj et al., 1972), FLA-63 or phenoxybenzamine (Maj et al., 1972) despite marked sympathomimetic signs.

However, clonidine (1-25 mg/kg) did potentiate the partial reversal of locomotor activity produced by apomorphine or piribedil in mice pretreated with reserpine (Anden et al., 1970a, 1973, 1976; Jenner and Marsden, 1975; Jenner and Pycock, 1976; Maj et al., 1972; Dolphin et al., 1976; Menon et al., 1977), alpha-methyl-paratyrosine (Anden et al., 1970a; Maj et al., 1972), and FLA-63 (Maj et al., 1972) at doses which do not interfere with the metabolism of apomorphine (Anden et al., 1973). Furthermore, increased locomotor activity induced by the dopamine receptor stimulant metatyrosine (Anden et al., 1973) or LSD (Menon et al., 1977) in reserpine-treated mice was enhanced by clonidine (1.0 mg/kg i.p.) pretreatment. Caffeine (25 mg/kg) produced a four-fold increase in the locomotor activity reversing effect of ET-495 plus clonidine in reserpinized mice (Waldeck, 1973). Subcutaneous administration of clonidine (0.125-0.5 mg/kg) promoted intense locomotor activity in rats pretreated with 6-hydroxydopamine plus reserpine (Zebrowska-Lupina et al., 1977). Similar but less intensive hyperactivity was observed when rats were given clonidine after combined pretreatment with 6-hydroxydopamine plus p-chlorophenylalanine plus alpha-methyl-p-tyrosine or with reserpine plus yohimbine (3 mg/kg) (Zebrowska-Lupina et al., 1977). Clonidine (5 and 25 mg/kg) did not potentiate the apomorphine antagonism of a phenoxybenzamine-induced decrease in locomotor activity but, on the contrary, decreased the effect of apomorphine (Maj et al., 1972).

Repeated administration of electroconvulsive shock (ECS) to mice enhanced the locomotor stimulatory effect of clonidine (1.5 mg/kg) in reserpinized mice treated with apomorphine (Modigh, 1975). Furthermore, administration of clonidine (1.5 mg/kg) to mice receiving only ECS pretreatment resulted in increased locomotor activity (Modigh, 1975), suggesting that repeated ECS increases the sensitivity of noradrenergic receptors.

Administration of clonidine (100 or 500 μg/kg but not 25 μg/kg) to mice during withdrawal from long-term haloperidol treatment resulted in marked locomotor stimulation as compared to vehicle-treated mice, suggesting that the long-term haloperidol treatment resulted in the development of supersensitive noradrenergic receptors (Dunstan and Jackson, 1976, 1977).

The potentiating effect of clonidine on apomorphine-induced locomotor stimulation in reserpine-treated mice was almost completely blocked by phenoxybenzamine (20 mg/kg), partially antagonized by tolazoline (50 mg/kg), and not significantly affected by yohimbine (3 and 10 mg/kg) (Anden et al., 1976) or FLA-63 (Dolphin et al., 1976). Similarly, Zebrowska-Lupina et al. (1977) reported that the alpha-receptor blockers phenoxybenzamine, phentolamine, aceperone, as well as yohimbine (10 mg/kg) antagonized the clonidine-induced locomotor stimulation of rats pretreated with 6-hydroxydopamine plus reserpine. The dopamine receptor antagonists spiroperidol and pimozide had no antagonist effect (Zebrowska-Lupina et al., 1977).

The reduction of locomotor activity in mice and rats by clonidine was antagonized by atropine and scopolamine (Maj et al., 1975). The peripheral cholinolytic agents atropine methyl nitrate and scopolamine butyl bromide were ineffective in mice and partly effective in rats in antagonizing the clonidine-induced decrease in locomotor activity (Maj et al., 1975).

In conclusion, these studies have demonstrated that clonidine causes a dose-dependent decrease in the locomotor activity of both mice and rats. However, clonidine may potentiate the increase in locomotor activity produced by other drugs under certain pharmacological conditions. Results of studies on the mechanism by which clonidine affects locomotor activity suggest the involvement of cholinergic (Maj et al., 1975) and noradrenergic (Anden et al., 1976; Zebrowska-Lupina et al., 1977) mechanisms. These studies also support the suggestion by Maj et al., (1972) that stimulation of both dopaminergic and noradrenergic systems is required for maximal stimulation of locomotor activity.

Exploratory Activity

The exploratory motor activity of laboratory animals is often measured in the open field and hole tests. In the open field situation, rats are placed individually in a circular arena and the frequency of diameter crossings ("ambulation score") and of rearings ("rearing score") is recorded. Similarly, the number of fecal pellets excreted over the observation period is recorded ("defecation score") (Janssen et al., 1960). In the hole test, laboratory animals are placed in a box containing several round holes. The number of times the animals put their heads in the holes ("peeping") is recorded as a measure of exploratory activity (File and Pope, 1974).

Dandiya and Patni (1973) reported that intraventricular administration of clonidine decreased the ambulation and rearing of rats in an open field situation. Similarly, Herman et al., (1976) found that clonidine (0.1 mg/kg but not 0.05 mg/kg) decreased ambulation, rearing, and defecation in the open field and reduced the peeping of rats in the hole test. Intracerebroventricular administration of 6-hydroxydopamine potentiated the depressant action of clonidine (Herman et al., 1976).

Strombom (1975) reported that clonidine (0.025-0.8 mg/kg) depressed the exploratory behavior of mice in a Y-shaped runway maze and appeared to break the pattern of adaptation.

These data suggest that norepinephrine may be of importance for exploratory behavior.

Rotorod Test

Rotorod performance is measured by the ability of an animal to stay on a revolving drum or cylinder over a period of time. Clonidine (1.0 mg/kg, i.p.)

reduced rotorod performance in rats (Laverty and Taylor, 1969) and mice (ED_{50} 0.24 mg/kg S.C.) (Cornfeldt et al., 1978).

Circling

Circling or rotational behavior in rats with unilateral lesions of the nigrostriatal pathway is believed to be dopamine-dependent behavior. This assumption is based on the finding that drugs which increase dopaminergic activity in the central nervous system after the lesion provoke rotational behavior (Ungerstedt et al., 1969).

Using a rotometer measuring the number of full turns the subject makes per unit time, Satoh et al. (1976) found that in rats with unilateral 6-hydroxydopamine-induced lesions of the substantia nigra, intraventricular injection of apomorphine, dopamine, and norepinephrine in doses of 64 ug caused the rats to turn toward the intact side, whereas intraventricular injection of methamphetamine (250 ug) caused them to turn toward the damaged side. On the other hand, intraventricular injection of clonidine (64 μg) did not induce any turning. It was suggested by Satoh et al. that dopamine, norepinephrine, and apomorphine directly stimulate the supersensitive dopamine receptors on the side of the lesion, whereas methamphetamine indirectly stimulates dopamine receptors on the intact side. Since clonidine is considered to be an alpha-noradrenergic agonist (Anden et al., 1970), norepinephrine-induced turning was attributed to a nonspecific stimulation of dopamine receptors.

Direct injection of clonidine (100 ug) into one striatum of rats with intact nigrostriatal systems did not cause circling, nor did this pretreatment result in circling after the subcutaneous administration of the dopamine agonist apomorphine (0.5 mg/kg) (Jenner and Pycock, 1976). However, circling behavior induced by either apomorphine (0.25 mg/kg S.C.) of d-amphetamine (3 mg/kg i.p.) in mice with unilateral lesions of the nigrostriatal pathway was potentiated by pretreatment with clonidine (0.06-2.0 mg/kg i.p.) (Jenner and Pycock, 1976; Pycock et al., 1977). In contrast to this latter finding, Cornfeldt et al. (1978) reported that clonidine (ED_{50} 0.08 mg/kg i.p.) blocked amphetamine-induced circling but did not block apomorphine-induced circling in rats with striatal lesions. Unilateral electrolytic destruction of the locus coeruleus in rats results in spontaneous ipsilateral turning behavior which is soon replaced by contralateral turning (Pycock et al., 1975). One week after locus coeruleus lesioning, when spontaneous turning had stopped, intraperitoneal administration of the dopamine agonists apomorphine, d-amphetamine, and piribedil, but not of the noradrenergic agonist clonidine (0.05-0.5 mg/kg), elicited contralateral circling (Donaldson et al., 1977). Donaldson et al. suggested that circling behavior seen after unilateral locus coeruleus lesions is caused by supersensitive striatal dopamine receptors in the nigrostriatal pathway on the side of the lesion.

The results of the above studies of the effects of clonidine on rotational behavior indicate that clonidine does not stimulate dopamine receptors and provide further evidence that rotational behavior depends on dopaminergic rather than on noradrenergic mechanisms. However, it appears that rotational behavior induced by dopaminergic agonists may be modified by clonidine (Jenner and Pycock, 1976; Pycock et al., 1977).

Stereotypy

Stereotypic behavior consists of repeated spontaneous motor responses which are within the animal's normal behavior pattern, such as licking, sniffing, gnawing, and head bobbing (Seiden and Dykstra, 1977). Stereotypic behavior is believed to be the result of heightened dopaminergic activity in the corpus striatum (Seiden and Dykstra, 1977). Both direct and indirect dopaminergic agonists, such as apomorphine and d-amphetamine, elicit stereotypic behavior (Seiden and Dykstra, 1977).

Intraperitoneal administration of clonidine (0.5 mg/kg) to rats did not produce stereotyped behavior and did not affect the stereotyped behavior induced by apomorphine (0.1-5.0 mg/kg S.C.) (Jenner and Pycock, 1976; Pycock et al., 1977). It appears, therefore, that clonidine does not stimulate striatal dopamine receptors.

Catalepsy

Catalepsy is generally defined as the condition of an animal that is amenable to being placed in awkward positions by an experimenter and maintains these postures until shifted by the experimenter (Rech and Moore, 1971). Catalepsy may be caused by decreased dopaminergic activity within the nigrostriatal system (Seiden and Dykstra, 1977). Neuroleptic drugs, such as haloperidol, which decrease dopaminergic activity induce catalepsy (Rech and Moore, 1971).

Clonidine (0.5 mg/kg i.p.) has been reported to potentiate the cataleptic action of haloperidol (0.1-2.0 mg/kg i.p.) in rats; however, this action is probably non-specific and related to the sedative effect of clonidine (Jenner and Pycock, 1976; Pycock et al., 1977).

Motor Dysfunctions (Body Shakes)

"Wet dog shakes" in rats have been ascribed to heat gain mechanisms (Wei et al., 1974). Clonidine has been reported to inhibit the "wet dog shakes" produced in rats by immersion in ice-cold water (Wei, 1975) or by administration of the drug AG-3-5 [1-(hydroxyphenyl)-4(3-nitrophenyl)-1,2,3,6 tetrahydropyrimidin-2-one] (Wei, 1976). Jahn and Mixich (1976) reported that clonidine (0.01-0.1 mg/kg S.C.) caused a dose-dependent reduction of "wet dog shakes" induced by the benzylideneaminoxycarbonic acid derivative Sqd 8473. The ability of clonidine to reduce "wet dog shakes" may be non-specific since several

OPERANT BEHAVIOR

Schedule Control

Clonidine (0.006-0.3 mg/kg) caused a dose-dependent suppression of operant behavior maintained by fixed-ratio (Colelli et al., 1976; Sparber and Meyer, 1978), fixed-interval (Harris et al., 1976, 1977), and differential reinforcement of low-rate (Tilson et al., 1977) schedules of food-reinforced responding. In one study, tolerance was found to develop to the behavioral depressant effect of clonidine on food-reinforced responding in five days of administration. No sedative effect of clonidine was seen after two weeks (Meyer et al., 1977). Termination of clonidine treatment in the tolerant rats resulted in a suppression of normal operant behavior for as long as one week (Meyer et al., 1977). Clonidine antagonized the disruption of fixed-ratio operant behavior produced by naloxone injection in morphine-dependent rats (Colelli et al., 1976; Sparber and Meyer, 1978).

Whereas the rate-decreasing effect of apomorphine in a fixed-interval schedule of food reinforcement was potentiated by naloxone, the effect of clonidine was unaltered (Harris et al., 1976, 1977). At doses capable of suppressing operant behavior in morphine-dependent rats (Gellert and Sparber, 1977), naloxone failed to disrupt operant behavior in clonidine-tolerant rats (Meyer et al., 1977).

Suppression of fixed-ratio food-reinforced operant behavior in rats caused by depletion of brain catecholamines with alpha-methyl-para-tyrosine or tetrabenazine was not antagonized by apomorphine or clonidine; however, L-dopa reversed the suppression caused by alpha-methyl-para-tyrosine but not that caused by tetrabenazine (Ahlenius et al., 1971).

A dose-dependent suppression of water-reinforced responding in rats trained on a fixed-interval schedule occurs after both apomorphine (0.25-10.0 mg/kg) and clonidine (0.002-0.1 mg/kg). Frontal cortical lesions increased the sensitivity to apomorphine but not to clonidine (Glick and Cox, 1976).

Intraventricular administration of 1-norepinephrine (10 μg), restored the dose-related decrease in the rate of substantia nigra self-stimulation caused by diethyldithiocarbamate inhibition of norepinephrine synthesis (Belluzi et al., 1975).

In sum, these findings indicate that clonidine suppresses operant behavior maintained by different schedules of food-reinforced responding and by a fixed-interval schedule of water-reinforced responding. Since clonidine also reduces food intake (Le Douarec et al., 1972), water intake (Le Douarec, 1971), and locomotor activity (Tilson et al., 1977) in rats, it is not certain whether clonidine suppresses operant behavior for food and water reinforcement by virtue of its anorexic and adipsic effect or its sedative effect. Inasmuch as a reduction in operant behavior is observed after a reduction in noradrenergic transmission (Belluzi et al., 1975), the suppressant effect of clonidine on operant behavior may be related to its stimulation of presynaptic alpha-adrenergic receptors, which reduces noradrenergic transmission. This assumption is supported by the finding that norepinephrine, but not clonidine (Belluzi et al., 1975), will restore operant behavior suppressed by inhibition of norepinephrine synthesis. Finally, the suppressant action of clonidine on operant responding is not related to any action on endorphin mechanisms since naloxone fails to alter the effect of clonidine (Harris et al., 1976, 1977; Gellert and Sparber, 1977).

Conditioned Avoidance Response

In the paradigm of conditioned avoidance responding (CAR), animals are trained to avoid an aversive consequence by responding to a stimulus preceding the onset of the aversive event. If the subject responds to the warning stimulus, this permits avoidance of the oncoming aversive events. Failing that, a response emitted to terminate the aversive stimulus is known as an escape response. Both dopamine and norepinephrine are considered to be involved in the mediation of an avoidance response (for review see Seiden and Dykstra, 1977). Neuroleptic drugs selectively disrupt avoidance responding at doses which do not disrupt escape behavior (for review see Seiden and Dykstra, 1977).

Laverty and Taylor (1969) reported that intraperitoneal administration of clonidine (0.1-1.0 mg/kg) to rats trained to climb a pole to avoid a shock caused a dose-dependent inhibition of the conditioned avoidance behavior. This may be a non-specific effect, however, and may be the result of sedation since these doses have been reported to decrease locomotor activity and operant responding (Maj et al., 1972; Tilson et al., 1977). Delbarre and Schmitt (1974) found that subcutaneous administration of clonidine (0.15 mg/kg) depressed an avoidance-conditioned reflex in the rat but did not influence the escape response. However, Izquierdo and Cavalhiero (1976) reported that clonidine (0.2 mg/kg i.p.) depressed both the avoidance and escape responding of rats in a two-way shuttle avoidance paradigm.

Pretreatment with atropine (10 mg/kg), yohimbine (1-2 mg/kg), and piperoxane (10 mg/kg) antagonized the depression of the conditioned avoidance reflex produced by clonidine (Delbarre and Schmitt, 1974). Phenoxybenzamine (10 mg/kg) blocked a clonidine-avoidance paradigm (Izquierdo and Cavalhiero, 1976); however, Delbarre and Schmitt (1974) reported that phenoxybenzamine alone also depressed the conditioned avoidance reflex.

In contrast to the above studies demonstrating a suppression of CAR by clonidine, Ruiz and Monti (1975) and Lenard and Beer (1975) reported that suppression of a previously learned conditioned avoidance response in rats produced by intraventricular administration of 6-hydroxydopamine was reversed by intraventricular administration of norepinephrine, dopamine, L-dopa, or by intraperitoneal administration of amphetamine, phenelzine, desipramine, apomorphine, and clonidine. Pretreatment with the neuroleptic spiroperidol prevented the recovery produced by the above drugs; however, clonidine-induced recovery was the least affected (Lenard and Beer, 1975).

In conclusion, these studies have demonstrated that clonidine may depress or restore conditioned avoidance responding, depending upon the pharmacological state of the subject. Furthermore, the action of clonidine on CAR appears to be mediated through catecholaminergic and cholinergic mechanisms.

Brain Self-Stimulation

It is well established that laboratory animals will press a lever to obtain electrical stimulation when electrodes are placed in various brain areas. Investigations of the neurochemical mechanisms underlying the reinforcing property of intracranial self-stimulation (ICSS) suggest that both dopaminergic and noradrenergic systems may be involved (for review see Seiden and Dykstra, 1977). On the other hand, it has recently been reported that a stronger case can be made for the involvement of dopaminergic mechanisms (for review see Fibiger, 1978).

Utilizing a shuttle-box technique that provides a rate-dependent index of the rewarding and aversive components of ICSS, Hunt et al. (1976) found that intraperitoneal administration of clonidine (0.004-0.063 mg/kg) led to a dose-dependent increase in the latency of initiation of lateral hypothalamic ICSS, whereas the latency of escape from ICSS was largely unaffected except at doses which depressed performance. The peripheral alpha-adrenergic agonist 1-phenylephrine (0.05-1.0 mg/kg) was ineffective in this regard, indicating that inhibition of reward by clonidine was a central effect (Hunt et al., 1976). Clonidine acted in a synergistic manner with the catecholamine synthesis inhibitor alpha-methyl-para-tyrosine (250 mg/kg), greatly increasing (>500 percent) the magnitude of the latency of initiation and prolonging the duration of inhibition of reward while leaving the magnitude of the escape latency largely unaffected (Hunt et al., 1976). Whereas administration of clonidine (0.016-0.064 mg/kg) or alpha-methyl-para-tyrosine alone 24 hours before testing had no effect, their concomitant administration resulted in complete elimination of the initiating behavior, while escape behavior remained unaffected (Hunt et al., 1976). High-rate lateral hypothalamic ICSS in squirrel monkeys was blocked by clonidine (0.1 mg/kg), whereas in the same animal caudate ICSS was much less affected at this dose (Spencer and Revzin, 1976). A higher dose of clonidine (0.25 mg/kg) which produced sedation depressed ICSS to equal degrees at both sites (Spencer and Revzin, 1976). In contrast, amphetamine (10 mg/kg) and chlorpromazine

(0.5 or 1.0 mg/kg) had significantly greater effects on caudate ICSS than on lateral hypothalamic ICSS (Spencer and Revzin, 1976).

Depression of lateral hypothalamic ICSS by clonidine (0.15 mg/kg) was antagonized by doses of piperoxane (1.7-15.0 mg/kg) which selectively block presynaptic alpha-adrenergic or epinephrine receptors, while higher doses of piperoxane (45 mg/kg), pentolamine (0.55-15.0 mg/kg), and phenoxybenzamine (0.1-10.0 mg/kg), which block both pre- and post-synaptic receptors, were ineffective (Franklin and Herberg, 1977).

Vetulani et al. (1977) reported that intraperitoneal administration of clonidine to rats in doses producing no motor deficits (0.05-0.20 mg/kg) resulted in a dose-dependent depression of medial forebrain bundle ICSS. Furthermore, clonidine (0.10 mg/kg) blocked the facilitation of medial forebrain bundle ICSS by d-amphetamine (0.5 mg/kg) (Vetulani et al., 1977). Since d-amphetamine has been reported to release norepinephrine, it was suggested that the blockade of medial forebrain bundle ICSS by clonidine is due to its stimulatory action at presynaptic alpha-noradrenergic receptors or its blockade of postsynaptic noradrenergic receptors (Vetulani et al., 1977).

In view of the demonstration of suppression of ICSS by clonidine in the above experiments, it is not surprising that inhibition of substantia nigra ICSS in rats by the norepinephrine synthesis inhibitor diethyl-dithiocarbamate (Belluzi et al., 1975) or inhibition of lateral hypothalamic ICSS by the norepinephrine synthesis inhibitor disulfiram (Shaw and Rolls, 1976) was not restored by clonidine (0.5-3.0 µg intraventricularly or 0.037-3.0 mg/kg i.p.).

In conclusion, the findings on ICSS suggest that clonidine attenuates the rewarding component of ICSS. Furthermore, this action appears to be mediated through its stimulatory action at central presynaptic alpha-noradrenergic receptors, which decreases noradrenergic transmission (Hunt et al., 1976; Franklin and Herberg, 1974; Vetulani et al., 1977). This suggestion is supported by other investigators (Wise et al., 1973; Hastings and Stutz, 1973; Franklin and Herberg, 1974; German and Bowden, 1974; Belluzi et al., 1975; Shaw and Rolls, 1976) who showed that reduced noradrenergic transmission inhibits self-stimulation. It must be noted, however, that although inhibition of ICSS has been reported at doses which do not produce motor deficits, equal doses were observed to decrease locomotor activity measured in an activity chamber (Tilson et al., 1977).

Conflict-Induced Suppression

The Geller conflict procedure consists of a punishment component and a non-punishment component (Seiden and Dykstra, 1977). In the punishment component of this procedure, punishment (usually an electric grid shock) is superimposed upon ongoing behavior (usually lever pressing for food reward); in the non-punishment component, no punishment is superimposed. Behavior is usually inhibited in the punishment component. Anxiolytic drugs restore behavior which has been suppressed by punishment (for review see Seiden and Dykstra, 1977), and the Geller conflict procedure is therefore widely used to evaluate potentially anxiolytic drugs.

Bullock et al. (1978) have reported that intraperitoneal administration of clonidine (0.025-0.10 mg/kg) to rats led to a significant increase in responding during the punishment phase of the Geller conflict procedure, whereas responding during the non-punishment phase was relatively unaffected except at the highest dose (0.1 mg/kg), at which sedation was observed. These data suggest a possible anxiolytic effect of clonidine.

AGGRESSIVE BEHAVIOR

It has been suggested that central catecholamines and serotonin are involved in the mediation of aggressive behavior (for review see Seiden and Dykstra, 1977). Morpurgo (1968) was the first to report that intraperitoneal administration of high doses (10 and 50 mg/kg) of clonidine induced aggression (biting attacks) in mice but not in rats or rabbits. This behavior was also produced when clonidine was administered orally, intravenously, or subcutaneously. Intracerebral injection of a 0.5 percent solution of clonidine immediately elicited biting attacks (Morpurgo, 1968). More recently, Pazzak et al. (1975) also reported that clonidine (50 mg/kg i.p.) induced automutilation in mice; however, this behavior occurred only when mice were housed individually in the absence of objects to bite. Ozawa et al. (1975) reported that clonidine (40 mg/kg) induced aggressive behavior in mice without altering the brain levels of serotonin, norepinephrine, or dopamine. By contrast, Pazzak et al. (1977) reported that a large dose of clonidine which induced automutilation in mice markedly increased brain norepinephrine, slightly increased brain dopamine levels, and did not change cerebral serotonin levels. The results of these studies suggest that the effect of clonidine on cerebral neurotransmitter levels and their turnover in relation to aggression induced by this drug should be investigated further.

Other imidazoline derivatives (naphazoline, oxymetazoline) with peripheral sympathomimetic effects similar to those of clonidine did not induce biting even when administered intracerebrally (Morpurgo, 1968). This is particularly interesting in view of the finding that the imidazoline derivatives, including naphazoline and oxymetazoline, which do not cross the blood-brain barrier, cause analgesia when administered intracerebroventricularly (Schmitt et al., 1974).

Pretreatment with neuroleptic drugs (*e.g.,* haloperidol, ED_{50} 1.6 mg/kg) inhibited clonidine-induced biting attacks. However, pretreatment with the alpha-adrenergic blocking agent phentolamine or the anticholinergic drug atropine was ineffective in preventing aggressive behavior (Morpurgo, 1968). Since the sympathomimetic effects of clonidine were still evident following neuroleptic pretreatment, the findings of Morpurgo (1968) suggest that clonidine-induced aggression in mice is independent of its alpha-adrenergic action. Ozawa et al. (1975), however, have reported that aggressive behavior in mice induced by intraperitoneal administration of clonidine (40 mg/kg) was markedly inhibited by intraperitoneal pretreatment with the alpha-blocking agent phenoxybenzamine (20 mg/kg). Similarly, Razzak et al. (1977), reported that automutilation induced by a large dose of clonidine was inhibited by prior treatment with reserpine, alpha-methyl-para-tyrosine, phenoxybenzamine, phentolamine, or chlorpromazine.

Pretreatment with amitriptyline, para-chlorophenylalanine, L-dopa, 5-hydroxy-tryptophan, or glycine had no effect on the clonidine-induced aggression and self-mutilation (Ozawa et al., 1975; Stern and Catovic, 1975; Razzak et al., 1977).

Aggression and automutilation induced by clonidine were reported to be potentiated by disulfiram, lithium chloride (Ozawa et al., 1975), nalorphine, maphensin (Stern and Catovic, 1975), methamphetamine, caffeine, and theophylline (Razzak et al., 1977).

These results imply that central noradrenergic mechanisms are involved in the mediation of aggression and automutilation by clonidine.

In rats, aggression can be induced by sufficiently high doses of the dopaminergic agonist apomorphine (McKenzie, 1971) or by termination of chronic narcotic administration (Lal, 1975). It has been suggested that both these forms of aggression are due to hyperstimulation of dopaminergic neurons in the central nervous system (Lal, 1975; Lal et al., 1975). Clonidine by itself administered subcutaneously in doses of 0.25 and 0.5 mg/kg did not cause aggression in drug-naive rats; however, it enhanced aggression caused by a subthreshold (for aggression) dose (2.5 mg/kg) of apomorphine, in dose-dependent fashion (0.0625-0.25 mg/kg), and it enhanced aggression when administered to rats from which morphine had been withdrawn 72 hours previously (Gianutsos et al., 1976).

It has also been reported that irritability and violent aggressive behavior occur in rats after chronic treatment with clonidine (Laverty and Taylor, 1969; Paalzow, 1979) and that rats become irritable and aggressive while receiving clonidine (5 μg/ml) in their drinking water (Dix and Johnson, 1977).

While all of the above studies suggest that clonidine may promote aggressive behavior in mice and rats, Laverty and Taylor (1969) reported that subcutaneous administration of clonidine (0.2-1.0 mg/kg) resulted in a dose-dependent inhibition of aggressive behavior induced by application of painful electric shocks to the grid floor of a cage in which a pair of rats were placed. Cornfeldt et al. (1978), reported that clonidine (ED_{50} 3.8 mg/kg orally) inhibited foot shock-induced aggression in mice. However, clonidine is known to produce analgesia (see Analgesia section) as measured by an increase in the threshold for vocalization (Paalzow, 1974; Schmitt et al., 1974) and vocalization after discharge (Paalzow, 1974; Paalzow and Paalzow, 1976) following electrical stimulation of the rat's tail and several other procedures (Fielding et al., 1978). Therefore, clonidine-induced inhibition of fighting induced by application of an electrical shock to the grid floor may be due to its analgesic action rather than to an ability to modulate aggressive behavior. However, Buss-Lassen (1978) reported that clonidine (0.05-0.16 mg/kg) inhibited aggressive behavior in mice produced by isolation. Simultaneous administration of the alpha-antagonist piperoxane at a dose (5 mg/kg) which selectively blocks presynaptic alpha-adrenergic receptors prevented the antiaggressive effect of clonidine, suggesting that the antiaggressive action of clonidine is mediated by its stimulatory action at presynaptic alpha-adrenergic receptors (Buss-Lassen, 1978).

In conclusion, it has been demonstrated that clonidine may promote, inhibit, or have no effect on aggressive behavior. Its effect on aggressive behavior appears to depend on several factors, including species, dose, treatment regimen (acute vs. chronic), and the method of inducing aggression. Aggressive behavior induced by clonidine appears to be dependent on the postsynaptic stimulation of both dopaminergic and noradrenergic receptors (Morpurgo, 1968; Ozawa et al., 1975; Razzak et al., 1977), while aggressive behavior inhibited by clonidine appears to be dependent on presynaptic noradrenergic stimulation (Buss-Lassen, 1978).

DRUG DISCRIMINATION

It is now widely established that drugs of several pharmacological classes can function experimentally as discriminative stimuli (for review see Lal, 1977). Usually, laboratory animals are trained to emit one response when treated with a drug and an alternate response when treated with the drug vehicle, another dose of the same drug, or a different drug. When such response differentiation is reliably achieved, the drug is said to produce a discriminative stimulus that determines the differential response of the trained subjects.

Miksic et al. (1978), trained rats to discriminate between morphine and saline and tested their rats for generalization of the morphine stimulus to clonidine. They reported that intraperitoneal administration of clonidine (0.08-0.64 mg/kg) failed to generalize with morphine (10 mg/kg). The rats injected with clonidine selected the lever appropriate for saline. Since the discriminative stimulus produced by morphine is considered to be related to its subjective effect in man (Lal and Gianutsos, 1976; Lal et al., 1977), this observation suggests that clonidine has no morphine-like subjective effects. In view of the fact that clonidine produces analgesia (see Analgesia section) and reduced narcotic withdrawal symptoms in animals and humans (see Antiwithdrawal section), these data become particularly important, for they imply that clonidine may provide a non-narcotic treatment for opiate addiction, without producing the psychotomimetic effects of morphine or possessing any potential for morphine-like abuse. This suggestion was recently supported by Washton et al. (1980), who found that clonidine lacks euphorigenic acitivty in individuals maintained on methadone.

LEARNING AND MEMORY

While an important role in learning and memory processes has been postulated for each of the central neurotransmitters, the exact role of each remains unclear. Furthermore, studies measuring the effect of pharmacological agents on learning and memory processes must be interpreted with caution since factors such as sedation and impairment of motor function can affect the results.

Gazzani and Izquierdo (1976) reported that post-trial intraperitoneal administration of clonidine (0.1 mg/kg) or haloperidol (0.5 mg/kg) to rats trained in a shuttle-avoidance paradigm resulted in a lower retention of this task in a retest session carried out seven days later, as compared with animals that received a post-trial saline injection. This effect of clonidine was prevented by pretreatment with either phenoxybenzamine (10 mg/kg) or phentolamine (10 mg/kg), while the effect of haloperidol was prevented by pretreatment with apomorphine (4 mg/kg, but not 0.5 mg/kg). These data suggest that clonidine may either impair memory consolidation or produce state-dependent learning.

In contrast to the above study, however, McEntee and Mair (1978) reported that administration of clonidine to patients with Korsakoff's syndrome (who had low CSF levels of methoxyhydroxyphenylglycol, which correlated with memory impairment) resulted in a consistent improvement of memory function. Since clonidine is presumed to be an alpha-noradrenergic agonist in the central nervous system, improvement of memory by clonidine (McEntee and Mair, 1978) provides additional evidence of an important role of norepinephrine in learning and memory processes. It may be pointed out that in the same study other CNS stimulants such as amphetamine or methylphenidate were inactive.

SELF-ADMINISTRATION OF DRUGS

Investigations of the neurochemical basis of reinforcement resulting from the self-administration of narcotics (Davis and Smith, 1972, 1973a; Glick et al., 1973) and psychomotor stimulants (Davis and Smith, 1972, 1973b) have implicated central catecholaminergic systems. Attempts to differentiate between noradrenergic and dopaminergic mechanisms have led to the conclusion that both dopaminergic and noradrenergic mechanisms appear to be involved in self-administration behavior.

Davis and Smith (1977) have reported that clonidine (15 but not 1 μg/kg injection) was self-administered by rats when administration required the pressing of a lever. The reinforcing effect of clonidine was attributed to its stimulatory action at postsynaptic alpha-noradrenergic receptors since intraperitoneal pretreatment with the alpha-blocking agent phenoxybenzamine (15 mg/kg) prevented the reinforcement associated with clonidine administration (Davis and Smith, 1977). Furthermore, intraperitoneal pretreatment with phenoxybenzamine (15 mg/kg) but not with haloperidol (5 mg/kg) prevented the application of a stimulus paired with injections of clonidine as a conditioned reinforcer (Davis and Smith, 1977). These findings indicate that it is the stimulation of the alpha-noradrenergic receptors by clonidine which yields positive reinforcement.

In rats self-administering the synthetic analgesic fentanyl (1 μg/kg injection), substitution of clonidine (15 but not 1 μg/kg injection) for the fentanyl solution did not attenuate continued self-administration (Shearman et al., 1977). Since an activation of noradrenergic systems is believed to be involved in the mediation of narcotic reinforcement (Davis et al., 1975), the maintenance of fentanyl-reinforced responses by clonidine may be attributable to its ability to stimulate central noradrenergic receptors.

SLEEP AND AROUSAL

Clonidine has been found to have somnifacient and sedative effects when administered by several routes to young chicks, mice, rats, cats, rabbits, and man (Zaimis, 1970; Delbarre and Schmitt, 1971; Holman et al., 1971, 1971a; Florio et al., 1975; Marley and Nistico, 1974, 1975; Walland, 1977; Autret et al., 1976, 1977; Ashton and Rawlins, 1978). Sleep induced by clonidine given intravenously was considered similar to normal sleep or sleep induced by intravenous epinephrine or norepinephrine (Holman et al., 1971, 1971a).

The somnifacient effect of clonidine has been reported to be antagonized by the following alpha-noradrenergic receptor blocking agents; phentolamine (Delbarre and Schmitt, 1971; Holman et al., 1971; Fugner, 1971; Marley and Nistico, 1974; Drew et al., 1977), tolazoline (Delbarre and Schmitt, 1971; Drew et al., 1977), yohimbine (Delbarre and Schmitt, 1973; Drew et al., 1977), piperoxane (Delbarre and Schmitt, 1971; Drew et al., 1977), and dibenamine (Delbarre and Schmitt, 1971). However, several alpha-adrenergic blockers including dibozane, ethoxane, azapetine, mosixylite (Delbarre and Schmitt, 1973), thymoxamine and labetalol (Drew et al., 1977) did not antagonize the sleep-inducing effect of clonidine. Since postsynaptic alpha-adrenoreceptors are more sensitive to the antagonistic effects of thymoxamine and labetalol (Drew, 1977), Drew et al. (1977) suggested that the alpha-adrenoreceptors which moderate the clonidine-induced sedation more closely resemble the peripheral presynaptic alpha-receptors than the postsynaptic alpha-receptors. Whereas Marley and Nistico (1974) reported that phenoxybenzamine antagonized the sedative effect of clonidine, Delbarre and Schmitt (1971) and Fugner (1971) noted that phenoxybenzamine did not antagonize the action of clonidine. These discrepant findings may be related to procedural differences.

Sleep induced by clonidine was not antagonized by several beta-blockers (Delbarre and Schmitt, 1973; Marley and Nistico, 1974), atropine (Marley and Nistico, 1974), methysergide (Holman et al., 1971), or p-chlorophenylalanine (Holman et al., 1971, 1971a; Marley and Nistico, 1974). However, lysergic acid diethylamide (LSD) pretreatment effectively prevented clonidine-induced sleep (Holman et al., 1971).

Clonidine (1.0-2.5 mg/kg) prolonged the chloral hydrate sleeping time in rats (Laverty and Taylor, 1969), chickens and mice (Delbarre and Schmitt, 1971, 1973). Tolazoline, phentolamine, piperoxane, dibenamine (Delbarre and Schmitt, 1971), and yohimbine but not phenoxybenzamine antagonized this action (Delbarre and Schmitt, 1973).

Clonidine induced electroencephalographic (EEG) synchronization and increased spindle activity (Hukuhara et al., 1978, Tran Quang Loc et al., 1974). Kleinlogel et al. (1975) reported that clonidine abolished paradoxical sleep (PS) in rats and reduced slow-wave sleep (SWS). This report was confirmed by Putkonen et al. (1977) who found that clonidine (5-20 μg/kg i.p.) caused a dose-dependent inhibition of PS in cats, a depression of SWS, and a synchronized rhythmic EEG. Ashton and Rawlins (1978) also reported a dissociation of EEG and behavioral effects of clonidine. Yohimbine (2 mg/kg) pretreatment antagonized the PS-suppressing action of clonidine (10 μg/kg) (Putkonen et al., 1977).

Behavioral depression and EEG synchronization induced by clonidine (0.1 mg/kg) in rats, cats, and rabbits were attenuated by pretreatment with the alpha-noradrenergic receptor-blocking agents phentolamine (10 mg/kg), tolazoline (10 mg/kg), and yohimbine (0.5 mg/kg), but not by phenoxybenzamine (10 mg/kg).

Pretreatment with alpha-methyl-para-tyrosine ester (100 mg/kg, 3 days) or reserpine (2 mg/kg) potentiated the clonidine (0.1 mg/kg) induced sedation and EEG synchronization (Florio et al., 1975). Amphetamine (1 or 2 mg/kg) reversed the behavioral depression and EEG synchronization produced by clonidine (0.2 mg/kg) (Florio et al., 1975). Furthermore, clonidine abolished the behavioral activation and EEG desynchronization induced by amphetamine (Florio et al., 1975; Marley and Nistico, 1974, 1975) and methamphetamine (Gogolak and Stumpf, 1969); however, the EEG arousal produced by physostigmine was unaffected by clonidine (Gogolak and Stumpf, 1969).

Ponto-geniculo-occipital (PGO) waves induced by the benzoquinolizine derivative Ro4-1248 or the tryptophan hydroxylase inhibitor p-chlorophenylalanine (PCPA) were suppressed by clonidine (Ruth-Monachon et al., 1976).

Bilateral lesions of the locus coeruleus increased the density of the PGO waves induced by PCPA, suggesting that suppression by clonidine may be due to stimulation of locus coeruleus neurons which depress neurons in the pontine reticular formation involved in the generation of PGO waves (Ruth-Monachon et al., 1976).

Clonidine increased the threshold of the EEG arousal reaction caused by reticular stimulation (Gogolak and Stumpf, 1969). Behavioral and electrocortical sleep induced by intraventricular administration of clonidine (5-15 µg) was easily interrupted by an arousing stimulus (Holman et al., 1971) and presentation of sensory stimuli during clonidine-induced sleep caused behavioral and phasic electrocortical arousal (Marley and Nistico, 1975).

Fletcher (1974) observed that clonidine (0.125 or 0.25 mg/kg) depressed the amplitude of the acoustic startle response when administered to reserpinized rats. This observation was confirmed by Davis et al. (1977) who found that intraperitoneal administration of clonidine (0.01-2.0 mg/kg) led to a dose-dependent depression of startle amplitude when rats were presented with startle-eliciting tones. Pretreatment with piperoxane (10 mg/kg) antagonized this effect; however, phentolamine (10 mg/kg) did not (Davis et al., 1977). Clonidine also depressed startle in acutely decerebrate rats and in rats with bilateral lesions of the locus coeruleus, suggesting that clonidine may depress startle by stimulating central epinephrine rather than norepinephrine receptors (Davis et al., 1977). The depression of startle by clonidine was related to its ability to improve habituation rather than to a reduction of sensitization or impairment of motor function (Davis et al., 1977).

In conclusion, several studies have demonstrated a sedative or sleep-inducing action of clonidine. Indications are that the sleep-inducing effect of clonidine results from a stimulatory action of this drug at central alpha-noradrenergic receptors. The sleep-inducing action of clonidine does not seem to depend on serotonergic (Holman et al., 1971, 1971a) or cholinergic (Marley and Nistico, 1974) transmission.

SEXUAL BEHAVIOR

Ahlenius et al. (1971a) have suggested that the expression of sexual behavior is under the control of both catecholaminergic and serotonergic systems. Malmnas (1973) examined the effect of LSD, clonidine, and apomorphine on testosterone-activated heterosexual copulatory behavior in castrated male rats. The percentage of subjects that displayed copulatory behavior was decreased by LSD (30 and 100 µg/kg) and increased by apomorphine (30-300 µg/kg). Clonidine (3-30 µg/kg) did not change the percentage of subjects engaging in copulatory behavior. In a number of clinical studies of the use of clonidine in the treatment of hypertension, the incidence of male impotence has ranged from 0.1 percent to 5.0 percent (McMahon, 1978).

Crowley et al. (1978) found that clonidine facilitated lordotic behavior in female guinea pigs.

The available data do not allow any inferences to be drawn about a possible effect of clonidine on sexual behavior.

ANALGESIA

The antinociceptive activity of clonidine has been demonstrated in a variety of test procedures developed to measure pain in laboratory animals, including electrical stimulation of the tail, Charpentier's test (Paalzow, 1974, 1979; Paalzow and Paalzow, 1976; Schmitt et al., 1974), placing the animal on a hot (56°C) plate, hot plate test (Schmitt et al., 1974), immersion of the tail in water, tail withdrawal test (Sewell and Spencer, 1975; Fielding et al., 1977, 1978), exposure of the tail to radiant heat, tail flick test (Fielding et al., 1977, 1978; Speulding et al., 1978a), application of pressure to an inflamed paw, the Randall-Selitto test (Fielding et al., 1977, 1978), and intraperitoneal injection of phenyl-p-benzoquinone (Fielding et al., 1977, 1978), acetic acid, or acetylcholine, writhing tests (Bentley et al., 1977). In all of the above procedures except the tail withdrawal test in rats (Fielding et al., 1977, 1978), clonidine was found to be more potent than morphine.

Charpentier's Test

Paalzow (1974) measured the changes in the threshold for vocalization in mice and the threshold for motor response (spinal reflex), vocalization, and vocalization after discharge induced in mice and rats by electrical stimulation of the tail. Subcutaneous administration of clonidine (0.08-1.25 mg/kg) led to a dose-dependent increase (100-500 percent) of the threshold for vocalization and vocalization after discharge in rats, while the threshold for motor response was raised by 100 percent at a dose of 10 mg/kg; however, this dose caused sedation and marked sympathomimetic signs (Paalzow, 1974). Clonidine also increased the threshold for vocalization in mice; however, the dose was higher (2.5-10.0 mg/kg) than that required to cause a similar elevation in rats (Paalzow, 1974).

Tolerance to the antinociceptive action of clonidine in elevating the threshold for vocalization in rats was observed after chronic treatment (Paalzow, 1979).

Acute administration of clonidine (0.5 mg/kg S.C.) given simultaneously with morphine (5.0 mg/kg) greatly augmented the morphine-induced increase of the threshold for vocalization in rats (Paalzow, 1979).

Pretreatment with chlorpromazine (5 mg/kg S.C.), atropine (1 mg/kg S.C.), and p-chlorophenylalanine (400 mg/kg i.p.) increased the antinociceptive activity of clonidine (0.625 mg/kg S.C.) at both the threshold for vocalization and the threshold for vocalization after discharge, while pretreatment with phenoxybenzamine (10 mg/kg i.p.) and reserpine (10 mg/kg i.p.) increased the activity at the threshold for vocalization, only leaving the threshold for vocalization after discharge unaffected (Paalzow and Paalzow, 1976). Yohimbe (2 mg/kg i.p.) pretreatment decreased the antinociceptive activity of clonidine at both thresholds, while pretreatment with 5-hydroxytryptophan (50 mg/kg i.p.) and alpha-methyl-p-tyrosine (250 mg/kg i.p.) decreased the effects at the threshold for vocalization after discharge only (Paalzow and Paalzow, 1976). Naloxone (8 mg/kg S.C.) pretreatment or concomitant LSD (50 μg/kg S.C.) did not alter the antinociceptive activity of clonidine at either of the pain responses studied (Paalzow and Paalzow, 1976).

Schmitt et al. (1974) reported the effect of clonidine on four types of behavioral reaction to electrical stimulation of the rat tail: startle, flight, vocalization, and biting of the electrodes. Intraperitoneal administration of clonidine (0.5-3.0 mg/kg) resulted in a dose-dependent reduction of the startle, cry, and biting of electrodes; however, clonidine was weakly effective against flight (Schmitt et al., 1974). Intraventricular administration of clonidine (30 μg) reduced the vocalization and the biting of electrodes but was less effective in terms of startle and flight (Schmitt et al., 1974). Intraventricular clonidine was 5-7 times as potent as clonidine administered intraperitoneally (Schmitt et al., 1974).

Hot Plate Test

The hot plate test measures the ability of drugs to inhibit reflex responses of mice placed on a plate maintained at a constant temperature of 55°C. A drug is said to procduce analgesia if the time of reaction to the heat is significantly increased. Schmitt et al. (1974) observed that intraperitoneal (0.1 and 1.0 mg/kg) and intraventricular (0.3-1.0 μg) administration of clonidine increased the reaction time to heat. The antinociceptive activity of clonidine in Charpentier's test and the hot plate test appears to be mediated centrally since other alpha-sympathomimetics of the inidazoline series (naphazoline, tetryzoline, and oxymetazoline) which do not cross the blood-brain barrier exercise antinociceptive activity only when administered intracerebroventricularly (Schmitt et al., 1974).

Tail Withdrawal Test

The tail withdrawal test measures the ability of drugs to alter the time within which mice or rats withdraw their tails from hot water, usually maintained at 55°C. A drug is said to produce analgesia in this test if the delay in tail withdrawal is significantly increased (for details see Miksic and Lal, 1977). Using the tail withdrawal test in mice, Sewell and Spencer (1975) found that subcutaneous administration of clonidine (0.3 mg/kg) produced analgesia. However, when clonidine (0.5 mg) was injected intracerebroventricularly, it showed only marginal antinociceptive activity and, furthermore, substantially reduced the analgesic effect of morphine (3 mg/kg S.C.) when given concurrently (Sewell and Spencer, 1975). The antinociceptive activity of subcutaneously administered clonidine (0.3 mg/kg) was significantly antagonized by concurrent intraventricular administration of phentolamine (10 µg) (Sewell and Spencer, 1975). Intraventricular administration of propranolol (10 µg) did not potentiate the antinociceptive effect of concurrent S.C. administration of morphine (2.5 mg/kg), pentazocine (15 mg/kg), or clonidine (0.3 mg/kg) (Sewell and Spencer, 1975).

Intraperitoneal administration of clonidine (2.5 and 10.0 mg/kg) to rats was effective in inhibiting tail withdrawal from hot water (Fielding et al., 1977, 1978). Naloxone (5 mg/kg) did not antagonize the antinociceptive action of clonidine (2.5 mg/kg) (Fielding et al., 1977, 1978).

Tail Flick Test

The tail flick test measures the ability of drugs to alter the time in which mice or rats remove their tails from a radiant heat source. A drug is considered to produce analgesia in this test if the delay in removal of the tail from the heat is significantly increased.

Subcutaneous administration of clonidine was reported to result in a dose-dependent (ED_{50} 0.7 mg/kg) inhibition of the tail flick response in mice (Fielding et al., 1977, 1978). Whereas the ED_{50} of morphine for analgesia in mice in the tail flock was increased 4-7 times following spinal transection, the ED_{50} of clonidine was not significantly altered (Spaulding et al., 1978a). These data indicate that clonidine and morphine have different action sites in this test.

The antinociceptive action of clonidine in this test was not antagonized by naloxone (1.0 mg/kg) (Fielding et al., 1977, 1978) or phenoxybenzamine (10.0 mg/kg) (Fielding et al., 1978).

Subcutaneous administration of clonidine (0.016 mg/kg) increased the analgesic effect of morphine in the tail flick test approximately fivefold, while morphine (0.16 mg/kg) increased the antinociceptive effect of clonidine four times (Spaulding et al., 1978). Naloxone reversed the morphine-induced increase in the effect of clonidine (Spaulding et al., 1978).

No tolerance to the antinociceptive action of clonidine in the tail withdrawal and tail flick procedures has been observed (Fielding et al., 1977). Cross-tolerance to the antinociceptive action of clonidine in morphine-pelleted mice also has not been observed (Spaulding et al., 1978).

Randall-Selitto Test

The Randall-Selitto test measures the ability of drugs to alter the reaction to pressure applied to an inflamed paw by an "analgesia meter." A drug is considered to produce analgesia in this procedure if the amount of pressure required to induce a reaction is significantly increased.

In a modified version of the Randall-Selitto test, Fielding et al. (1977, 1978) found that subcutaneous administration of clonidine (0.125-1.0 mg/kg) produced a dose-dependent increase in the threshold for pain caused by pressure on an inflamed paw. It was concluded that clonidine may be effective in relieving pain association with inflammation.

Writhing Tests

Writhing tests measure the ability of drugs to alter writhing induced by other chemical agents. A drug is considered to produce analgesia in this test if the number of writhes induced by the chemical agent is significantly decreased.

Subcutaneous administration of clonidine (0.0125-0.05 mg/kg) to mice resulted in dose-dependent inhibition of writhing induced by phenyl-p-benzoquinone (Fielding et al., 1977, 1978). The anti-writhing action of clonidine was not antagonized by naloxone (1.0 mg/kg) (Fielding et al., 1977, 1978) or phenoxybenzamine (Fielding et al., 1977). Clonidine, oxymetazoline, and 1-norepinephrine bitartrate were equally effective in antagonizing the nociceptive action of acetic acid or acetylcholine when administered subcutaneously to mice, while phenylephrine was ineffective (Bentley et al., 1977). Piperoxane (8 and 16 mg/kg) antagonized the antinociceptive action of oxymetazoline and norepinephrine, and particularly antagonized the antinociceptive effect of clonidine, whereas phentolamine (16 mg/kg) had no antagonistic effect on any of the three drugs (Bentley et al., 1977). Clonidine and oxymetazoline were more potent when administered intracisternally; however, their antinociceptive effect when administered by this route was not antagonized by piperoxane (16 mg/kg) administered subcutaneously or (50 μg) intracisternally (Bentley et al., 1977).

In summary, these investigations have shown that clonidine produces a dose-dependent analgesia as measured by a variety of procedures for inducing pain in laboratory animals. Clonidine-induced analgesia does not seem to be the result of an impairment of motor function since the threshold for a motor response (Paalzow, 1974) or flight reaction (Schmitt et al., 1974) is unaffected at doses which produce analgesia. The analgesic action of clonidine appears to be mediated centrally since other alpha-sympathomimetics of the imidazoline series which do not cross the blood-brain barrier display antinociceptive activity only when administered intracerebroventricularly (Schmitt et al., 1974). However, the antinociceptive effect of clonidine in writhing tests may be due to its stimulatory action on alpha-adrenoreceptors located at sensory nerve endings in the peritoneum, inasmuch as other peripherally acting alpha-agonists are also antinociceptive in these tests (Bently et al., 1977). Depending on the dose, route of administration, and animal species, it appears that clonidine may increase (Spaulding et al., 1978; Paalzow, 1979) or decrease (Sewell and Spencer, 1975) the analgesic effect of morphine. Similarly, depending upon the procedures used to measure analgesia and produce tolerance, it appears that tolerance to the antinociceptive action of clonidine may (Paalzow, 1979) or may not (Fielding et al., 1977) develop. The absence of naloxone antagonism of the antinociceptive action of clonidine (Paalzow and Paalzow, 1976; Fielding et al., 1977, 1978) suggests that the analgesic effect of clonidine is not mediated by interaction with opiate receptors. In view of the results of studies on the effects of other drugs on clonidine-induced analgesia (Paalzow and Paalzow, 1976; Sewell and Spencer, 1975; Fielding et al., 1977, 1978; Bentley et al., 1977), it appears that several neurochemical systems may mediate the antinociceptive action of clonidine.

ANTIWITHDRAWAL

Wet dog-like body shakes are reliable signs, in the rat, of narcotic withdrawal which are widely used to evaluate the effectivness of new drugs against symptoms due to narcotic withdrawal. Using this sign and other observations, Fielding et al. (1977, 1978) noted that clonidine (0.01-0.16 mg/kg) given i.p. abolished narcotic withdrawal signs in a dose-dependent fashion. This effect of clonidine was not reversed by naloxone. Other investigators (Tseng et al., 1975; Vetulani and Bednarczyk, 1977) employed higher and more sedative doses (0.1-0.8 mg/kg) to block narcotic withdrawal signs precipitated by the administration of narcotic antagonists to rats. Lipman and Spencer (1978), who recently confirmed the above studies, also observed that clonidine at a high dose (0.8 mg/kg) caused stereotypy in narcotic withdrawn rats similar to the earlier observations of Gianutsos et al. (1976). These authors reported increased aggression in morphine-addicted but detoxified rats. Lipman and Spencer (1978) observed augmented morphine withdrawal signs after injecting clonidine directly into the ventricles. Redmond et al. (1976) and Redmond (1977), stimulating the locus coeruleus in the monkey, observed that some signs such as autonomic hyperactivity and ear reactions were similar to those observed in narcotic withdrawal animals although many other typical withdrawal signs were absent. The effects of locus coeruleus stimulation as simulated by piperoxane injection were antagonized by either clonidine or morphine, suggesting that certain of the withdrawal signs may be related to locus coeruleus activity.

Opiates administered systemically or applied microiontophoretically turn off the firing of locus coeruleus neurons (Korf et al., 1974). Tolerance can be developed to this effect of morphine and, in withdrawal, hyperactivity of the cells can be shown. Clonidine reverses this morphine withdrawal sign (Aghajanian, 1978) at the neuronal level.

The effectiveness of clonidine in relieving the withdrawal syndrome was recently confirmed in opioid-dependent patients by two independent research teams (Gold et al., 1978, 1978a, 1979; Washton et al., 1978, 1980). They reported that clonidine effectively blocks as well as reverses the heroin or methadone withdrawal symptoms with the use of a variety of rating scales and by physical examination of the patients. The syndrome induced by abrupt withdrawal of the narcotic is both prevented (Washton et al., 1980) and reversed (Gold et al., 1979) by a single dose of clonidine (about 0.005 mg/kg). This dose causes some hypotension in some patients. Both physical signs and the "affect" associated with narcotic withdrawal are relieved. Clonidine acts to relieve the high anxiety usually present during the drug-free detoxification procedures. Washton et al. (1980) have summarized several studies in which patients were maintained on clonidine alone for several days in order to achieve opioid-free detoxification as tested by the absence of naloxone-precipitated withdrawal signs at the end of this treatment. They found that clonidine proved effective in achieving complete detoxification from heroin or methadone. Similar results were recently reported by Gold et al. (1979).

The ability of clonidine to relieve symptoms of narcotic withdrawal does not seem to be directly related to action on opiate receptors. Naloxone, an effective opiate antagonist, did not inhibit the ability of clonidine to decrease withdrawal signs in animals (Fielding et al., 1978) or human patients (Washton et al., 1978). Similarly, the Narcan test does not promote the withdrawal syndrome in addicts who are maintained on clonidine (Washton et al., 1980). Clonidine does not show any affinity for opioid or endorphin receptors. The mechanism by which it relieves the narcotic withdrawal syndrome is not known at present.

In addition to relieving the symptoms of narcotic withdrawal, clonidine has been found to relieve sweating, tremors, and anxiety associated with alcohol withdrawal in humans (Bjorkqvist, 1975).

FOOD AND WATER CONSUMPTION

In dogs, clonidine increased food intake at low doses and reduced it at high doses (LeDouarec et al., 1972). In rats, parenteral administration of clonidine (0.15-0.3 mg/kg) reduced food intake (LeDouarec et al., 1972; Atkinson et al., 1978). However, chronic subcutaneous administration of clonidine (0.3 mg/kg/day) to rats had an appetite-stimulating effect, suggesting the development of tolerance to the anorectic effect of clonidine.

Piperoxane antagonized the inhibitory effect of clonidine on food intake in rats, while yohimbine and phentolamine proved partially antagonistic (LeDouarec et al., 1972). However, many alpha-adrenergic receptor blockers such as tolazoline, dibenamine, and phenoxybenzamine were ineffective, as were beta-adrenergic receptor blockers (LeDouarec et al., 1972).

Intrahypothalamic administration of clonidine (1 μg) strongly increased food consumption in satiated rats (LeDouarec et al., 1972; Broekkamp and Van

Rossum, 1972). The clonidine-induced eating response was completely blocked by the alpha-antagonist phentolamine (Broekkamp and Van Rossum, 1972).

Holman et al. (1971) reported that after intraventricular administration of clonidine (25-75 µg/kg) to rats, approximately one-third of the rats began eating continuously, and sometimes periods of eating alternated with periods of sleep. Ritter et al. (1975) also found that rats ate voraciously after intraventricular injection of clonidine (0.05-5 µg) and that clonidine facilitated feeding with a potency 100 times greater than that of norepinephrine. Intraventricular administration of clonidine reversed the anorectic effect of intraperitoneally administered d-amphetamine.

In an investigation of the effect of clonidine on behavior associated with food intake, Poignant and Rismondo (1975) observed that clonidine (0.05-0.2 mg/kg) increased the time for intake of standard alimentary material in hamsters without affecting the associated hoarding behavior. By contrast, amphetamine (1 and 2 mg/kg) modified both intake time and hoarding behavior (Poignant and Rismondo, 1975).

Clonidine (0.0375-0.3 mg/kg) reduced water intake and induced diuresis in water-deprived and water-satiated rats (LeDouarec et al., 1971; Atkinson et al., 1978). The antidipsogenic effect of clonidine was followed by a delayed increase in water consumption apparently due to the diuretic effect of the drug since this was suppressed by nephrectomy (Atkinson et al., 1978).

The reduction in water intake was antagonized by piperoxane, tolazoline, and phentolamine; however, other alpha-adrenergic receptor blockers such as dibenamine and phenoxybenzamine were ineffective (LeDouarec et al., 1971). Beta-adrenergic blockers as well as the anticholinergic drugs atropine and mecamylamine were devoid of any antagonistic activity (LeDouarec et al., 1971).

In conclusion, clonidine may increase or decrease food intake, depending on the dose, route of administration, and the animal's state of food deprivation (LeDouarec et al., 1972; Holman et al., 1971; Broekkamp and Van Rossum, 1972; Ritter et al., 1975; Atkinson et al., 1978). However, its effect on water intake seems to be solely inhibitory (LeDouarec et al., 1971; Atkinson et al., 1978). Feeding elicited by intrahypothalamic (especially the perifornical area) injection of norepinephrine in satiated rats is blocked by the administration of alpha-noradrenergic receptor blockers (for review see Seiden and Dykstra, 1977); therefore, the increase of food intake in satiated rats by clonidine may be a result of its stimulatory action at postsynaptic alpha receptors. However, the differential antagonism of the clonidine-induced decrease in food and water intake by alpha-adrenergic blocking agents makes it appear that the receptors involved in mediating these inhibitory effects of clonidine have some properties in common with classical alpha-adrenergic receptors but differ from them in other ways (LeDouarec et al., 1971, 1972). Stimulation of central alpha-adrenergic receptors is known to inhibit drinking (Setler, 1974); therefore, the clonidine-induced decrease in the water intake of water-deprived and water-satiated rats may be related to the stimulatory action of clonidine at postsynaptic alpha-adrenergic receptors.

BODY TEMPERATURE

Thermoregulation normally involves the integration of both behavioral and physiological mechanisms. Studies on the role of central neurotransmitters in thermoregulation point to involvement of both catecholamines and serotonin (Stricker and Zigmond, 1976; Cooper et al., 1978).

Wendt and Caspers (1968) reported a suppression of sweating in man during exposure to heat and exercise after oral administration of 75 and 150 μg (about 1 and 2 μg/kg) of clonidine, while Laverty and Taylor (1969) observed a fall in body temperature when clonidine (0.1-2.5 mg/kg) was subcutaneously administered to rats. Similarly, Tsoucaris-Kupfer and Schmitt (1972) found that subcutaneous or intraperitoneal administration of clonidine (0.5-1.5 mg/kg) induced hypothermia in rats, the intensity and duration of which was dose-dependent.

Maskrey et al. (1970) reported that intraventricular administration of clonidine (0.067-0.107 μg/kg) lowered or elevated body temperature in sheep and goats, depending on whether the ambient temperature was above or below thermoneutrality. Intraventricular injection of clonidine in a dose of 15 μg (Tseng et al., 1975), but not in doses of 2-3 μg (Rsoucaris-Kupfer and Schmitt, 1972), lowered body temperature in rats and produced a dose-dependent (0.02-0.4 μM) degree of hypothermia in young chicks and adult fowls (Marley and Nistico, 1974, 1975) at thermoneutrality. Intrahypothalamic administration of clonidine (3 μg or 0.04 μM) was also found to cause hypothermia (Tsoucaris-Kupfer and Schmitt, 1972; Marley and Nistico, 1975).

The hypothermia produced by clonidine administration was found to be antagonized by the alpha-blocking agents phentolamine, phenoxybenzamine, piperoxane, tolazoline, and dibenamine (Tsoucaris-Kupfer and Schmitt, 1972; Reid et al., 1975; Marley and Nistico, 1974, 1975). Piperoxane was the most effective antagonist (Tsoucaris-Kupfer and Schmitt, 1972). The beta-adrenergic receptor antagonists propranolol, pindolol, and bunitrolol were also reported to be effective in decreasing the hypothermic effect of clonidine (Tsoucaris-Kupfer and Schmitt, 1972). However, Reid et al. (1975) and Marley and Nistico (1974, 1975) observed that propranolol did not alter the hypothermic action of clonidine. Similarly, Tsoucaris-Kupfer and Schmitt (1972) noted that atropine and haloperidol were effective in decreasing the hypothermic effect of clonidine, while mecamylamine and imipramine were ineffective. Maj et al. (1975) and Marley and Nistico (1974, 1975), on the other hand, reported that atropine did not affect clonidine-induced hypothermia, and Reid et al. (1975) found that the relatively selective dopamine receptor antagonist, pimozide did not modify the hypothermic effect of clonidine. Marley and Nistico (1975) reported that haloperidol did not attenuate the hypothermic effect of clonidine. Other alpha-sympathomimetic imidazolines such as naphazoline, tetryzoline, and oxymetazoline, which do not cross the blood-brain barrier (Walland, 1977), were also effective in producing hypothermia after peripheral administration (Tsoucaris-Kupfer and Schmitt, 1972). Depletion of brain catecholamines by intracisternal administration of 6-OHDA failed to alter the hypothermic response to clonidine (Reid et al., 1975). Therefore, the hypothermic effect of clonidine may be due to action at both central and peripheral sites.

Scheel-Kruger and Hasselager (1974) found that the hypothermia induced by clonidine (0.5 mg/kg) in rats could be antagonized by apomorphine (2 x 2.5 mg/kg). These authors suggested that the hypothermic effect of clonidine may be due to its action on serotonin turnover since apomorphine also significantly antagonized the clonidine-induced decrease of 5-hydroxyindoleacetic acid levels and the time course of this action of apomorphine correlated with its antagonism of clonidine-induced hypothermia. However, Marley and Nistico (1974, 1975) found that intraventricular pretreatment with the serotonin receptor blocker methysergide (0.1 μM) or the serotonin depletor PCPA methyl ester did not attenuate the hypothermic effect produced by intraventricular injection of clonidine (0.05-0.2 μM).

Finally, Tseng et al. (1975) noted that intraperitoneal (0.1-0.4 mg/kg) or intraventricular (5 and 15 μg) administration of clonidine inhibited precipitated shakes and potentiated escape attempts induced by naloxone in morphine-dependent rats. These symptoms of morphine withdrawal were previously thought (Wei et al., 1974) to be related to heat gain and heat loss mechanisms, respectively.

In conclusion, these findings demonstrate that clonidine produced hypothermia via several routes of administration. In view of the antagonism of clonidine-induced hypothermia by alpha-adrenergic blocking agents, it appears that the hypothermic action of clonidine is mediated by its stimulatory action at alpha-adrenergic receptors. This assumption is supported by the finding that hypothermia induced by intraventricular administration of norepinephrine is antagonized by phentolamine (Burks, 1972). However, as suggested by Scheel-Kruger and Hasselager (1974), the hypothermic effect of clonidine may be secondary to its action on noradrenergic receptors and may be the result of the clonidine-induced decrease in serotonin turnover (Anden et al., 1970; Scheel-Kruger and Hasselager, 1974; Rochette and Bralet, 1975). According to Feldberg (1964), intraventricular administration of serotonin causes hyperthermia. It would follow, therefore, that a reduction in serotonin turnover by clonidine results in hypothermia. Lastly, we cannot be certain whether or not the hypothermic effect of clonidine is produced at central or peripheral alpha-adrenergic receptors, or both, since other imidazoline sympathomimetics that do not cross the blood-brain barrier also cause hypothermia when administered peripherally.

SUMMARY

Clonidine, a potent centrally-acting pharmacological agent, has been used for the treatment of hypertension. In addition to its antihypertensive property, clonidine exerts a variety of psychopharmacological effects. In this chapter we have reviewed these effects in the hope that they may be investigated further to determine potential clinical applications.

ACKNOWLEDGEMENTS

The editorial assistance of Debbie Bennett and the typographic services of Mrs. Edith Williams are greatly appreciated.

REFERENCES

Aghajanian, G.K. (1978): Tolerance of locus coeruleus neurons to morphine and suppression of withdrawal response by clonidine. *Nature 276:* 186-188.
Ahlenius, S., Anden, N.E., and Engel, J. (1971): Importance of catecholamine release by nerve impulses for free operant behavior. *Physiol. Behav. 7:* 931-934.
Ahlenius, S., Eriksson, H., Larsson, K., Modigh, K., and Sodersten, P. (1971a): Mating behavior in the male rat treated with p-chlorophenylalanine methyl ester alone and in combination with pargyline. *Psychopharmacol. 20:* 383-388.
Anden, N.E., Corrodi, H., Fuxe, K., Hokfelt, B., Rydin, C., and Svensson, T. (1970): Evidence for a central noradrenaline receptor stimulation by clonidine. *Life Sci. 9:* 513-523.
Anden, N.E., Butcher, S.G., and Engel, J. (1970a): Central dopamine and noradrenaline receptor activity of the amines formed from m-tyrosine, alpha-methyl-m-tyrosine and alpha-methyldopa. *J. Pharm. Pharmacol. 22:* 548-550.
Anden, N.E., Strombom, U., and Svensson, T.H. (1973): Dopamine and noradrenaline receptor stimulation: Reversal of reserpine-induced suppression of motor activity. *Psychopharmacologia 29:* 289-298.
Anden, N.E., Gabrowska, M., and Strombom, U. (1976): Different alpha adrenoceptors in the central nervous system mediating the biochemical and functional effects of clonidine and receptor blocking agents. *Naunyn–Schiedebergs Archives Pharmacol. 292:* 43-52.
Ashton, H., and Rawlins, M. (1978): Central nervous system depressant actions of clonidine and UK-14, 304; partial dissociation of EEG and behavioral effects. *Brit. J. Clin. Pharmacol. 5:* 135-140.
Atkinson, J., Kirchertz, E., and Peters-Haefeli, L. (1978): Effects of peripheral clonidine on ingestive behavior. *Physiol. Behav. 21:* 73-77.
Autret, A., Minz, M., Beillevaire, T., Cathala, H.P., Castaigne, P. (1976): Suppression of paradoxal sleep by clonidine in man. *C.R. Acad. Sci. D, 283:* 955-957.
Autret, A., Minz, M., Beillevaire, T., Cathala, H.P., and Schmitt, H. (1977): Effect of clonidine on sleep patterns in man. *Eur. J. Clin. Pharmacol. 12:* 319-322.

Belluzi, J.D., Ritter, S., Wise, C.D., Stein, L. (1975): Substantia nigra self-stimulation: dependence on noradrenergic pathways. *Behav. Biol. 13:* 103-111.

Bentley, G.A., Copeland, I. W., and Starr, J. (1977): The actions of some alpha-adrenoceptor agonists and antagonists in an antinociceptive test in mice. *J. Clin. Exp. Pharmacol. Physiol. 4:* 405-419.

Bjorkqvist, S.E. (1975): Clonidine in alcohol withdrawal. *Acta Psych. Scand. 52:* 256-263.

Broekkamp, C., and Van Rossum, J. (1972): Clonidine induced intrahypothalamic stimulation by eating in rats. *Psychopharmacol. 25:* 162-168.

Bullock, S.A., Kruse, H., and Fieldings, S. (1978): The effect of clonidine on conflict behavior in rats: Is clonidine an anxiolytic agent? *Pharmacologist 20:* 223.

Burks, R.F. (1972): Central alpha-adrenergic receptors in thermoregulation. *Neuropharmacol. 11:* 615-624.

Buus–Lassen, J. (1978): Piperoxane reduces the effects of clonidine on aggression in mice and on noradrenaline dependent hypermotility in rats. *Eur. J. Pharmacol. 47:* 4549.

Colelli, B., Meyer, D.R., and Sparber, S.B. (1976): Clonidine antagonizes disruption of fixed ratio operant behavior in morphine pelleted rats given naloxone. *Pharmacologist 18:* 236.

Cooper, J.R., Bloom, F.F., and Roth, R.H. (1978): *The Biochemical Basis of Neuropharmacology.* Oxford University Press, New York.

Cornfeldt, M.L., Fielding, S., Kruse, H., Billey-Nichuck, J., Dobson, C., and Wilker, J. (1978): Clonidine: Inhibition of amphetamine-induced circling and other psychopharmacological effects. *Pharmacologist 20:* 162.

Crowley, W., Nock, B., and Feder, H. (1978): Facilitation of lordosis behavior by clonidine in female guinea pigs. *Pharmacol. Biochem. Behav. 8:* 207-209.

Dandiya, P., and Patni, S. (1973): Influence of substances acting on the central adrenergic receptor on open field behavior in rats. *Indian J. Med. Res. 61:* 891-895.

Davis, W.M., and Smith, S.G. (1972): Alpha-methyl-tyrosine to prevent self-administration of morphine and amphetamine. *Curr. Ther. Res. 14:* 814-819.

Davis, W.M., and Smith, S.G. (1973a): Blocking of morphine based reinforcement by alpha-methyltyrosine. *Life Sci. 12:* 185-191.

Davis, W.M., and Smith, S.G. (1973b): Blocking effect of alpha-methyltyrosine on amphetamine based reinforcement. *J. Pharm. Pharmacol. 25:* 174-177.

Davis, W.M., and Smith, S.G. (1975): Effect of haloperidol on (+) amphetamine self-administration. *J. Pharm. Pharmacol. 27:* 540-542.

Davis, W.M., and Smith., S.G. (1977): Catecholaminergic mechanisms of reinforcement: direct assessment by drug self-administration. *Life Sci. 20:* 483-492.

Davis, W.M., Cedarbaum, J., Aghajanian, G., and Gendelman, D. (1977): Effects of clonidine on habituation and sensitization of acoustic startle in normal decerebrate and locus coeruleus lesioned rats. *Psychopharmacol. 51:* 243-253.

Davis, W.M., Smith, S.G., and Khalsa, J.H. (1975): Noradrenergic role in the self-administration of morphine and amphetamine. *Pharmacol. Behav. 3:* 477-484.

Delbarre, B., and Schmitt, H. (1971): Sedative effects of alpha-sympathomimetic drugs and their antagonism by adrenergic and cholinergic blocking drugs. *Eur. J. Pharmacol. 13:* 356-363.

Delbarre, B., and Schmitt, H. (1973): A further attempt to characterize sedative receptors activated by clonidine in chickens and mice. *Eur. J. Pharmacol. 22:* 355-359.

Delbarre, B., and Schmitt, H. (1974): Effects of clonidine and some alpha-adrenoreceptor blocking agents on avoidance conditioning reflexes in rats: Their interactions and antagonism by atropine. *Psychopharmacol. 35:* 195-202.

Dix, R., and Johnson, E., Jr. (1977): Withdrawal syndrome upon cessation of chronic clonidine treatment in rats. *Eur. J. Pharmacol. 44:* 153-159.

Dolphin, A., Jenner, P., and Marsden, C. (1976): The relative importance of dopamine and noradrenaline receptor stimulation for the restoration of motor activity in reserpine or alpha-methyl-p-tyrosine pre-treated mice. *Pharmacol. Biochem. Behav. 4:* 661-670.

Donaldson, I., Dolphin, A., Jenner, P., Marsden, C., and Pycock. C. (1976): The roles of noradrenaline and dopamine in contraversive circling behavior seen after unilateral electrolytic lesions of the locus coeruleus. *Eur. J. Pharmacol. 39:* 179-191.

Drew, G.M. (1977): Pharmacological characterization of pre-synaptic alpha adrenoceptors which regulate cholinergic activity in the guinea pig ileum. *Brit. J. Pharmacol. 59:* 513.

Drew, G., Gower, A., and Marriott, A. (1977): Pharmacological characterization of alpha-adrenoceptors which mediate clonidine-induced sedation. *Brit. J. Pharmacol. 61:* 468.

Dunstan, R., and Jackson, D.M. (1976): The demonstration of a change in adrenergic receptor sensitivity in the central nervous system of mice after withdrawal from long-term treatment with haloperidol. *Psychopharmacol. 48:* 105-114.

Dunstan, R., and Jackson, D. (1977): The effect of apomorphine and clonidine on locomotor activity in mice after long term treatment with haloperidol. *Clin. Exp. Pharmacol. Physiol. 4:* 131-141.

Fechter, L. (1974): The effects of 1-dopa, clonidine, and apomorphine on the acoustic startle reaction in rats. *Psychopharmacol. 39:* 331-344.

Feldberg, W., and Myers, R.D. (1964): Effects on temperature of amines injected into the cerebral ventricles. A new concept of temperature regulation. *J. Physiol. 173:* 226-237.

Fibiger, H.C. (1978): Drugs and reinforcement mechanisms. A Critical review of the catecholamine theory. *Ann. Rev. Pharmacol. Tox. 18:* 37-56.

Fielding, S., and Lal, H. (1980): Clonidine: New research in psychotrophic drug pharmacology. *Medicinal Res. Rev., 1:* 97-123.

Fielding, S., Wilker, J., Hynes, M., Szewzak, M., Novick, W. and Lal, H. (1977): Antinociceptive and withdrawal actions of clonidine: A comparison with morphine. *Fed. Proc. 36:* 1024.

Fielding, S., Wilker, J., Hynes, M., Szewczak, M., Novick, W. and Lal, H. (1978): A comparison of clonidine with morphine for antinociceptive and antiwithdrawal actions. *J. Pharmacol. Exp. Ther. 207:* 899-905.

File, S.E., and Pope, J. H. (1974): The action of chlorpromazine on exploration in pairs of rats. *Psychopharmacol. 37:* 249-254.

Florio, V., Bianchi, L., and Lonogo, V.G. (1975): A study of the central effects of sympathomimetic drugs: EEG and behavioral investigations of clonidine and naphazoline. *Neuropharmacol. 14:* 707-714.

Franklin, K.B.J., and Herberg, L.J. (1974): Self-stimulation and catecholamines: Drug-induced mobilization of the "reserve" pool re-established responding in catecholamine-depleted rats. *Brain Res. 67:* 429-437.

Franklin, K.B.J., and Herberg, L.J. (1977): Presynaptic alpha-adrenoceptors: The depression of self-stimulation by clonidine and its restoration by piperoxane but not by phentolamine or phenoxybenzamine. *Eur. J. Pharmacol. 43:* 33-38.

Fugner, A. (1971): Antagonism of the drug-induced behavioral sleep in chicks. *Arzneim. Forsch. 71:* 1350-1356.

Gazzani, J.L., and Izquierdo, I. (1976): Possible peripheral adrenergic and central dopaminergic influences on memory consolidation. *Psychopharmacol. 49:* 109-112.

Gellert, V.F., and Sparber, S.B. (1977): A comparison of the effects of naloxone upon body weight loss and suppression of fixed-ratio operant behavior in morphine-dependent rats. *J. Pharmacol. Exp. Ther. 201:* 44-54.

German, D.C., and Bowden, D.M. (1974): Catecholamine systems as the neural substrate for intracranial self-stimulation: A hypothesis. *Brain Res. 73:* 381-419.

Gianutsos, G., Hynes, M.D., and Lal, H. (1976): Enhancement of morphine-withdrawal and apomorphine-induced aggression by clonidine. *Psychopharm. Comm. 2:* 165-171.

Glick, S.D., Zimmerberg, B., and Charap, A.D. (1973): Effects of alpha-methyl-para-tyrosine on morphine dependence. *Psychopharmacol. 32:* 365-371.

Glick, S.D., and Cox, R. (1976): Differential sensitivity to apomorphine and clonidine following frontal cortical damage in rats. *Eur. J. Pharmacol. 36:* 241-245.

Gogolak, V.G., and Stumpf, Ch. (1966): The effects of 2-(2,6-dichloro-phenylamino)-2-imidazoline hydrochloride on the EEG-arousal reaction in rabbits. *Arzneim. Forsch. 16:* 1050-1052.

Gold, M.A., Redmond, D.E., Jr., and Kleber, H.D. (1978): Clonidine in opiate withdrawal. *Lancet 1:* 929-930.

Gold, M.A., Redmond, D.E., Jr., and Kleber, H.D. (1978a): Clonidine blocks acute opiate-withdrawal symptoms. *Lancet 2:* 599-602.

Gold, M.A., Redmond, D., and Kleber, H. (1979): Noradrenergic hyperactivity in opiate withdrawal supported by clonidine reversal of opiate withdrawal. *Am. J. Psychiat. 136:* 100-102.

Harris, R.A., Snell, D., Loh, H.H., and Way, E.L. (1976): Behavioral interactions of apomorphine, clonidine and naloxone: possible presynaptic involvement. *Proc. West. Pharmacol. Soc. 19:* 448-451.

Harris, R.A., Snell, D., Loh, H.H., and Way, E.L. (1977): Behavioral interactions between naloxone and dopamine agonists. *E. J. Pharmacol. 43:* 243-246.

Hastings, L., and Stutz, R.M. (1973): The effect of alpha- and beta-adrenergic antagonists on the self-stimulation phenomenon. *Life Sci. 13:* 1253-1259.

Herman, Z.S., Brus, R., Drybanski, A., Szkilnik, R., and Slominska-Zurek, J. (1976): Influence of 6-hydroxydopamine on the behavioral effects induced apomorphine or clonidine in rats. *Psychopharmacol. 50:* 73-80.

Hill, R.T., and Tedeschi, D.H. (1971): Animal testing and screening procedures in evaluating psychotropic drugs. In: *An Introduction to Psychopharmacology.* Raven Press, New York, p. 237-279.

Holman, R.B., Shillito, E.E., and Vogt, M. (1971): Sleep produced clonidine (2-(2,6-dichlorophenylamino)-2-imidazoline hydrochloride). *Brit. J. Pharmacol. 43:* 685-695.

Holman, R.B., Shillito, E., and Vogt, M. (1971a): Sleep elicited by clonidine and its relation to new ones containing 5-hydroxytryptamine. *J. Physiol. (Lond.) 217:* 51P-52P.

Hukuhara, R., Jr., Otsuka, Y., Takeda, R., and Sakai, F. (1968): Synchronization of EEG and increased spindle activity following clonidine in cats. *Arzneim.-Forsch. 18:* 1147.

Hunt, G.E., Atrens, D.M., Chechet, G.B., and Becker, F.T. (1976): A noradrenergic modulation of hypothalamic self-stimulation: studies employing clonidine, 1-phenylephrine and alpha-methyl-p-tyrosine. *Eur. J. Pharmacol. 37:* 105-111.

Izquierdo, I., and Cavalhiero, E.A. (1976): Three main factors in rat shuttle behavior: their pharmacology and sequential entry in operation during a two-way avoidance session. *Psychopharmacol. 49:* 145-157.

Jahn, U., and Mixich, G. (1976): Wet dog shake behavior in normal rats elicited by benzylidenamino-oxycarbonic acid derivatives. *Psychopharmacol. 46:* 191-196.

Janssen, P.A.J., Jageneau, A.H.M., and Schelledens, K.H.L. (1960): Chemistry and pharmacology of compounds related to 4/4-hydroxyphenyl-piperidino-butyropheone. Part IV. Influence of haloperidol (R 16251) and chlorpromazine on the behavior of rats in an unfamiliar "open field" situation. *Psychopharmacol. 1:* 389-392.

Jenner, P.G., and Marsden, C.D. (1975): The influence of piribedil (ET 495) on components of locomotor activity. *Eur. J. Pharmacol. 33:* 211-216.

Jenner, P.G., and Pycock, C.J. (1976): Interaction of clonidine with dopamine dependent behaviors in rodents. *Brit. J. Pharmacol. 58:* 469.

Kleinlogel, H., Scholtysik, G., and Sayer, A. (1975): Effects of clonidine and BS 100-41 on the EEG sleep pattern in rats. *Eur. J. Pharmacol. 33:* 159-163.

Korf, J., Bunney, B.S., and Aghajanian, G.K. (1974): Noradrenergic neurons: morphine inhibition of spontaneous activity. *Eur. J. Pharmacol. 25:* 165-169.

Lal, H. (1975): Morphine-withdrawal aggression. In: S. Ehrenpreis and E.A. Neidle (Eds.), *Methods in Narcotic Research.* Marcel Dekker, New York. pp. 149-169.

Lal, H. (Ed.) (1977): *Discriminative Stimulus Properties of Drugs.* Plenum Press, New York.

Lal, H., and Gianutsos, G. (1976): Discriminable stimuli produced by narcotic analgesics. *Psychopharmacol. Comm. 2:* 311-314.

Lal, H., Gianutsos, G., and Puri, S.K. (1975): Comparison of narcotic analgesics with neuroleptics on behavioral measures of dopaminergic activity. *Life Sci. 17:* 29-34.

Lal, H., Gianutsos, G., and Miksic, S. (1977): Discriminable stimuli produced by analgesics. In: H. Lal (Ed.), *Discriminative Stimulus Properties of Drugs.* Plenum Press, New York.

Lal, H., and Shearman, G.T. (1981): Psychotrophic actions of clonidine. *Prog. Clin. Biol. Res. 71:* 99-145.

Laverty, R., and Taylor, K.M. (1969): Behavioral and biochemical effects of 2-(2,6-dichlorophenylamino-2-imidazoline hydrochloride (ST 155) on the central nervous system. *Brit. Pharmac. 35:* 253-264.

LeDouarec, J.C., Schmitt, H., and Lucet, B. (1971): Effect of clonidine and alpha-sympathomimetics on water intake in rats deprived of water. *J. Pharmacol.* (Paris) *2:* 435-444.

LeDouarec, J.C., Schmitt, H., and Lucet, B. (1972): Effects of clonidine and other alpha-sympathomimetic agents on food intake: Antagonism by adrenolytics. *J. Pharmacol.* (Paris) *3:* 187-198.

Lenard, L.G., and Beer, B. (1975): Modification of avoidance behavior in 6-hydroxydopamine-treated rats by stimulation of central noradrenergic and dopaminergic receptors. *Pharmacol. Biochem. Behav. 3:* 887-893.

Lipman, J., and Spencer, P. (1978): Clonidine and opiate withdrawal. *Lancet 2:* 521.

Maj, J., Sowinska, H., Baran, L., and Kapturkiewicz, Z. (1972): The effect of clonidine on locomotor activity in mice. *Life Sci. 11:* 483-491.

Maj, J., Baran, L., Sowinska, H., and Zielinski, M. (1975): The influence of cholinolytics on clonidine action. *Pol. J. Pharmacol. 27:* 17-26.

Malmnas, C. (1973): Monoaminergic influence on testosterone-activated copulatory behavior in the castrated male rat: IV. Effects of LSD-25, clonidine and apomorphine on copulatory behavior in the male rat. *Acta. Physiol. Scand. Suppl. O:* 1-128.

Marley, E., and Nistico, G. (1974): Sleep and hypothermic effects of clonidine in fowls. *Brit. J. Pharmacol. 52:* 434-435.

Marley, E., and Nistico, G. (1975): Central effects of clonidine, (2-(2,6-dichlorophenylamino)-3-imidazoline hydrochloride) in fowls. *Brit. J. Pharmacol. 55:* 459-473.

Maskrey, M., Vogt, M., and Bligh, J. (1977): Central effects of clonidine (2-(2,6-dichlorophenylamino)-2-imidazoline hydrochloride, ST 155) upon thermoregulation in the sheep and goat. *Eur. J. Pharmacol. 12:* 297-302.

McEntee, W.J., and Mair, R.G. (1978): Korsakoff's amnesia: A noradrenergic hypothesis. *A.C.N.P. Abstracts.*

McKenzie, G.M. (1971): Apomorphine-induced aggression in the rat. *Brain Res. 34:* 323-330.

McMahon, F.G. (1978): Clonidine (Catapres). In: *Management of Essential Hypertension.* Futura, New York. pp. 151-174.

Menon, M.K., Clark, W.G., and Masvoka, D.T. (1977): Possible involvement of the central dopaminergic system in the antireserpine effect of LSD. *Psychopharmacol. 52:* 291-297.

Meyer, D.R., El-Azhary, R., Bierer, D., Hanson, S.K., Robbins, M.S., and Sparber, S.B. (1977): Tolerance and dependence after chronic administration of clonidine to the rat. *Pharmacol. Biochem. Behav. 7:* 227-231.

Miksic, S., and Lal, H. (1977): Tolerance to morphine-produced discriminative stimuli and analgesia. *Psychopharmacol. 54:* 217-221.

Miksic, S., Shearman, G., and Lal, H. (1978): Generalization study with some narcotic and non-narcotic drugs in rats trained for morphine-saline discrimination. *Psychopharmacol. 60:* 103-104.

Modigh, K. (1975): Electroconvulsive shock and postsynaptic catecholamine effects: increased psychomotor stimulant action of apomorphine and clonidine in reserpine pretreated mice by repeated ECS. *J. Nueral Transm. 36:* 19-32.

Morpurgo, C. (1968): Aggressive behavior induced by large doses of 2-(2,6-dichlorophenyl-amino)-2-imidazoline hydrochloride (ST155) in mice. *Eur. J. Pharmacol. 3:* 374-377.

Ozawa, H., Miyanchi, T., and Sugawara, K. (1975): Potentiating effect of lithium chloride on aggressive behavior induced in mice by nialamide plus L-Dopa and by clonidine. *Eur. J. Pharmacol. 34:* 169-179.

Paalzow, L. (1974): Analgesia produced by clonidine in mice and rats. *J. Pharm. Pharmacol. 26:* 361-363.

Paalzow, G. (1979): Development of tolerance to the analysis effect of clonidine in rats: Cross-tolerance to morphine. *Nauyn-Schmiederberg Arch. Pharmacol. 304:* 14.

Paalzow, G., and Paalzow, L. (1976): Clonidine antinociceptive activity: Effects of drugs influencing central monoaminergic and cholinergic mechanisms in the rat. *Nauyn-Schmiederberg Arch. Pharmacol. 292:* 119-126.

Pijneberg, A., Honig, W., Van Der Heyden, J., and Van Rossum, J. (1976): Effects of chemical stimulation of the mesolimbic dopamine system upon locomotor activity. *Eur. J. Pharmacol. 35:* 45-58.

Pijneberg, A., Honig, W., Boudier, H., Cools, A., Van Der Heyden, J., and Van Rossum, J. (1976a): Further investigations on the effects of ergometrine and other ergot derivatives following injection into the nucleus accumbens of the rat. *Arch. Int. Pharmacodyn. Ther. 222:* 103-115.

Poignant, J.C., and Rismondo, N. (1975): Influence of the administration of psychopharmacological compounds on the take-up time of an alimentary material in the hamster and a study of the associated behavior. *Psychopharmacol. 43:* 47-52.

Putkonen, P., Leppavour, A., and Stenberg, D. (1977): Paradoxical sleep inhibition by central alpha-adrenoceptor stimulant clonidine antagonized by alpha-receptor blocker yohimbine. *Life. Ace. 21:* 1059-1065.

Pycock, C.J., Donaldson, I. MacG., and Marsden, C.D. (1975): Circling behavior produced by unilateral lesions of the locus coeruleus in rats. *Brain Res. 97:* 317-323.

Pycock, C.J., Jenner, P.G., and Marsden, C.D. (1977): The interaction of clonidine with dopamine-dependent behavior in rodents. *Naunyn-Schmiederberg Arch. Pharmacol. 297:* 133-141.

Razzak, A., Fujiwara, M., and Veki, S. (1975): Automutilation induced by clonidine in mice. *Eur. J. Pharmacol. 30:* 356-360.

Razzak, A., Fujiwara, W., Oishi, R., and Veki, S. (1977): Possible involvement of a central noradrenergic system in automutilation induced by clonidine in mice. *Jap. J. Pharmacol. 27:* 145-152.

Redmond, D.E., Jr., Huang, Y.H., Snyder, D.R., and Maas, J.W. (1976): Behavioral effects of stimulation of the nucleus locus coeruleus in the stump-tailed monkey Macaca arctoides. *Brain Res. 116:* 502-510.

Redmond, D.E., Jr. (1977): Alterations in the function of the nucleus locus coeruleus: A possible model for studies of anxiety. In: I. Hanin and E. Usdir (Eds.) *Animal Models in Psychiatry and Neurology*. Pergamon Press,Oxford. pp. 293-305.

Reid, J.L., Lewis, P.J., and Meyers, M.G. (1975): Role of contral dopaminergic mechanisms in piribedil and clonidine induced hypothermia in the rat. *Neuropharmacol. 14:* 215-220.

Ritter, S., Wise, D., and Stein, L. (1975): Neurochemical regulation of feeding in the rat: Facilitation by alpha-noradrenergic but not dopaminergic, receptor stimulants. *J. Comp. Physiol. Psych. 88:* 778-784.

Rochette, L., and Bralet, J. (1975): Effect of the norepinephrine receptor stimulating agent "clonidine" on the turnover of 5-hydroxytryptamine in some areas of rat brain. *J. Neural Trans. 37:* 259-267.

Ruiz, M., and Monti, J.M. (1975): Reversal of the 6-hydroxydopamine-induced suppression of CAR by drugs facilitating central catecholaminergic mechanisms. *Pharmacol. 13:* 281-286.

Ruth-Monachon, M., Jaffre, M., and Haefely, W. (1976): Drugs and PGO waves in the lateral gericulate body of the curarized cat. III. PGO wave activity and brain catecholamines. *Arch. Int. Pharmacodyn. Ther. 219:* 287-307.

Satoh, J., Satoh, Y., Notsu, Y., and Honda, F. (1976): Adenosine 3',5'-cyclic monophosphate as a possible mediator of rotational behavior induced by dopaminergic receptor stimulation in rats lesioned unilaterally in the substantia nigra. *Eur. J. Pharmacol. 39:* 365-377.

Scheel-Kruger, J., and Hasselager, E. (1974): Studies of various amphetamines, apomorphine and clonidine on body temperature and brain. *Psychopharmacologia 36:* 189-202.

Schmitt, H., LeDouarec, J.C., and Petillot, N. (1974): Antinociceptive effects of some alpha-sympathomimetic agents. *Neuropharmacol. 13:* 289-294.

Seiden, L.S., and Dykstra, L.A. (1977): Dopamine, norepinephrine and behavior. In: *Psychopharmacology: A Biochemical and Behavioral Approach*. Van Nostrand Reinhold Co., New York. pp. 117-171.

Sewell, R.D.E., and Spencer, P.S.J. (1975): Antinociceptive activity in mice after central injections of alpha- and beta-adrenoceptor antagonists. *Brit. J. Pharmacol. 54:* 256-257.

Shaw, S.G., and Rolls, E.T. (1976): Is the release of noradrenaline necessary for self-stimulation of the brain. *Pharmacol. Biochem. Behav. 4:* 375-379.

Shearman, G., Hynes, M., Fielding, S., and Lal, H. (1977): Clonidine self-administration in the rat: A comparison with fentanyl self-administration. *Pharmacologist 19:* 171.

Skolnick, P., Daly, J., and Segal, D. (1978): Neurochemical and behavioral effects of clonidine and related imidazolines: interaction with alpha-adrenoceptors. *Eur. J. Pharmacol. 47:* 451-455.

Sparber, S., and Meyer, D. (1978): Clonidine antagonizes naloxone induced suppression of conditioned behavior and body weight loss in morphine-dependent rats. *Pharmacol. Biochem. Behav. 9:* 319-325.

Spaulding, T.S., Venafro, J., Ma, M., Cornfeldt, M., and Fielding, S. (1978): Interaction of morphine and clonidine in the tail flick test: potentiation studies. *Pharmacologist 20:* 269.

Spaulding, T.S., Venafro, J.J., Ma., M.G., and Fielding, S. (1978a): The dissociation of the antinociceptive effect of clonidine from supraspinal structures. *Neuropharmacol.* 103-105.

Spencer, J., and Revzin, A. (1976): Amphetamine, chlorpromazine and clonidine effects on self-stimulation in caudate or hypothalamus of the squirrel monkey. *Pharmacol. Biochem. Behav. 5:* 149-156.

Stern, P., and Catovic, S. (1975): Brain glycine and aggressive behavior. *Pharmacol. Biochem. Behav. 3:* 723-726.

Stricker, E.M., and Zigmond, M.J. (1976): Recovery of function following damage to central catecholamine-containing neurons: A neurochemical model of the lateral hypothalamic syndrome. In: J.M. Sprague and A.N. Epstein (Eds.) *Progress in Psychobiology and Physiological Psychology.* Academic Press, New York.

Strombom, U. (1975): Effects of low doses of catecholamine receptor agonists on exploration in mice. *J. Neural Transm. 37:* 229-235.

Strombom, U. (1976): Catecholamine receptor agonists: Effects on motor activity and rate of tyrosine hydroxylation in mouse brain. *Naunyn-Schmied. Arch. Pharmacol. 292:* 167-176.

Strombom, U., Svensson, T., Carlsson, A. (1977): Antagonism of ethanol's central stimulation in mice by small doses of catecholamine-receptor agonists. *Psychopharmacol. 51:* 293-299.

Tilson, H.A., Chamberlain, J.H., Gylys, J.A., and Boyniski, J.P. (1977): Behavioral suppressant effects of clonidine in strains of normotensive and hypertensive rats. *Eur. Pharmacol. 43:* 99-105.

Tran Quang Loc, D., Tscovcaris-Kupfer, Y., Bogaievsky, D., Delbarre, B., and Schmitt, H. (1974): Antagonisme de l'action sedative de la clonidine par quelques -adrenolytiques: etude electrocorticographique et comportement ale chez le lapin et le chat. *J. Pharmacol.* (Paris) *5:* 51-55.

Tseng, L.F., Loh, H.H., and Wei, E.T. (1975): Effect of clonidine on morphine withdrawal signs in the rat. *Eur. Pharmacol. 30:* 93-99.

Tsoucaris-Kupfer, D., and Schmitt, H. (1972): Hypothermic effect of alpha-sympathomimetic agents and their antagonism by adrenergic and cholinergic blocking drugs. *Neuropharmacol. 11:* 625-635.

Urgerstedt, U., Butcher, L.L., Butcher, S.G., Anden, N.E., and Fuxe, K. (1969): Direct chemical stimulation of dopaminergic mechanism in the neostriatum of the rat. *Brain Res. 14:* 461-468.

Vetulani, J., and Bednarczyk, B. (1977): Depression by clonidine of shaking behavior elicited by nalorphine in morphine-dependent rats. *J. Pharm. Pharmacol. 29:* 567-568.

Vetulani, J., Leith, N.J., Stawarz, R.J., and Sulser, F. (1977): Effect of clonidine on the noradrenergic cyclic AMP generating system in the limbic forebrain and on medial forebrain self-stimulation behavior. *Experientia 33:* 1490-1491.

Waldeck, B. (1973): Sensitization by caffeine of central catecholamine receptors. *J. Neural Transm. 34:* 61-72.

Walland, A. (1977): Clonidine. In: M.E. Goldberg (Ed.), *Pharmacological and Biochemical Properties of Drug Substances.* Association American Pharmaceutical, Washington, D.C. pp. 67-107.

Washton, A.M., Resnick, R.B., and LaPlaca, R.A. (1978): Clonidine hydrochloride: A nonopiate treatment for opiate withdrawal. *Abstract ACNP.*

Washton, A.M., Resnick. R.B., and Rawson, R.A. (1980): Clonidine hydrochloride: A nonopiate treatment for opiate withdrawal. Proceedings of the 41st Annual Scientific Meeting of the Committee on Problems of Drug Dependence, Philadelphia., NIDA Research Monograph, U.S. Govt. Printing Office.

Wei, E. (1975): Resemblance of morphine antinociception to the central depressant actions of norepinephrine. *Life Sci. 17:* 17-18.

Wei, E. (1976): Chemical stimulants of shaking behavior. *J. Pharm. Pharmacol. 28:* 722-723.

Wei, E., Tseng, L-F., Loh, H.H., and Way, E.L. (1974): Morphine abstinence signs: similarity to thermoregulatory behavior. *Nature 247:* 398-400.

Wendt, F., and Caspers, I. (1968): Koppertemperateur und schweiss-sekretin vei koperlicker belastung unter dem einflurs von 2-(2,6-dichlorophenylamino)-2-imidazolin hydrochlorid. In: L. Heilmeyer, H.J. Holtmeier, and E.F. Pfeiffer (Eds.), *Hochdruck-Therapie, Symposium uben 2(2,6-dichlorophenylamino)-2-imidazolin hydrochlorid.* George Thieme, Stuttgart.

Wise, C.D., Bergen, B.P., and Stein, L. (1973): Evidence of alpha-noradrenergic reward receptors and serotonergic punishment receptors in the rat brain. *Biol. Psychiat. 6:* 3-11.

Zaimis, E. (1970): The Pharmacology of Catapres (ST 155). In M.E. Conolly (Ed.), *Catapres in Hypertension.* Butterworth, London. pp. 9-22.

Zebrowska-Lupina, I., Pregdinski, E., Sloniec, M., and Kleinrok, Z. (1977): Clonidine-induced locomotor hyperactivity in rats. The role of central postsynaptic alpha-adrenoceptors. *Naunyn-Schmiedegergs Arch. Pharmacol. 297:* 227-231.

10

The Clinical Profile of Psychotropic Drugs

Frans de Jonghe
Jacob A.C. Bleeker
Eliza D.J. Lindenbergh

INTRODUCTION

A large and growing variety of psychotropic drugs is available to the physician seeking the proper drug for his patient. One might think that this provides him with the opportunity to choose the most appropriate one. However, choosing implies the comparing of alternatives, which in this case are the drugs. Unfortunately, they are hardly comparable. The explosive increase of the literature about them has generated so much unsystematic and contradictory information that confusion rather than knowledge has been the result. The here proposed "Clinical Profile of Psychotropic Drugs" (CPPD) is a tool for the multidimensional description of the clinical actions of psychotropic drugs. It is intended as a conveyor of condensed and systematic information about the similarities and differences existing between drugs.

It is not the first time that this has been attempted. However, first, the existing systems are often conceptually unclear. Bobon, *e.g.*, confuses an antimanic action pertaining to a syndrome, an antidelusional one pertaining to a symptom, and an antiautistic one pertaining to the hazy concept of autism (Bobon et al., 1972). Secondly, the systems have been constructed for drugs belonging to a certain traditional class, *i.e.*, the major tranquillizers (Delay, 1959; Lambert et al., 1959; Pichot, 1960; Bobon et al., 1965) or the antidepressants (Kielholz, 1963). As such, they do not allow the comparison of drugs belonging to different traditional classes, *e.g.*, chlorpromazine and imipramine. Finally and most importantly, these taxonomies reflect the opinions of clinicians, based on their personal experience. Considering that this clinical experience is undoubtedly large, these judgments may carry authority, especially when experts agree.

However, even the shared subjective estimations of experienced clinicians remain impressionistic. The controlled data of double blind research deserve the last say in the matter.

THE CLINICAL ACTIONS

Nine pathological phenomena or dysfunctions, pertaining to five psychic and to two neurologic activities, lie at the basis of the CPPD. They are indicated in Table 1.

TABLE 1. The Clinical Profile of Psychotropic Drugs (CPPD): Functions, Dysfunctions and Actions

Functions	Dysfunctions	Actions Inducing	Reducing
Cognition	Psychotic cognition	Psychotogenic	Antipsychotic
Emotion	Pathological anxiety	Anxiogenic	Anxiolytic
Psychomotor activity	Agitation	Stimulating	Sedative
Sleep	Insomnia	Insomnia inducing	Hypnogenic
Mood	Pathological euphoria	Euphorizing	Anti-euphoric
	Pathological depression	Depression inducing	Antidepressive
Extrapyramidal activity	Extrapyramidal dysfunction	Extrapyramidal	Anti-extrapyramidal
Autonomic activity	Parasympathetic hyperactivity	Parasympathico-mimetic	Parasympathicolytic
	Sympathetic hyperactivity	Sympathicomimetic	Sympathicolytic

On each of the nine dysfunctions an inducing and a reducing effect can be exercised. This leads to the distinctions of eighteen actions, grouped in nine pairs of opposites (the inducing and the reducing ones). The nine phenomena and the eighteen actions are described as follows (examples are given in Figures 1 through 7):

1. *Psychosis* is the generic indication of severe pathological phenomena in the realm of cognition, *i.e.*, dysfunctional perception and/or thinking with loss of reality testing (*e.g.*, hallucinations). A *Psychotogenic* action induces these phenomena, an *Antipsychotic* one reduces them. Excluded from the psychosis category are the cognitive disturbances of the so-called affective psychoses (mania and melancholia), which are regarded as secondary to the pathological mood.
2. *Anxiety* refers to a pathological emotional state, both as the experience of danger and as the concomitant bodily reactions. An *Anxiogenic* action induces these phenomena, an *Anxiolytic* one reduces them. It must be added that drugs with an anxiolytic action have a reducing effect not only on pathological but also on normal anxiety, eventually leading to an abnormal absence of anxiety reactions.
3. *Agitation* is the description of a state of psychomotor hyperactivity. A *Stimulating* action induces these phenomena, a *Sedative* one reduces them. Drugs with a sedative action reduce normal activity also, eventually leading to a state of psychomotor hypoactivity. Drugs with a stimulating action may activate retarded patients to normal activity levels.
4. *Insomnia* is the qualitative and/or quantitative reduction of normal sleep. An *Insomnia Inducing* action induces these phenomena, a *Hypnogenic* one reduces them. Hypnogenic drugs may cause hypersomnia, insomnia inducing drugs may relieve it.

It has to be stressed that in the literature the important distinction between an anxiolytic, sedative and hypnogenic action is poorly made (Delay, 1959; Lambert et al., 1959; Kielholz, 1965). All these actions are reducing, but the first one reduces anxiety, the second agitation and the third insomnia, respectively bearing upon emotions, psychomotor activity and sleep.

5. *Euphoria* indicates the pathological mood state of elation. An *Euphorizing* action induces these phenomena, an *Anti-Euphoric* one reduces them.
6. *Depression* indicates a pathologically low mood state. A *Depression Inducing* action induces these phenomena, an *Anti-Depressive* one reduces them.
7. *Extrapyramidal Dysfunction* refers to the pathological motor phenomena controlled by the extrapyramidal system: tremor, hypertonia, hypokinesia, hyperkinesia and dyskinesia. An *Extrapyramidal* action induces these phenomena, and *Anti-Extrapyramidal* one reduces them.
8. *Parasympathetic Hyperactivity* regards the manifold pathological phenomena caused by relative hyperfunction of the parasympathetic part of the peri-

pheral efferent autonomic system (*e.g.,* hypersalivation, accelerated intestinal passage). A *Parasympathicomimetic* action induces these phenomena, a *Parasympathicolytic* one reduces them. Parasympathicolytic drugs not only reduce hyperactivity to normal levels but also normal activity to hypofunction, causing a state of parasympathetic hypofunction. Parasympathicomimetic drugs may relieve such a hypofunction.

9. *Sympathetic Hyperactivity* means relative hyperfunction of the orthosympathetic part of the peripheral efferent autonomic system (*e.g.,* tachycardia, increase in blood pressure). A *Sympathicomimetic* action induces these phenomena, a *Sympathicolytic* one reduces them. Sympathicolytic drugs can cause a state of orthosympathetic hypoactivity, sympathicomimetic drugs may relieve it.

THE QUANTIFICATION OF THE ACTIONS

Each of the eighteen actions of the profile is quantified on a five point scale, with scores from zero up to four corresponding with the quantification: none, weak, moderate, strong and very strong. The following definitions for the scores are proposed:

Score 0 (not demonstrated): this statement refers to two different conditions: (a) the action has not been studied; (b) it has been studied and has been found comparable to, *i.e.,* not differentiable from, the action of a placebo. Therefore, in the following text score 0 means either "unknown" or "absent."

Score 2 (moderate action): an action comparable to, *i.e.,* not differentiable from, the action of the standard given in Table 2. Drugs typical for the action concerned have been selected. On the other hand thrift has been strived for. The bulk of evidence from double-blind studies favour the drugs over placebos, so it can be asserted that drugs display the action concerned beyond reasonable doubt.

Score 4 (very strong action): an action which surpasses beyond reasonable doubt the standard given for moderate action. This cannot be assumed on account of just one study, therefore a statistically significant stronger action than that scored as moderate must have been repeatedly demonstrated. For example, a drug, which has been shown over and over again to surpass significantly 15 mg diazepam in anxiety reduction, attains a score of four for its anxiolytic action.

As a result of the foregoing, the *Scores 1* (weak action) and *3* (strong action) are self-evident: they are attributed when doubt is reasonable.

TABLE 2. The Clinical Profile of Psychotropic Drugs (CPPD): Standards for Moderate Action (Score 2)

Action	Standard drug	Oral daily dosage
Antidepressive	Imipramine	150 mg
Anti-euphoric	Chlorpromazine	300 mg
Anti-extrapyramidal	Orfenadrine	150 mg
Antipsychotic	Chlorpromazine	300 mg
Anxiogenic	Detroamphetamine	30 mg
Anxiolytic	Diazepam	15 mg
Depression inducing	Reserpine	3 mg
Euphorizing	Dextroamphetamine	30 mg
Extrapyramidal	Chlorpromazine	300 mg
Hypnogenic	Chlorpromazine	300 mg
Insomnia inducing	Dextroamphetamine	30 mg
Parasympathicolytic	Chlorpromazine	300 mg
Parasympathicomimetic	Physostigmine	3 mg
Psychotogenic	Dextroamphetamine	30 mg
Sedative	Chlorpromazine	300 mg
Stimulating	Dextroamphetamine	30 mg
Sympathicolytic	Chlorpromazine	300 mg
Sympathicomimetic	Dextroamphetamine	30 mg

THE EMPIRICAL BASIS

One could use the system described in order to express his views concerning the actions of a drug based on his personal clinical experience. At any rate this would receive the benefit of concreteness and explicitness. As such it could be useful for every doctor to draw a profile of the drugs he prescribes. However, research data are more reliable and should form the grounds for a profile agreed to on all accounts. It is rather discouraging to realize that thousands of publications about one drug are no exception. Fortunately, the student soon realizes how vast the wasteland of irrelevant information is. The purpose of the profile is to enhance the comparability of drugs. Consequently, the best material available are double-blind comparative studies. This selection remarkably reduces the overwhelming amount of literature. The drugs show impressive differences in the number of times they appear to have been tested on a double-blind comparative basis, some of them dozens of times and others, among which are many widely used drugs, scarcely or not at all. Thus, in the approach proposed here, the first step in profiling a drug is to make a thorough investigation of its double-blind literature.

THE CONTROL OF SOME SOURCES OF VARIANCE

Mode and duration of administration of a drug as well as its dosage may influence the profile greatly. Therefore, a profile of a drug is drawn pertaining only to a well-defined dosage (or perhaps plasmaconcentration in the future), mode of administration and period of time (*e.g.*, the first four weeks of administration). Of course profiles can be drawn of the same drug for different dosage regimens, modes of administration or time periods.

DISCUSSION

a. The profile claims a fair allowance of objectivity, drawn from double-blind research. However, the objectivity of double-blind studies is not unquestioned. Furthermore, the profile does not automatically result from the scrutiny of the outcomes of double-blind literature, which first have to be converted to scores by judgments. The existing studies have not been carried out with the CPPD in mind. The definitions used for clinical actions are often quite different. It is not unusual to find that an antipsychotic action is attributed to a drug on account of changes in the sum-score of the Brief Psychiatric Rating Scale (Overall and Gorham, 1962) of a group of schizophrenic patients. The same applies to an antidepressive action alleged on the grounds of changes in the sum-score of the Hamilton Rating Scale (Hamilton, 1960) of patients with a depression. These scales permit one to conclude whether schizophrenic or depressive patients get better or not, but only some of their items pertain to an antipsychotic or antidepressive action of a drug as defined here. Another major problem is the fact that the studies using different populations, experimental designs, measurement methods and statistics are hardly comparable. Since an action can be taken for granted only after having been demonstrated repeatedly, one is often tempted to conclude that nothing in this realm has been proved, thus providing us only with shared ignorance. Undoubtedly, our knowledge of the clinical actions of psychotropic drugs is grossly overestimated by most people. Still, unless we are willing to accept that nothing can be said about these drugs, some estimation has to be made based on general trends in the results of double-blind studies. These trend-indicating evaluations are the judgments reflected in the scores. They are more subjective in nature than the data of the double-blind studies themselves. In short, treated this way, there is a hard core of objectivity at the basis of the profile, but obviously its Achilles heel is the jump from the objective data to the more subjective estimations of the raters in defining their scores. The profile has to be read as consisting of tentatively attributed scores, not as *ex cathedra* proclaimed truth.

b. The profile is essentially a sort of summary. It therefore cannot surpass the quality of what is summarized, in this case the scientific literature. As far as concerns its proving clinical actions, much has to be done. It is hoped that the profile will stimulate the research worker sharply to differentiate its eighteen actions and systematically to investigate them all. The profile of a drug is dated. New information may lead to revisions in an existing profile. Thus, the CPPD has to be understood as a living document, not as fossilized, once-and-forever, established knowledge.

c. The profile regards clinical actions resulting in clinical effects. Effect and action must be clearly discriminated. For example, a hypnogenic effect is not necessarily due to a hynogenic action: a drug with an anxiolytic action can promote sleep in an anxious patient as a result of anxiety reduction very much as an analgetic drug can do this in a person sleepless from toothache. However, a drug with a hypnogenic action shows this effect independently of anxiety reduction or analgesia. It is crucial to distinguish primary from secondary effects. An effect is primary if it is not a result of another one. An antidepressive effect is primary when it is not due to an anxiolytic, sedative or hypnogenic effect. Actually, most of the effects described here can be primary or secondary. Only in the first case a corresponding action is attributed to the drug concerned. Anxiety reduction may be a primary effect of a drug, which is then considered as having an anxiolytic action. But anxiety reduction may be consequent to the fading of hallucinations and delusions, due to a drug with an antipsychotic action which is not entitled to an anxiolytic action. On the other hand, a drug with an anxiolytic action will probably have many secondary effects, *e.g.*, on sleep and agitation, without deserving credit for these specific actions.

d. The definitions used are undoubtedly inaccurate. One might wish more refinement, *e.g.*, distinguishing neurotic from psychotic anxiety, discriminating several types of insomnia, differentiating sorts of depression. It is not unlikely that in the future refinements will be made, *e.g.*, based on a biochemical typology of depressions or based on a biochemical typology of extrapyramidal phenomena (probably caused by a contrary biochemical imbalance, some of them are induced by haloperidol whereas other are reduced by it). With respect to the sympathicolytic action, it must be specified whether an alpha- or a beta-blockade is meant. However, generally speaking, further division of the categories mentioned is for the moment premature and would be mixing hypotheses with established facts.

e. A distinction between wanted and unwanted actions, leading to so-called effects and side-effects, is not made. An action (*e.g.*, a hypnogenic one) can be wanted or unwanted, depending upon the symptomatic state of the patient, the intensity of the action, the time of day, etc.

f. It should be clear that the information provided by the profile is far from being exhaustive. Out of the manifold clinical actions of psychotropic drugs an arbitrary (but not unfounded) selection has been made. The profile has to be read as containing necessary but not sufficient information for the clinician.

g. It must be stressed that the profile neglects very important aspects of the clinical situation, the so-called nondrug factors. Patient response to drug administration is determined not only by the characteristics of the drug but also by those of the patient, the doctor, the setting and the concomitant therapies. In order to say something distinctive about a certain drug, these factors have to be eliminated from consideration, *e.g.*, by considering the drug actions in a group of patients.

h. The profile facilitates the comparison of drugs belonging to different traditional classes. The borders between these classes have never been very clear and are becoming more and more blurred. Some major tranquillizers are used as sedatives, hypnotics, ataractics and even as antidepressants. Certain minor tranquillizers are considered the drug of choice for symptomatic psychotic states. Several antidepressants are said to possess neuroleptic qualities or are used in the treatment of phobias. As a matter of fact, the use of the CPPD could render the traditional classification of drugs out of date.

i. For clinical use the drug profile requires a patient profile as its counterpart. Only then will the physician be able to select the most appropriate drug by matching the individual clinical profile of his patient with the drug profiles available to him. For this purpose a patient profile has to be worked out based on the same pathological phenomena underlying the drug profile.

EXAMPLES

Chlorpromazine

The CPPD of chlorpromazine at an oral daily dosage of 300 mg is shown in Figure 1.

FIGURE 1. The CPPD of Chlorpromazine

Daily Dosage   : 300 mg (100 mg t.i.d.)
Mode of Administration : per os
Period of Administration : first four weeks

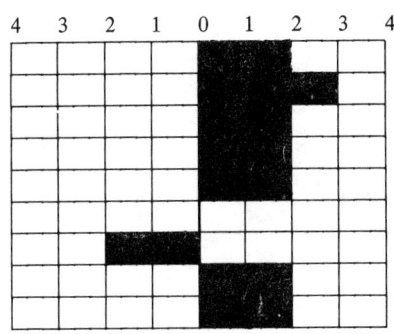

	4	3	2	1	0	1	2	3	4	
Psychotogenic										Antipsychotic
Anxiogenic										Anxiolytic
Stimulating										Sedative
Insomnia inducing										Hypnogenic
Euphorizing										Anti-euphoric
Depression inducing										Antidepressive
Extrapyramidal										Anti-extrapyramidal
Parasympathicomimetic										Parasympathicolytic
Sympathicomimetic										Sympathicolytic

The psychotogenic, anxiogenic, stimulating, insomnia inducing, euphorizing, anti-extrapyramidal, parasympathicomimetic and sympathicomimetic actions of chlorpromazine are easily scored (scores being "zero") for no one has ever claimed the drug to display them. On the contrary, the antipsychotic, sedative, extrapyramidal, parasympathicolytic and sympathicolytic actions have been demonstrated too often to mention (Klein and Davis, 1969). By definition these scores are "two." The hypnogenic action of chlorpromazine is well documented (Toyoda, 1961; Itil, 1968, 1969; Sagale et al., 1969; Feinberg et al., 1969; Lester et al., 1971; Kupfer et al., 1971; Hartman and Cravens, 1973: Kaplan et al., 1974). The same holds well for the anti-euphoric action (Platman, 1970; Spring et al., 1970; Johnson et al., 1971; Prien et al., 1972; Takashi et al., 1975; Shopsin et al., 1975). Both scores are "two" by definition. Much confusion exists about the depression inducing and antidepressive actions. Chlorpromazine is often said to induce depression although this action is not evidenced by double-blind studies. On the other hand, the drug has been favourably compared with imipramine in the treatment of depression (Fink et al., 1964, 1965; Klein, 1966; Paykel et al., 1968; Raskin, 1968, 1971, 1974, 1975; Raskin et al., 1970, 1971). Both actions are claimed but are not sufficiently demonstrated; the scores are "zero." Finally, the unquestioned anxiolytic action has to be scored. Chlorpromazine at the dosage of 75 mg has been shown to be equivalent to 15 mg diazepam or to 75 mg chlordiazepoxide, which are comparable (Hare, 1963; Smith and Chassan, 1964; Yamamoto et al., 1973). At the fourfold dosage of 300 mg, chlorpromazine obtains a score of "three." This profile gives us a good opportunity to call attention to a possible faulty interpretation. In analyzing the profile one could conclude that chlorpromazine is more anxiolytic than antipsychotic. This comparison is as senseless as saying that a banana is more yellow than long.

Dextroamphetamine

The CPPD of dextroamphetamine at an oral daily dosage of 30 mg is shown in Figure 2.

FIGURE 2. The CPPD of Dextroamphetamine

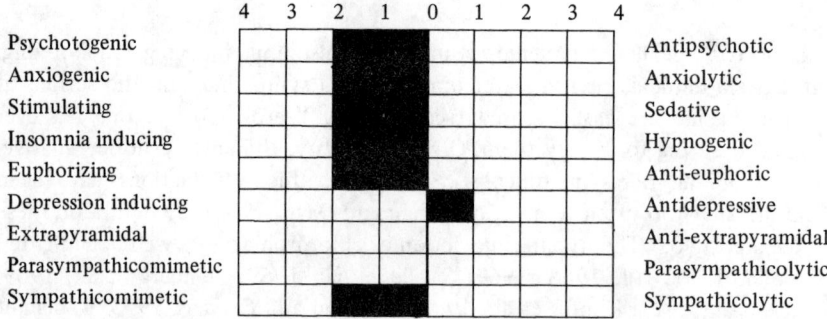

As far as the clinical actions of dextroamphetamine are concerned, the literature is almost unanimous. The antipsychotic, anxiolytic, sedative (except for hyperactive children with minimal brain damage), hypnogenic, anti-euphoric, depression-inducing, parasympathicomimetic, parasympathicolytic and sympathicolytic actions are not claimed. On the contrary, the psychotogenic, anxiogenic, stimulating, insomnia inducing, euphorizing and sympathicomimetic actions are uncontested. By definition, the scores of the latter actions are "two." Dextroamphetamine has also widely been used as an antidepressant drug. However, the scarce double-blind literature casts doubt on the alleged antidepressive action (Miller et al., 1960; Overall et al., 1962; Hare et al., 1962; Gen. Pract. Res. Gr., 1964; Malitz and Kanzler, 1971). Hence the score is "one." The profile of dextroamphetamine appears to be the reverse of the chlorpromazine profile, which is not to be wondered at.

Imipramine

The CPPD of imipramine at an oral daily dosage of 150 mg is shown in Figure 3.

FIGURE 3. The CPPD of Imipramine

Daily Dosage : 150 mg (50 mg t.i.d.)
Mode of Administration : per os
Period of Administration : first four weeks

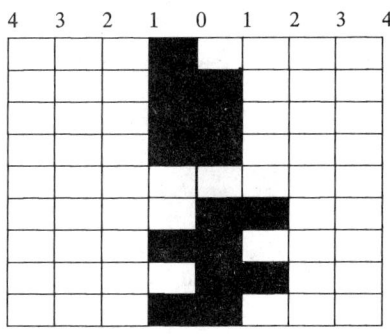

Several reviews exist of the extensive double-blind literature on imipramine (Toyoda, 1964; Klerman and Cole, 1965; Davis, 1965, 1976; Morris and Beck, 1974; Rogers and Clay, 1975). It has been demonstrated beyond reasonable doubt that the drug has an antidepressive action, by definition scored "two." An antipsychotic, anti-euphoric, depression-inducing and parasympathicomimetic action has never been claimed. Apart from the occasional provoking of a manic state, the drug has no euphorizing action. Therefore all these actions are scored "zero." On the contrary, there exist several reports of a slight psychotogenic action (Schover, 1960; Kramer, 1963; Kane and Keeler, 1964; Klein, 1965; Schulterbrandt et al., 1974), thus scored "one." Effects on anxiety, agitation, insomnia and extrapyramidal phenomena are reported regularly. Unfortunately, the only consistency of these reports is in their contradictory character. That the drug displays these effects can hardly be doubted. That the intensity of the actions meets the standards of diazepam, chlorpromazine and dextroamphetamine can hardly be asserted. Each action achieves the score "one." It might seem nonsensical to attribute two contradictory actions to the same drug, for instance an anxiolytic and an anxiogenic one. One should of course bear in mind that the drug does not exert both actions in the same individual at the same moment, but rather either in different individuals or at different moments. The impact of imipramine on the peripheral efferent autonomic system must be taken for granted. Compared with the standard chlorpromazine, the parasympathicolytic action seems to be at least equally outspoken and the sympathicolytic action, on the contrary, probably less (Schulterbrandt et al., 1974). Thus the scores are respectively "two" and "one." Finally, imipramine can display some sympathicomimetic action (Lapierre, 1974), hence scored "one."

Diazepam

The CPPD of diazepam at an oral daily dosage of 15 mg is shown in Figure 4.

FIGURE 4. The CPPD of Diazepam

Daily Dosage : 15 mg (5 mg t.i.d.)
Mode of Administration : per os
Period of Administration : first four weeks

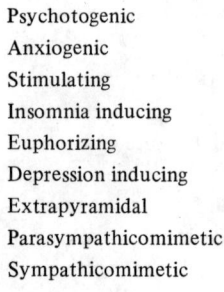
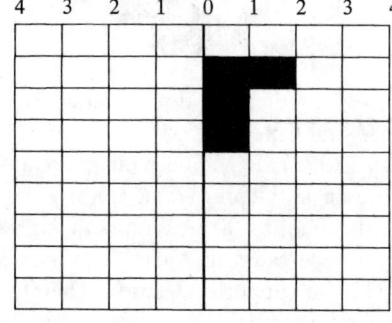

Only three actions obtain a score higher than zero. Some of the other ones have been claimed now and then, but none of them has been proved. The review of double-blind literature (Greenblatt, 1974) demonstrates undebatably the anxiolytic action of the drug, scored "two" by definition. The hypnogenic and sedative action as well are beyond doubt. In this respect, 15 mg of diazepam corresponds to 75 mg of chlorpromazine (Hare, 1963; Smith and Chassan, 1964). Therefore these actions are scored "one."

Haloperidol

The CPPD of haloperidol at an oral daily dosage of 5 mg is shown in Figure 5.

FIGURE 5. The CPPD of Haloperidol

Daily Dosage   : 5 mg ± 1.5
Mode of Administration : per os
Period of Administration : first four weeks

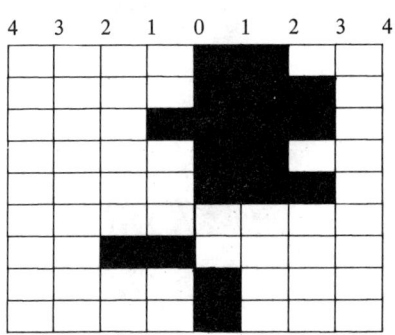

It is based on all double-blind placebo studies and double-blind comparisons with the standard drugs (a total of 40 publications) published between 1960 and March 1978. In 12 studies a significant antipsychotic action was reported, but there is insufficient evidence to call haloperidol 5 mg more antipsychotic than chlorpromazine 300 mg. (Azima et al., 1960; Brandrup and Kristjansen, 1961; Howard, 1974; Lafave et al., 1967; Madalena, 1964; Ota and Kurland, 1973; Rees and Davies, 1965; Selman et al., 1976; Serafetinides et al., 1972; Simpson et al., 1967; Sugerman et al., 1964; Vichaiya, 1971). Anxiolytic (Azima et al., 1960; Deberdi, 1972; Finnerty, 1976, Fyro et al., 1974; Janke and Debus,

1972; Rogerson and Butler, 1971; Samuels, 1961; Serafetinides et al., 1972), sedative (Craft, 1965; Cunningham et al., 1968; Deberdi, 1972, Janke and Debus, 1972, Rogerson and Butler, 1971; Serafetinides et al., 1972; Serafetinides and Clark, 1973; Simpson et al., 1967; Sugerman et al., 1964) and anti-euphoric (Serafetinides et al., 1972; Wald et al., 1978) actions are all outspoken and probably stronger than in the standard drugs, resp. diazepam 15 mg and chlorpromazine 300 mg, (Man and Chen, 1973; Shopsin et al., 1975; Singh et al., 1975; Stevenson, 1976). There is some evidence for a stimulating, a parasympatholytic and a sympatholytic action. A hypnogenic action was twice proved and often mentioned as a side effect. The extrapyramidal action is undisputed.

Pimozide

The CPPD of pimozide, based on 21 double-blind studies, is shown in Figure 6.

FIGURE 6. The CPPD of Pimozide

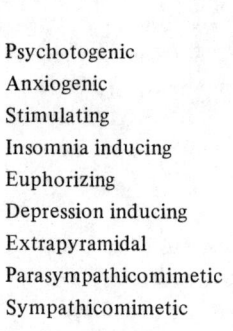
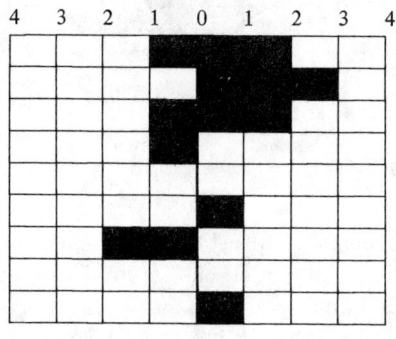

The antipsychotic action of pimozide 7.5 mg has been proved in 9 studies (Chouinard et al., 1970; Clark et al., 1975; Gross, 1974; Janssen et al., 1972; Mahal and Janakiramaiah, 1975; Shridhar Sharma and Dipali Dutta, 1976; Sugerman, 1971; Pinard et al., 1972; Denijs and Vereecken, 1973). A psychotogenic action is mentioned by six authors, but without reaching significance. The anxiolytic action is well documented (8 studies) (Goldberg and Kurland,

1974; Gross, 1974; Holmgren, 1975; Janke and Debus, 1972; Janssen et al., 1972; Reyntjens and Van Mierlo, 1972; Campos Cervera, 1974; Denijs and Vereecken, 1973); compared to diazepam 15 mg, it sometimes appeared to be superior. The sedative action has been proved in at least four studies (Gross, 1974; Holmgren, 1975; Huber et al., 1971; Denijs and Vereecken, 1973). A stimulating, insomnia inducing, antidepressive and sympatholytic action has been mentioned in different studies. The extrapyramidal action is undisputed.

Trifluoperazine

The CPPD of trifluoperazine based on 35 double-blind studies is shown in Figure 7.

FIGURE 7. The CPPD of Trifluoperazine

Daily Dosage   : 20 mg
Mode of Administration : per os
Period of Administration : first four weeks

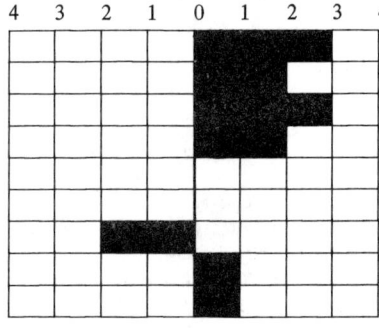

Both antipsychotic and sedative action of trifluoperazine 20 mg are well established in eleven studies (Childers and Therrien, 1961; Clark et al., 1975; Hamilton et al., 1963; Howell et al., 1961; Oybir, 1962; Prien et al., 1969; Reardon and Abrans, 1966; Sarada Menon and Ramachandran, 1972; Weckowics and Ward, 1960; Pinard et al., 1972; Lafave et al., 1967) and three studies (Hunter and Stephenson, 1963; Prien et al., 1969; Sharpe, 1962), respectively. Compared to chlorpromazine 300 mg it appears to have a superior antipsychotic and sedative action in several studies, however in higher doses than 20 mg, which justifies score 3 instead of 4 (Childers and Therrien, 1961; Reardon and Abrans, 1966;

Teja et al., 1975; Bishop and Gallant, 1965; Claghorn, 1970; Hollister et al., 1960; Platz et al., 1967; Smith and Chassan, 1964; Wilson et al., 1961). The anxiolytic action has been reported in five studies (Burt and Bressler, 1961; Howell et al., 1961; May et al., 1959; Reardon and Abrams, 1966; Gross, 1974). In two studies (Smith and Chassan, 1964; Vilkin, 1964) it was found to be less anxiolytic than diazepam. The hypnogenic and the extrapyramidal actions are well documented. The parasympathicolytic and sympathicolytic actions are often mentioned as side effects.

PRECIS

The authors propose a "Clinical Profile of Psychotropic Drugs" (CPPD): a system for the multidimensional description of the clinical actions of psychotropic drugs. Nine opposite pairs of inducing and reducing action are distinguished and quantified. Scores are attributed according to the results of double-blind comparative studies. As example, the system is applied to chlorpromazine, dextroamphetamine, imipramine, diazepam, haloperidol, pimozide and trifluoperazine. Being applicable to a large variety of drugs, the system makes the comparison of drugs belonging to different traditional classes possible. This drug profile requires a patient profile as its counterpart.

REFERENCES

Azima, H., et al. (1960): The effect of R 1625 (haloperidol) in mental syndromes: a multiblind study. *Am. J. Psychiatry 117:* 546-547.

Bishop, M.P., and Gallant, D.M. (1965): Trifluoperidol in "paranoid" and "non-paranoid" schizophrenics. *Curr. Ther. Res. 7:* 96-101.

Bobon, J., Bobon, D.P., Pinchard, A., et al. (1972): A new comparative physiognomy of neuroleptics. *Acta Psychiat. Belg. 72:* 542-554.

Bobon, J., Pinchard, Breulet, M., et al. (1965): Physionomie compareé des principaux thymanaleptiques actuels. *Acta Neurol. Belg. 65:* 659-666.

Brandrup, E., and Kristjansen, P. (1961): A controlled clinical test of a new psycholeptic drug (haloperidol). *J. Ment. Sci. 107:* 778-782.

Burt, O.P. and Bressler, F.D. (1961): Trifluoperazine in postoperative gynecological patients. *Ohio State Med. J. 57:* 1008-1009.

Campos Cervera, H. (1974): Evaluation clinia del pimozide en pacientes neuroticos. *Acta Psiquiat. Psicol. Amer. Lat. 20:* 418.

Childers, R.T., and Therrien, R. (1961): A comparison of the effectiveness of trifluoperazine and chlorpromazine in schizophrenia. *Amer. J. Psychiatry 118:* 552-554.

Chouinard, G., Lehmann, H.E., and Ban, T.A. (1970): Pimozide in the treatment of chronic schizophrenic patients. *Curr. Ther. Res. 12:* 598-603.

Claghorn, J. (1970): Differential drug effects on social and symptomatic behaviours. *Curr. Ther. Res. 12:* 580-584.

Clark, M.L., Huber, W.K., Hill, D., Wood, F., and Costiloe, J.P. (1975a): Pimozide in chronic schizophrenic outpatients. *Dis. Nerv. Syst. 36:* 137-141.

Clark, M.L., Paredes, A., Costiloe, J.P., Wood, F., and Barrett, A. (1975b): Loxapine in newly admitted chronic schizophrenic patients. *J. Clin. Pharmacol. 15:* 286-294.
Craft, M. (1965): A trial of haloperidol in schizophrenia. *Clinical Trials J.:* 140-142.
Cunningham, M.A., Pillai, V., and Blachford Rogers, W.J. (1968): Haloperidol in the treatment of children with severe behaviour disorders. *Brit. J. Psychiatr. 114:* 845-854.
Davis, J.M. (1965): Efficacy of tranquillizing and antidepressant drugs. *Arch. Gen. Psychiat. 13:* 552-572.
Davis, J.M. (1976): Tricyclic antidepressants. In: L.L. Simpson (Ed.), *Drug Treatment of Mental Disorders.* Raven Press, New York. pp. 127-146.
Deberdi, R. (1972): Low doses of haloperidol in anxiety-tension states. *Psychiatria Neurologia, Neurochirugia 75:* 317-324.
Delay, J. (1959): Classification and terminology of psychotropic drugs. In: N.S. Kline (Ed.), *Psychopharmacology Frontiers.* Churchill, London. pp. 426-428.
Denijs, E.L., and Vereecken, J.L.T.M. (1973): Pimozide (Orap R 6238) in residual schizophrenia: A clinical evaluation with long-term double-blind follow-up. *Psych. Neur. Neurchirurgia.* Elsevier Publishing Company, Amsterdam.
Feinberg, I., Wender, P.H., Koresko, R.L., et al. (1969): Differential effects of chlorpromazine and phenobarbital on EEG sleep patterns. *J. Psychiat. Res. 7:* 101-109.
Fink, M., Klein, D., and Kramer, J.C. (1965): Clinical efficacy of chlorpromazine-procyclidine combination, imipramine and placebo in depressive disorders. *Psychopharmacologia 7:* 27-36.
Fink, M., Pollack, M., Klein, D.F., et al. (1964): Comparative studies of chlorpromazine and imipramine. In: P.B. Bradley, et al. (Eds.), *Neuropsychopharmacology 3.* Elsevier Publishing Company, Amsterdam. pp. 370-372.
Finnerty, R.J., et al. (1976): Haloperidol in the treatment of psychoneuric anxious outpatients. *Dis. Nerv. Syst.* 621-624.
Fyro, B., Beck-Friis, J., and Sjostrand, E.G. (1974): A comparison between diazepam and haloperidol in anxiety states. *Acta Psychiat. Scand. 50:* 586-595.
Gen. Pract. Res. Group Rep. Number 51 (1964): Dexamphetamine comapred with an inactive placebo in depression. *Practioner 192:* 151-154.
Goldberg, J.B., and Kurland, A.A. (1974): Pimozide in the treatment of behaviour disorders of hospitalized adolescents. *J. Clin. Pharmacol. 14:* 134-139.
Greenblatt, D.J., and Shader, R.I. (1974): *Benzodiazepines in Clinical Practice.* Raven Press, New York.
Gross, H.S. (1974): A double-blind comparison of once-a-day pimozide, trifluoperazine, and placebo in the maintenance care of chronic schizophrenic outpatients. *Curr. Ther. Res. 16:* 696-705.
Hamilton, M. (1960): A rating scale for depression. *J. Neurol. Neurosurg. Psychiat 23:* 56-62.
Hamilton, M., Hordern, A., Waldrop, F.N., and Lofft, J. (1963): A controlled trial on the value of prochlorperazine trifluoperazine and intensive group treatment. *Brit. J. Psychiat. 109:* 510-522.
Hare, E.H., Dominian, J., and Sharpe, L. (1962): Pheneizine and dexamphetamine in depressive illness: a comparative trial. *Brit. Med. J. 1:* 9-12.
Hare, H.P. (1963): Comparison of diazepam, chlorpromazine and a placebo in psychiatric practice. *I. New Drug 3:* 233-240.
Hartman, E., and Cravens, J. (1963): The effects of long term administration of psychotropic drugs on human sleep: IV. The effects of chlorpromazine. *Psychopharmacologia 33:* 203-218.
Hollister, L.E., Erickson, E.V., and Mazzenlecker, F.P. (1960): Trifluoperazine in chronic psychiatric patients. *J. Clin. Exp. Psychopath. 21:* 15-22.

Holmgren, S. (1975): Pimozide in the treatment of stress-induced psychic and functional disorders. A double-blind comparison with clopoxide and palcebo. *Nord. Psykiat. Tidsskr. 29:* 577-584.

Howard, J.S. (1974): Haloperidol for chronically hospitalized psychotics: a double-blind comparison with thiothixine and placebo; a follow-up open evaluation. *Dis. Nerv. Syst. 35:* 458-463.

Howell, R.J., Brown, H.M., and Beaghler, H.E. (1961): A comparison of fluphenazine trifluoperazine and a placebo in the context of an active treatment unit. *J. Nerv. Mental. Dis. 6:* 522-530.

Huber, W., Serafetinides, E.A., Colmore, J.P. (1971): Pimozide in chronic schizophrenic patients. *J. Clin. Pharm. 11:* 304-309.

Hunter, H., and Stephenson, G.M. (1963): Chlorpromazine and trifluoperazine in the treatment of behavioural abnormalities in the severely subnormal child. *Brit. J. Psychiat. 109:* 411-417.

Itil, T.M. (1968): Human Psychopharmacology and functional electroencephalography. In: D.H. Efron, et al. (Eds.), *Psychopharmacology: A Review of Progress 1957-1967.* Government Printing Office, Washington, D.C. pp. 509-522.

Itil, T.M. (1969): Digital computer "sleep prints" and psychopharmacology. *Biol. Psychiat. 1:* 91-95.

Janke, W., and Debus, G. (1972): Double-blind psychometric evaluation of pimozide and haloperidol versus placebo in emotionally labile volunteers under two different work load conditions. *Pharmakopsychiatr. 1:* 34-51.

Janssen, P., Brugmans, J., Dony, J., and Schuermans, V. (1972): An international doubleblind clinical evaluation of pimozide. *J. Clin. Pharm. 12:* 26-34.

Johnson, G., Gershon, S., Burdock, E.I., et al. (1971): Comparative effects of lithium and chlorpromazine in the treatment of acute manic states. *Brit. J. Psychiat. 119:* 267-276.

Kane, F.J., and Keeler, M.H. (1964): Visual hallucinosis while receiving imipramine. *Amer. J. Psychiat. 121:* 611-612.

Kaplan, J., Dawson, S., Vaughan, T., et al. (1974): Effect of prolonged chlorpromazine administration on the sleep of chornic schizophrenics. *Arch. Gen. Psychiat. 31:* 62-66.

Kielholz, P. (1963): Gegenwärtiger stand und zukünftige Möglichkeiten der pharmakologischen Depressionsbehandlung. *Nervenarzt 34:* 181-183.

Kielholz, P. (Ed.) (1965): *Psychiatrische Pharmakotherapie in Klinik und Praxis.* Huber, Bern.

Klein, D.F. (1966): Chlorpromazine-procyclidine combination, imipramine and placebo in depressive disorders. *Canad. Psychiat. Ass. J. 11:* spec. suppl. 146-149.

Klein, D.F. (1965): Visual hallucination with imipramine. *Amer. J. Psychiat. 121:* 911-914.

Klein, D.F., and Davis, J.M. (1969): *Diagnosis and Drugs Treatment of Psychiatric Disorders.* Williams and Wilkins, Baltimore.

Klerman, G.L., and Cole, J.O. (1965): Clinical pharmacology of imipramine and related antidepressant compounds. *Pharmacol. Rev. 17:* 101-141.

Kramer, M. (1963): Delirium as a complication of imipramine therapy in the aged. *Amer. J. Psychiat. 120:* 502-503.

Kupfer, D.J., Wyatt, R.J., Snijder, F., et al. (1971): Chlorpromazine and sleep in psychiatric patients. *Arch. Gen. Psychiat. 24:* 185-189.

Lafave, H.G., Steward, A., and Segovia, G. (1967): Haloperidol. New addition to the drug treatment of schizophreniz. *Can. Psych. Ass. J. 12:* 597-602.

Lambert, P.A., Perring, J., Revol, L., et al. (1959): Essai de classification des neuroleptiques d'aprés leurs activités psychopharmacologiques et cliniques. In: P.B. Bradley, et al. (Eds.), *Neuro-Psychopharmacology 1.* Elsevier, Amsterdam. pp. 619-624.

Lapierre, Y.D. (1974): The comparative anxiolytic effects of placebo, imipramine and chlorpromazine using psychiatric and psychophysiological measurement. *Int. J. Clin. Pharmacol. 9:* 16-22.

Lester, B.K., Coulter, J.D., Cowden, L.C., et al. (1971): Chlorpromazine and human sleep. *Psychopharmacologia 20:* 280-287.

Madalena, J.C. (1964): Avaliacao de um novo derivado benzoquinolizinoco, O RO 4-6451 na esquizofrenia cronica. *A Folha Medica 48:* 33-41.

Mahal, A.S., and Janakiramaiah, N. (1975): A double-blind placebo controlled trial of pimozide (R 6238) on 49 hospitalized chronic schizophrenics. *Indian J. Psychiat. 17:* 45-56.

Malitz, S., and Kanzier, M. (1971): Are antidepressants better than placebo? *Amer. J. Psychiat. 127:* 41-47.

Man, P.L., and Chen, C.H. (1973): Rapid tranquillization of acutely psychotic patients with intramuscular haloperidol and chlorpromazine. *Psychosomatics 14:* 59-63.

May, A.R., Stuart Whiteley, J., and Gradwell, B.G. (1959): Trifluoperazine (stelazine) in psychoneuroses. A clinical assessment. *J. Mental Sci. 115:* 1059-1063.

Miller, A., Baker, E.F.W., Lewis, D., et al. (1960): Imipramine a clinical evaluation in a variety of settings. *Canad. Psychiat. Ass. J. 5:* 150-160.

Morris, J.B., and Beck, A.T. (1974): The efficacy of antidepressant drugs. *Arch. Gen. Psychiat. 30:* 667-674.

Ota, K.Y., and Kurland, A.A. (1973): A double-blind comparison of haloperidol oral concentrate, haloperidol solutabs and placebo in treatment of chronic schizophrenia. *J. Clin. Pharm. 13:* 99-110.

Overall, J.E., and Gorham, D.R. (1962): The brief psychiatric rating scale. *Psychol. Rep. 10:* 799-812.

Overall, J.E., Hollister, L.E., Pokorny, A.D., et al. (1962): Drug therapy in depressions. *Clin. Pharm. Ther. 3:* 16-22.

Oybir, F. (1962): Trifluoperazine in chronic, withdrawn schizophrenics. *Dis. Nerv. Syst. 23:* 348-350.

Paykel, E.S., Price, J.S., Gillan, R.V., et al. (1968): A comparative trial of imipramine and chlorpromazine in depressed patients. *Brit. J. Psychiat. 114:* 1281-1287.

Pichot, P. (1960): Modèle factoriel de représentation de l'action des neuroleptiques. *Rev. Lyon Méd. 56:* n⁰ special: 56-57.

Pinard, G., Prenoveau, Y., Fliesen, W., Elie, R., Bielmann, P., Lamontagne, Y., and Tetreault, L. (1972): Pimozide: a comparative study in the treatment of chronic schizophrenic patients. *Int. J. Clin. Pharm. Ther. Toxicol. 6:* 22-27.

Platman, S.R. (1970): A comparison of lithium carbonate and chlorpromazine in mania. *Amer. J. Psychiat. 127:* 127-129.

Platz, A.R., Klett, C.J., and Caffey, E.M. (1967): Selective drug action related to chronic schizophrenic subtype (A comparative study of carphanzine, chlorpromazine and trifluoperazine). *Dis. Nerv. Syst. 28:* 601-605.

Prien, R.F., Caffey, E.M., Jr., and Klett, C.J. (1972): Comparison of litium carbonate and chlorpromazine in the treatment of mania. *Arch. Gen. Psychiat. 26:* 146-153.

Prien, R.F., Levine, J., and Cole, J.O. (1969): High dose trifluoperazine therapy in chronic schizophrenia. *Amer. J. Psychiat. 126:* 305-313.

Raskin, A. (1968): High dosage chlorpromazine alone and in combination with an antiparkinsonia agent (procyclidine) in the treatment of hospitalized depressions. *J. New Ment. Dis. 147:* 184-195.

Raskin, A. (1971): Drugs and depression subtypes. In: R. Fieve (Ed.), *Depression 1970.* Excerpta Medica, New York. pp. 87-95.

Raskin, A. (1974): Age-sex differences in response to antidepressant drugs. *J. Nerv. Ment. Dis. 159:* 120-130.

Raskin, A. (1975): Antidepressants in black and white patients. *Arch. Gen. Psychiat. 32:* 643-649.

Raskin, A., Schulterbrandt, J.G., Reatig, N., et al. (1970): Differential response to chlorpromazine, imipramine and placebo. *Arch. Gen. Psychiat. 23:* 164-173.

Raskin, A., and McKeon, J.J. (1971): Super factors of psychopathology in hospitalized depressed patients. *J. Psychiat. Res. 9:* 11-19.

Reardon, J.D., and Abrams, S. (1966): Acute paranoid schizophrenia. *Dis. Nerv. Syst. 27:* 265-270.

Rees, L., and Davies, B. (1965): A study of the value of haloperidol in the management and treatment of schizophrenic and manic patients. *In. J. Neuropsychiat. 1:* 263-266.

Reyntjens, A.M., and Van Mierlo, F.P. (1972): A comparative double-blind trial of pimozide in stress-induced psychic and functional disorders. *Curr. Med. Res. and Opinion 1:* 116-122.

Rogers, S.C., and Clay, P.M. (1975): A statistical review of controlled trials of imipramine and placebo in the treatment of depressive illness. *Brit. J. Psychiat. 127:* 599-603.

Rogerson, R., and Butler, J.K. (1971): Assessment of low dosage haloperidol in anxiety state. *Brit. J. Psychiat. 119:* 169.

Sagales, T., Erill, S., and Domino, E.F. (1969): Differential effects of scopalamine and chlorpromazine on REM and NREM sleep in normal male subjects. *Clin, Pharmacol. Ther. 10:* 522-529.

Samuels, A.S. (1961): A controlled study of haloperidol: the effects of small dosage. *Am. J. of Psychiat. 118:* 253-254.

Sarada Menon, and Ramachandran, V. (1972): A controlled clinical trial of trifluoperidol on a group of chronic schizophrenic patients. *Curr. Ther. Res. 14:* 17-21.

Schover, C.E. (1960): Report of hypomanic excitement with imipramine treatment of depression. *Am. J. Psychiat. 116:* 844-845.

Schulterbrandt, J.C., Raskin, A., and Reatig, N. (1974): True and apparent side effects in a controlled trial of chlorpromazine and imipramine in depression. *Psychopharmacologia 38:* 303-331.

Selman, F.B., McClure, R.F., and Helwig, H. (1976): Lozapine succinate: a double-blind comparison with haloperidol and placebo in acute schizophrenics. *Curr. Ther. Res. 19:* 645-652.

Serafetinides, E.A., Colins, S., and Clark, M.L. (1972): Haloperidol, clopenthixol and chlorpromazine in chronic schizophrenia. *J. Nerv. Ment. Dis. 154:* 31-42.

Serafetinides, E.A., and Clark, M.L. (1973): Psychological effects of single-dose antipsychotic medication. *Biol. Psychiatry 7:* 263-267.

Sharpe, D.S. (1962): A controlled trial of trifluoperazine in the treatment of the mentally subnormal patient. *J. Ment. Sci. 108:* 220-224.

Shopsin, B., Gershon, S., and Thompson, H. (1975): Psychoactive drugs in mania. *Arch. Gen. Psychiat. 32:* 34-42.

Shridhar Sharma, and Dipali Dutta, (1976): Double-blind study of pimozide in the treatment of schizophrenic patients. *Indian J. Psychiat. 18:* 34-37.

Simpson, G.M., et al. (1969): A controlled study of haloperidol in chronic schizophrenia. *Curr. Ther. Res. 9:* 407-412.

Singh, M.M., et al. (1975): A longitudinal therapeutic comparison between two prototypic neuroleptics (haloperidol and chlorpromazine) in matched groups of schizophrenics. Non-therapeutic interactions with trihexypehenidyl. Theoretical implications for potency differences. *Psycho-pharmacologia 43:* 115-123.

Smith, M.E., and Chassan, J.B. (1964): Comparisons of diazepam, chlorpromazine and trifluoperazine in a double-blind clinical investigation. *J. Neuropsychiat. 5:* 593-600.
Spring, G., Schweid, D., Steinberg, J., et al. (1970): A double-blind comparison of litium and chlorpromazine in the treatment of manic states. *Amer. J. Psychiat. 126:* 140-143.
Stevenson, J. (1976): Comparison of low doses of haloperidol and diazepam in anxiety states. *Med. J. Aust. 1:* 451-452.
Sugerman, A.A. (1971): A pilot of pimozide in chronic schizophrenic patients. *Curr. Ther. Res. 13:* 706-713.
Sugerman, A.A., Williams, B.H., Adlerstein, A.A. (1964): Haloperidol in the psychiatric disorders of old age. *Am. J. Psychiat. 120:* 1190-1192.
Takahashi, R., Sakuna, A., Itoh, K., et al. (1975): Comparison of efficacy of litium carbonate and chlorpromazine in mania. *Arch. Gen. Psychiat. 32:* 1310-1318.
Teja, J.S., Grey, W.H., et al. (1975): Tranquillizers or antidepressants for chronic schizophrenics: a long term study. *Aust. NZ. J. Psychiatry 9:* 241-247.
Toyoda, J. (1964): The effects of chlorpromazine and imipramine on the human nocturnal sleep electroencephalogram. *Folia Psychiat. Neurol. Jap. 18:* 198-221.
Vichaiya, V. (1971): Clinical trial of haloperidol in schizophrenia. *J. Psychiatr. Ass. of Thailand 16:* 31-43.
Vilkin, M.I. (1964): Comparative chemotherapeutic trial in treatment of chronic borderline patients. *Amer. J. Psychiat. 120:* 104.
Wald, D., Ebstein, R.P., and Belmaker, R.H. (1978): Haloperidol and litium blocking of the mood response to intravenous methyphenidate. *Psychopharmacology 57:* 83-87.
Weckowics, T.E., and Ward, R.F. (1960): Clinical trial "stelazine" on apathetic chronic schizophrenics. *J. Ment. Sci. 106:* 1008-1015.
Wilson, I.C., McKay, J., Sandifer, M.G. (1961): A double-blind trial to investigate the effects of thorazine (largactil, chlorpromazine), compazine (stemetil, prochlorperazine) and stelazine (trifluoperazone) in paranoid schizophrenia. *J. Ment. Sci. 107:* 90-99.
Yamamoto, J., Kline, F.M., and Burgoyne, R.W. (1973): The treatment of severe anxiety in outpatients: a controlled study comparing chlordiazepoxide and chlorpromazine. *Psychosomatics 24:* 46-51.

11

Clinical and Psychopharmacological Evaluation of L-5HTP in Depression

Motohisa Kaneko
Hisashi Kumashiro

The present paper reviews an outline of the antidepressant and related psychopharmacological actions of the serotonin precursor, L-5HTP, used to test the validity of the indoleamine hypothesis of depression.

At present there have been 17 papers concerning the antidepressant efficacy of L-5HTP, including four double blind studies. L-5HTP has been proven to be effective in approximately half of the cases of endogenous depression. Three out of four double blind studies reported that L-5HTP was either superior to placebo, or equal to imipramine in its antidepressant action. L-5HTP responders were found to be anxious, irritable, and showed a decreased cerebrospinal fluid level of 5HIAA prior to treatment. After the administration of L-5HTP the depressive episodes disappeared initially, and this effect was rapid in onset. The most prominent side-effects were observed in the gastro-intestinal system, although these symptoms can be averted. L-5HTP produces euphoria in some normal subjects, suggesting that in depressive patients it may selectively improve depressive mood. The presumed mechanism of this action is to increase 5HT release into the synaptic cleft of 5HT neuron in the brain. Also, the effect of L-5HTP on the catecholaminergic system and neuroendocrine function must be considered.

INTRODUCTION

Two major pharmacological observations have suggested the importance of brain biogenic amines in the pathogenesis of manic-depressive psychosis. One is the fact that reserpine, a drug which lowers brain biogenic amine levels induces severe depression. The other is that monoamine oxidase (MAO) inhibitors, which raise the brain levels of biogenic amines, can improve naturally occurring or reserpine-induced depression. Based on these findings the biogenic amine hypothesis that depression is caused by a deficiency of brain biogenic amines was advanced. Currently, two distinct aminergic hypotheses are offered, namely, the catecholamine (CA) (Schildkraut, 1965; Bunney and Davis, 1965) and the indoleamine hypotheses (Coppen, 1967; Lapin and Oxendrug, 1969) have been proposed. The former emphasizes the role of CA, while the latter attaches importance to the role of serotonin (5HT). There have already been voluminous studies in support of each of these two hypotheses. However, the fact that they may contradict one another indicates that both of them are far from being satisfactory. In recent years criticisms (Baldessarini, 1975; Luchins, 1976) and modifications (Ashcroft et al., 1972; Mendels and Frazer, 1975; Aprison et al., 1978) of both hypotheses have been made, and numerous attempts have also been made to classify depression into subgroups from either a pathophysiological or a genetic viewpoint (Asberg et al., 1973; Maas, 1975; Van Praag, 1977; Taylor and Abrams, 1973; Winokur and Cadoret, 1977).

It therefore seems worthwhile to evaluate the efficacy of L-5-hydroxytryptophan (L-5HTP), the direct 5-HT precursor, in relieving depression to test the legitimacy of the indoleamine hypothesis, with the purpose of clarifying the antidepressant and the related psychopharmacological actions of L-5HTP.

CURRENT STATUS OF THE INDOLEAMINE HYPOTHESIS

Before dealing with the main subject, it seems pertinent to review those studies on which the indoleamine hypothesis is based.

In recent years, biochemical and pharmacological approaches to the problem have been explored. Biochemical research has been directed mainly at the measurement of the amine concentrations and their metabolic products in body fluids of patients with manic-depressive psychosis. A diffuse trend in the pharmacological apporach has been that of evaluating symptomatic responses to the administration of drugs known to have a specific action on brain amines.

Biochemical studies indicating a decreased brain tissue level of 5HT in depressive patients who committed suicide are already available. Shaw et al. (1967), Pare et al. (1969), and Lloyd et al. (1974) have reported a decreased content of 5HT in the hindbrain, brainstem and raphe nuclei, respectively, of suicides, and Bourne et al. (1968) reported a decreased level of the main metabolite of 5HT, 5-hydroxyindoleacetic acid (5HIAA), in their hindbrain. On the other hand, it is widely known that the 5HIAA content of the cerebrospinal fluid (CSF) is reduced in patients with depression. Although it is still uncertain whether the 5HIAA in CFS obtained by lumbar puncture derives from the brain or from neurons of the spinal cord, the CSF level of this substance is considered to provide an indication of the serotoninergic activity in the central nervous system (CNS). Numerous investigators (Ashcroft et al., 1966; Dencker et al., 1966; Coppen et al., 1972; Sjöström and Roos, 1972; Bowers et al., 1969; Papeschi and McClure, 1971; Goodwin et al., 1973) reported a variably significant decrease of 5HIAA level in the CSF of depressed patients. Other studies on body fluids demonstrated a decreased blood level of 5HT (Sarai and Kayano, 1968; Kaneko, 1975; Banki, 1978) and of free tryptophan (Coppen et al., 1973; Kishimoto, 1977) which is said to control the metabolism of 5HT in the brain. With regard to the decreased brain 5HT level among depressive suicides however, several factors remain to be studied, *e.g.,* the influence of medication prior to suicide, the period of time elapsed from death to autopsy, and the time-span of specimens stored in a frozen state (Bourne et al., 1968). As for the 5-HIAA level in CSF, Ashcroft and Glen (1974) found an upward tendency in bipolar depression. All the aforementioned studies seem to provide sufficient evidence to suggest the functional reduction of 5HT in brain tissues of depressive individuals.

From the pharmacological standpoint, it has been suggested that the mechanism of antidepressant action of imipramine, amitriptyline and clomipramine (which represent tertiary amines among the tricyclic antidepressants) is to enhance the biological activity of 5HT by inhibiting its reuptake into the serotoninergic neurons (Carlsson et al., 1969). Para-chlorophenylalanine (PCPA), which specifically depletes 5HT, is known to reverse the remission of depression produced by the use of a MAO inhibitor or imipramine (Shopsin et al., 1975; Shopsin et al., 1976). However, even greater importance should be attached to the antidepressant potential of tryptophan (TP) and 5HTP, in examining the legitimacy of the indoleamine hypothesis from the pharmacological viewpoint. These two substances, because of their capability to cross the blood-brain barrier and capacity to raise the brain level of 5HT, are of great help in the study of physiological and pharmacological actions of 5HT in the brain. There are already a number of reports in favor of a potential antidepressant activity of TP, but its efficacy is still a matter of controversy, since some studies in the field failed to afford good evidence in support of an indoleamine hypothesis. In a retrospective study undertaken to search for evidence of the antidepressant effect of TP, only those double-blind controlled trials in which the concomitant use of drugs with antidepressant properties have been reviewed; *e.g.,* MAO inhibitors and tricyclic antidepressants, were clearly avoided. These trials are listed in Table 1. As can be seen, some of the studies (Coppen et al., 1972; Jensen et al., 1975; Rao and Broadhurst, 1976; Herrington et al., 1976) showed that the antidepressant efficacy of TP is comparable to that of tricyclic antidepressants, while others (Bunney et al., 1971; Murphy et al., 1974; Dunner and Fieve, 1975; Mendels et al., 1975) failed to reach the same conclusion. Accordingly, this series of studies does not allow any definite statement as to

TABLE 1. Clinical Evaluation of L-Tryptophan by Double-Blind Method in Depression

Authors	Patients Number	Diagnosis	Dose of L-TP (g/day)	Other drugs	Duration (day)	Design	Results
Bunney, Brodie, Murphy and Goodwin, 1971	8	depressed patients	8		16	vs. placebo	no significant effect
Coppen, Whybrow, Noguera, Maggs and Prange, 1972	15	primary depression	9	ascorbic acid	28	vs. imipramine	L-TP as effective as imipramine
Murphy, Baker, Goodwin, Miller, Kotin and Bunney, 1974	24	depressed patients	9.6	pyridoxine; ascorbic acid	20±2	vs. placebo	no significant effect
Mendels, Stinnett, Burns and Frazer, 1975	6	depressed patients	3 -16	pyridoxine	42	vs. placebo	some improvement in 1 of 6 patients
Dunner and Fieve, 1975	7	primary affective disorder	8.4- 9	pyridoxine; ascorbic acid	10-18	vs. placebo	improvement in 1 of 7 patients
Jensen, Fruengaard, Ahlfors, Pihkanen, Tuomikoski, Ose, Dencker, Lindberg and Nagy, 1975	22	endogenous depression	3 - 6		21	vs. imipramine	L-TP as effective as imipramine, but the reduction of symptoms was more rapid in imipramine group

TABLE 1. Clinical Evaluation of L-Tryptophan by Double-Blind Method in Depression (Continued)

Authors	Patients Number	Diagnosis	Dose of L-TP (g/day)	Other drugs	Duration (day)	Design	Results
Rao and Broadhurst, 1976	9	depressive illness	6	pyridoxine; ascorbic acid	28	vs. imipramine	L-TP as effective as imipramine
Herrinton, Bruce, Johnstone and Lader, 1976	20	depression	6 - 8	pyridoxine	28	vs. amitriptyline	L-TP as effective as amitriptyline

the antidepressant efficacy of TP, unless TP is effective only in very limited types of depression, and its effect is less favorable than that of imipramine.

Concerning the antidepressant effect of L-5HTP, the number of pertinent studies amounts to 17, four of which were conducted on a double-blind basis. Again, however, no consistent results were obtained. Thus, it may be said that no convincing evidence in support of the indoleamine hypothesis of depression has so far been provided.

ANTIDEPRESSANT EFFECT OF 5HTP

Antidepressant Effect of D,L-5HTP

Table 2 lists the available studies concerned with the antidepressant effect of D,L- and L-5HTP. The first attempt to treat depression with 5HTP was made by Pare and Sandler (1959). Probably because at that time 5HTP was exclusively available in racemic form and was used in small doses, no noteworthy effect was obtained. In their open study Klein and Sacks (1963) reported an antidepressant effect of D,L-5HTP, but they (Klein et al., 1964) subsequently failed to confirm this result in a double-blind trial. In contrast, Van Praag et al. (1972), reported that they found D,L-5HTP to be effective in three out of five depressed patients in a double-blind controlled study.

Antidepressant Effect of L-5HTP

Reports in favor of the antidepressant effect of L-5HTP may be traced back to Persson and Roos (1967), who found intravenously administered L-5HTP to be effective in a single case of therapy-resistant depression. Subsequently Sano (1971, 1972) reported that the oral administration of L-5HTP proved to be effective in more than half of 104 cases of endogenous depression and the effect was rapid in onset. Since then, there have been over 14 reports showing the antidepressant efficacy of L-5HTP and none contradicting them.

A study of the rate of improvement (the ratio of the number of cases showing a marked-moderate improvement to the total number of cases treated) by L-5HTP was made, selecting those reports in which the therapeutic effect was tested in more than five cases. The results are summarized in Table 3. As can be seen, although the figures are quite variable, an improvement rate in excess of 50 percent was achieved in 8 out of 12 series, indicating the potential usefulness of L-5HTP. Similar studies carried out in Japan seemed to match better among them than those from abroad, since they were all performed on an open basis by using relatively similar criteria for the assessment of 5-HTP efficacy, the majority of the subjects being patients with endogenous depression. According

TABLE 2. Clinical Effect of 5-Hydroxytryptophan in Depression

Authors	Patients Number	Diagnosis (no./cases)	Dose of 5HTP (mg/day)	Other drugs	Duration (day)	Design	Results
Pare and Sandler, 1959	6	not defined	D,L 12.5-150 iv or SC	with/without MAO inhibitor	iv.-single dose SC.-14	open	no improvement
Kline and Sacks, 1963	50	classical, pure dep. (20); schizo-affective dep. (30)	D,L. 25-50 iv	MAO inhibitor	single dose	open	18/20 marked response in classical, pure dep.; 7/30 marked response in schizo-affective dep.
Kline, Sacks and Simpson, 1964	37	primary dep.	D,L. 25-50 iv	MAO inhibitor	single dose	double-blind vs. placebo	8/37 marked improvement with 25 mg; 3/21 marked improvement with 50 mg; no significant difference between 5HTP and placebo
Praag, Korf, Dols and Schut, 1972	5	endogenous dep.	D,L. 200-3000 oral		21	double-blind vs. placebo	3/5 improvement
Persson and Roos, 1967	1	therapy-resistant, psychotic dep.	L. 10-50 iv	barbiturates diazepam	14	open	remission within 2 weeks

TABLE 2. Clinical Effect of 5-Hydroxytryptophan in Depression (Continued)

Authors	Patients Number	Diagnosis (no./cases)	Dose of 5HTP (mg/day)	Other drugs	Duration (day)	Design	Results
Sano, 1971, 1972	107	endogenous dep. unipolar (60); bipolar (47)	L.50-300 oral	trihexyphenidyl or metoclopramide	7-35	open	20/60 marked improvement within a week and 23/60 marked improvement within 2 weeks in unipolar type; 20/47 marked improvement within a week and 11/47 marked improvement within 2 weeks in bipolar type
Brodie, Sack and Siever, 1973	7	psychotic dep. (6); schizo-affective dep. (1)	L.250-3250 oral	with/without carbidopa	1-15	double-blind vs. placebo	1/7 modest improvement
Barlet and Paillard, 1973	25	melancholic syndrome (4); involutional dep. (7); reactive dep. (8); depressive state of neurosis or psychosis (6)	L.200-800 oral	sleep-inducer	10 days-8 months	double-blind vs. placebo	19/25 marked improvement
Fujiwara and Otsuki, 1974	20	endogenous dep. unipolar (4); bipolar (8); involutional (6); not defined (2)	L.50-200 oral		7-28	open	1/4 effective in unipolar type; 5/8 effective in bipolar type; 4/6 effective in involutional type

TABLE 2. Clinical Effect of 5-Hydroxytryptophan in Depression (Continued)

Authors	Patients Number	Diagnosis (no./cases)	Dose of 5HTP (mg/day)	Other drugs	Duration (day)	Design	Results
Matussek, Angst, Benkert, Gemür, Papousek, Rüther and Woggon, 1974	23	unipolar dep. (13); bipolar dep. (1); involutional dep. (8); schizo-affective dep. (1)	L.100-300 oral	with/without benserazide	4-20	open	2/15 symptom free within 5 days and 4/15 good improvement with Ro 4-4602; 1/8 symptom free within 3 days without Ro 4-4602
Sarai, 1974	19	endogenous dep. (18); neurotic dep. (1)	L. 120-150 oral	metoclopramide pherphenazine	10-91	open	3/19 marked improvement; 9/19 good improvement
Praag, Burg, Bos and Dols, 1974	5	endogenous dep. first episode (3); unipolar (1); bipolar (1)	L. 200-400 oral	carbidopa in beginning 2 weeks and added clomipramine to carbidopa in last 2 weeks	28	open	4/5 improvement. enhancement of the effect in 2 of 4 improved cases with addition of clomipramine
Aussilloux, Castelnau, Chiariny and Fraissinet, 1975	2	decompensatory dep. (1); chronic dep. (1)	L. 200-600 oral		20-25	open	2/2 improvement
Takahashi, Kondo and Kato, 1975	24	unipolar dep. (20); involutional dep. (2); neurotic dep. (1); psychotic dep. (1)	L. 300 oral	metoclopramide	14	open	7/20 marked improvement in unipolar type

TABLE 2. Clinical Effect of 5-Hydroxytryptophan in Depression (Continued)

Authors	Patients Number	Diagnosis (no./cases)	Dose of 5HTP (mg/day)	Other drugs	Duration (day)	Design	Results
Alino, Gutierrenz and Iglesias, 1976	15	endogenous dep. retarded (5); anxious (6); obsessive (4)	L. 50-300 oral	nialamide	15-20	double-blind vs. nialamide + placebo	9/15 complete remission; 3/15 definite improvement
Pühringer, Wirz-Justice, Graw, Lacoste and Gastpar, 1976	13	primary affective disorder unipolar (8); bipolar (5)	L. 200 iv	benserazide	single dose	open	3/13 short-term improvement
Takahashi, Takahashi, Masumura and Miike, 1976	14	endogenous dep. first episode (5); unipolar (7); involutional (1); neurotic dep. (1)	L. 150 oral	sleep-inducer	7	open	1/14 moderate improvement
Angst, Woggon Schoepf, 1977	10	tricyclic antidepressant resistant dep. (10)	L. 190 oral	benserazide	20–	open	improvement of somato-depressive syndrome, but no significant improvement of depression
	11	not defined	L. 1200 oral	benserazide	20–	open	highly significant improvement
	15	not defined	L. 800 oral	benserazide	20–	double-blind vs. imipramine	highly significant improvement as effective as imipramine

TABLE 2. Clinical Effect of 5-Hydroxytryptophan in Depression (Continued)

Authors	Patients		Dose of 5HTP (mg/day)	Other drugs	Duration (day)	Design	Results
	Number	Diagnosis (no./cases)					
Praag, 1977	5	endogenous dep. unipolar (2); bipolar (3)	L. 200 oral		one year	open	no recurrence in one year
Nakajima, Kudo and Kaneko, 1978	59	first episode dep. (3); unipolar dep. (17); bipolar dep. (21); mixed state of manic-depressives (2); presenile or senile dep. (9); neurotic dep. (4); reactive dep. (2); schizophrenic dep. (1)	L. 150-300 oral	metoclopramide trihexyphenidyl diazepam sleep-inducer	21 –	open	13/59 marked improvement 19/59 moderate improvement
Kaneko, Kumashiro, Takahashi and Hoshino, 1978	18	endogenous dep. first episode (3); unipolar (12); bipolar (3)	L. 150-300 oral	metoclopramide trihexyphenidyl sleep-inducer	10-28	open	2/18 very much improved 8/18 much improved

TABLE 3. The Rate of Improvement by L-5HTP Treatment in Depression

Authors*	Number of patients	Therapeutic effects				Rate of improvement (%)**
		Markedly improved	Moderately improved	Slightly improved	Unchanged or aggravated	
Sano, 1972	107	40	34	22	11	71.1
Sarai, 1974	19	3	9	4	3	63.1
Kaneko, Kumashiro, Takahashi and Hoshino, 1978	18	2	8	3	5	55.5
Nakajima, Kudo and Kaneko, 1978	59	13	19	8	19	54.2
Fujiwara and Otsuki, 1974	20	4	6	2	8	50.0
Takahashi, Kondo and Kato, 1975	24		7	2	15	29.1
Takahashi, Takahashi, Masumura and Miike, 1976	14		1	6	7	7.1
Alino, Gutierrenz and Iglesias, 1976	14	9	3	1	1	85.7
Praag, Burg, Bos and Dols, 1974	5		4		1	80.0
Barlet and Pallard, 1974	25	11	8	4	2	76.0
Matussek, Angst, Benkert, Gemür, Papousek, Rüther, and Woggon, 1974	23	3	4	4	12	30.4
Brodie Sack and Siever, 1973	7		1		6	14.2
	335	—	189	56	90	56.4

*Authors in this table reported the therapeutic effects of L-5HTP in more than 5 cases of depression.
**The rate of improvement was expressed as percent of markedly improved and moderately improved cases to total cases.

to these Japanese studies, the improvement rate with L-5HTP ranged from 7.1 percent to 71.1 percent, an amazingly striking difference. Roughly speaking, they as a whole indicated that approximately half of the patients with endogenous depression improved from the use of L-5HTP.

Four double-blind trials to assess the antidepressant efficacy of L-5HTP have been so far reported. Brodie et al. (1973), who were the first to conduct a double-blind study of L-5HTP, compared L-5HTP and placebo in seven cases of therapy-resistant depression by sequential analysis. They recognized moderate improvement in only one case and failed to substantiate the therapeutic usefulness of L-5HTP.

Barlet and Paliard (1974) compared 25 L-5HTP-treated cases with 25 cases receiving placebo and found L-5HTP to be definitely superior to placebo. They reported further that L-5HTP proved effective in involutional melancholia, markedly effective in depressive moods but had no demonstrable antianxiety action.

Alino et al (1976) treated 30 cases of endogenous depression either with L-5HTP plus nialamide or with placebo plus nialamide in a study to assess the efficacy of L-5HTP. The results indicated that the rate of improvement for the former combination regimen was 85.7 percent in comparison to the 40 percent improvement rate with the latter drug regimen. The fact that the combination of L-5HTP and nialamide (which is a MAO inhibitor in current use) far exceeded the activity shown by the MAO inhibitor alone, can undoubtedly be interpreted as a salient antidepressant effect of L-5HTP, even though a potentiating effect must also be taken into account.

Angst et al. (1977) performed a well-controlled double-blind comparative trial of L-5HTP and imipramine as active control. Thirty untreated patients with depression were involved in this study. They were divided into two groups, one of which was treated with 800 mg of L-5HTP and 375 mg of benzerazide (Ro4-4602), a peripheral decarboxylase inhibitor, while the other group received 150 mg of imipramine daily. Both treatments were given for more than 20 days. The results were consistent with those of two open studies carried out by the same authors, showing that L-5HTP has an antidepressant acitivity comparable to that of imipramine.

Dosage of L-5HTP and Concomitant Drugs

The dosage of L-5HTP varies widely with different investigators. Thus, doses from 50 to 3250 mg daily have been given by oral route, and 10 to 200 mg by intravenous administration.

Sano (1972) studies the relationship between the therapeutic effect of L-5HTP and its dosage level. No substantial difference can be noted in the rate of improvement of patients receiving 50 to 60 mg daily and those treated with 400 to 800 mg daily. We, too (Kaneko et al., 1978), do not detect significant difference in the therapeutic effect of L-5HTP given at two different dosage levels of 150 and 300 mg. Although the optimal dosage of L-5HTP in treating depression is not yet definitely established, it seems that oral administration produces essentially the same effect as dosage levels above 3 mg/kg daily.

Among drugs to be associated with L-5HTP, either MAO inhibitors (Alino et al., 1976) or clomipramine, a tricyclic antidepressant (Van Praag et al., 1974), were found to potentiate the effect of L-5HTP. Peripheral decarboxylase inhibitors, such as benserazide (Matussek et al., 1974; Pühringer et al., 1976; Angst et al., 1977) and carbidopa (Brodie, et al., 1973), did not potentiate an antidepressant effect to any appreciable extent, although they seemed to avoid some unwanted side-effects.

Characteristic Features of the Antidepressant Action of L-5HTP

It should be initially mentioned that L-5HTP rapidly exerts its antidepressant action. Sano (1972) reported that remission or marked improvement was obtained within one week after initiation of an L-5HTP regimen in 40 (37.3 percent) of 107 cases. Fujiwara and Otsuki (1974), Sarai (1974), Kaneko et al. (1976), independently reported that the effect of L-5HTP became manifest within four days following the drug administration with clear-cut improvement by the seventh to ninth day of treatment.

Van Praag (1977) classifed depression into two types, *i.e.*, one due to deficiency of 5HT and the other due to deficiency of noradrenaline (NA) and stated that no symptomatological distinction can be made between the two types. Fujiwara and Otsuki (1974) also classifed endogenous depression into 5HTP and DOPA responding, assuming the former as depression of an indoleamine type and the latter depression of a CA type, and described their clinical characteristics, which are reported in Table 4. We too, studied the clinical picture of 5HTP responders (Kaneko et al., 1978), obtaining results in agreement with those obtained by Fujiwara and Otsuki (1974). Favorable responses were more frequently elicited in female cases and cases of bipolar depression. It should also be noted that in our experience, depressive mood, and then anxiety and irritation in this descending order, are the depressive symptoms more responsive to L-5HTP administration, while psychomotor retardation and insomnia respond poorly. Fujiwara et al. (1974) state that in 5HTP responders, insomnia does not improve, but rather tends to worsen: in a typical case the patient did not sleep at all for two days following the administration of L-5HTP and later recovered from this condition after a brief period of hypomania.

TABLE 4. Characteristics of Indoleamine Type Depression
and Catecholamine Type Depression
(Fujiwara and Otsuki*)

	Indoleamine type	Catecholamine type
effective amine precursor	L-5HTP	L-DOPA
onset of improvement	1-3 days	2-7 days
appearance of maximum effect	within 7 days	within a month
subtypes according to nosological classification	bipolar and involutional types of endogenous depression	bipolar type of endogenous depression
symptoms before treatment	anxiety, agitation and insomnia	muteness, absence of motor activity and hypersomnia
side effect in responder	insomnia	
biochemical findings	decrease of CSF 5HIAA	increase of CSF 5HIAA
percent appearance in endogenous depression	50%	29%

*Foria Psychiatrica et Neurologica Japonica 28: 93-100 (1974).

Side-Effects

Table 5 lists the reported adverse side-effects of L-5HTP. Obviously, gastrointestinal symptoms occurred most frequently. Davidson et al. (1957) noted that when they administered D,L-5HTP to humans for the first time, intense gastrointestinal symptoms (e.g., nausea, vomiting, diarrhea and abdominal pain) occurred. Thus, the gastrointestinal side-effects are of greatest concern to physicians administering L-5HTP. To prevent these side-effects, various drugs, such as carbidopa (Brodie et al., 1973), benserazide (Matussek et al, 1974; Pühringer et al., 1976; Angst et al., 1977), metoclopramide (a gastric antacid: Sano, 1972; Sarai, 1974: Takahashi et al., 1975; Nakajima et al., 1978; Kaneko et al., 1978) and trihexyphenidyl (an anticholinergic agent: Sano, 1972; Nakajima et al., 1978; Kaneko et al., 1978) were used successfully together with L-5HTP. Whereas an increased level of 5HT in the gastrointestinal tissues has been implicated as a cause of these adverse reactions, an action of 5HTP on the stomach

TABLE 5. Side-Effects of L-5HTP

gastrointestinal	central nervous
nausea	headache
vomiting	drowsiness
diarrhea	insomnia
obstipation	dizziness
abdominal pain	euphoria
	acute brain syndrome
cardiovascular	neuromuscular
palpitation	tremor
	ataxia
skin	
flushing	
sweating	
urticaria	

and intestine can be directly responsible for them. In an experimental study on this argument, a single subcutaneous administration of L-5HTP in rabbits increases the concentration of 5HT in the duodenum, liver and kidney (Unno et al., 1977). However, such an increase is only 1.3-fold in the duodenum 2 hours after the administration, an increment too small to account for the clinically observed gastrointestinal symptoms. In striking contrast, the 5HT level of the kidney increased by as much as 83-fold one hour after the administration, indicating the likelihood of renal impairment following the long-term administration of L-5HTP.

Among the possible CNS side-effects of L-5HTP, insomnia, euphoria and acute brain syndromes deserve particular note. Of these, the former two will be further examined in the next section because of their presumed relationship with the action mechanism of L-5HTP.

Concerning the drug-induced acute brain syndrome, Angst et al. (1977) noted a syndrome of several days' duration consisting of mania, disorientation and deliriant overactivity in a depressed patient who was on a combined regimen of 375 mg of benserazide and 1500 mg of L-5HTP. Similarly, Pühringer et al. (1976) reported the occurrence of an acute brain syndrome in a normal volunteer given 300 mg L-5HTP intravenously following an oral 375 mg dose of benserazide. These authors warned of the possibility that L-5HTP in large doses tends to give rise to the syndrome.

Takahashi et al. (1976), reported tremors and ataxia as neuromuscular side-effects of L-5HTP, and available evidence indicates that either the choreiform movements of Huntington's chorea (Lee et al., 1968) or the bradykinesia and muscular rigidity of Parkinson's disease (Chase et al., 1972) are aggravated by the administration of 5HTP. It has been assumed that this action of L-5HTP on the extrapyramidal system depends on its effect on the CA system (Chase et al., 1976).

These side effects were all those encountered in depressed patients. Wyatt and Vaughan (1973) described a case in which a grand mal seizure occurred on abrupt discontinuance of L-5HTP therapy for schizophrenia; MacIndoe and Turkington (1973) also reported a case of psychomotor seizure occurring with L-5HTP. We observed a case of intractable epilepsy in which the use of L-5HTP was followed by a frequent appearance of epileptiform EEG discharges (Kumashiro et al., 1977). However, L-5HTP is known to be beneficial in some types of myoclonus (Growdon et al., 1976). In our experience (Kumashiro et al., 1977), L-5HTP administration in kindled animals was shown to have an inhibitory action on convulsions. However, the available information does not afford any definitive evidence for the anticonvulsant efficacy of L-5HTP. In any event, it should be taken into account that L-5HTP may give rise to convulsive seizures, in its clinical use.

MECHANISM OF ACTION

Metabolism of L-5HTP in Depressive Patients

Biochemical evidence suggests a deficiency of 5HT in brain tissues of 5HTP responders prior to the administration of L-5HTP. Fujiwara and Otsuki (1974) noted a decreased concentration of 5HIAA in the CSF of 5HTP responders before treatment with L-5HTP. Van Praag (1977) recognized that probenecid loading produced a decreased accumulation of 5HIAA in the CSF of 5HTP responders and stated the L-5HTP, when administered during a period of remission in such L-5HTP responders, may be anticipated to prove of value in the prevention of recurrence. Brodie et al. (1973), who failed to confirm the antidepressant effect of L-5HTP, as mentioned earlier, observed a decreased CSF level of homovanillic acid (HVA) with normal 5HIAA levels in the same depressed patients. In view of the aforementioned findings of Fujiwara and Otsuki, and of Van Pragg, it seems justifiable to infer that the cases of Brodie et al. would pertain to that category of depressed patients who cannot be ameliorated by L-5HTP administration. Table 6 lists the biochemical studies performed on L-5HTP-treated depressive patients. As can be seen in Table 6 (1), the CSF level of 5HIAA, the blood level of 5HT and urinary output of 5HIAA were all increased after the administration of L-5HTP, clearly indicating an increase in the 5HT content of the brain and of the peripheral tissues of depressed patients.

TABLE 6. Biochemical Findings in the Depressed Patients Administered L-5HTP

Authors	Biochemical findings
\multicolumn{2}{c}{Findings after administration of L-5HTP}	
Persson and Roos, 1967	increase of CSF 5HIAA
Brodie, Sack and Siever, 1973	increase of CSF 5HIAA, decrease of CSF HVA and decrease of urinary 17 OHCS
Fujiwara and Otsuki, 1974	increase of CSF 5HIAA and increase of urinary 5HIAA
\multicolumn{2}{c}{Findings after acute loading dose of L-5HTP}	
Coppen, Shaw and Malleson, 1965	reduction of the expiratory rate of $^{14}CO_2$ after an intravenously loading dose of D,L-5HTP labeled with 14C
Sarai, Amamoto, Iseki, Nomura, Tubokura, Sugimoto and Nishio, 1973	delay of the increase of serum 5HT level after an orally loading dose of L-5HTP
Gaillard, Eisenring and Tissot, 1973	increase of the uptake of L-5HTP in both brain and peripheral organs after an intravenously loading dose of L-5HTP
Takahashi and Kondo, 1973	decrease of the secretion of growth hormone after an orally loading dose of L-5HTP
Kaneko, Kumashiro and Takahashi, 1978	delay of the increase of serum 5HT level after an orally loading dose of L-5HTP
\multicolumn{2}{c}{Findings in L-5HTP responders}	
Takahashi, Kondo and Kato, 1975	increase of CSF HVA only in 5HTP responder
Takahashi, Takahashi, Masumura and Miike, 1976	more marked increase of blood 5HT and urinary 5HT and 5HIAA in 5HTP responder, compared with non-responder
Kaneko, Kumashiro, Takahashi and Hoshino, 1978	more marked increase of serum 5HT in 5HTP responder, compared with non-responder

On the other hand, however, there is also an indication that there are different processes of conversion from 5HTP to 5HT for depressed and normal individuals. As is apparent from Table 6 (2), Gaillard et al. (1973) measured the 5HTP concentration of the arterial and venous blood in patients with mania, depression, chorea or alcoholism in an effort to investigate the uptake of L-5HTP by the brain and peripheral tissues. They found an increased 5HTP uptake by brain and peripheral tissues in depressive subjects as compared with other patients. In our recent study (Kaneko et al., 1978), the serum 5HT level was determined over a 24-hour schedule in manic or depressive patients and in normal volunteers after an oral loading the L-5HTP. The results are reported in Figure 1. As can be seen, the serum level of 5HT had a tendency to increase to a lesser extent, to reach a peak in a longer time span and, moreover, to return back to the pre-loading level in a shorter time in depressive patients than in normal subjects. This finding, apparently in contradiction to Gaillard's, suggests that depression is associated with a reduced uptake of L-5HTP from the gastrointestinal tract, and probably decreased decarboxylase activity and increased MAO activity. In a similar investigation Sarai et al. (1973) obtained results consistent with ours. Coppen et al. (1965) observed that the intravenous administration of C^{14}-labelled D,L-5HTP is followed by a reduction of the excretion rate of C^{14}-labelled CO_2 in the air expired by depressed patients, suggesting that decarboxylase activity is diminished in depression.

A comparison of the biochemical findings of responding and non-responding patients after treatment with L-5HTP is given in Table 6 (3). Takahashi et al. (1975) noted that following L-5HTP administration, the CSF content of HVA increased only in responders, whereas the CSF level of 5HIAA was elevated to essentially the same extent in responders as in non-responders. This led the authors to surmise that in responders L-5HTP may be altered by the same enzyme system that is active in dopamine (DA) metabolism. Furthermore, Takahashi et al. (1976) also found that increments of serum 5HT and urine levels of 5HT and 5HIAA following the administration of L-5HTP were definitely smaller in non-responders than in responders, suggesting that non-responders might be unable to utilize 5HTP properly. It should be noted that in our study (Kaneko et al., 1978) comparing serum levels of 5HT prior to, and one week after, the administration of L-5HTP, in responding and non-responding patients, the former showed an elevation of serum 5HT level, whereas the latter did not show any change, the results thus being in agreement with those obtained by Takahashi et al. (1976).

Metabolism of L-5HTP in the Brain

The metabolism of brain L-5HTP as resulting from animal experiments may be considered.

FIGURE 1. Serum 5HT Level in Manic, Depressed and Normal Groups After a Loading Dose of L-5HTP

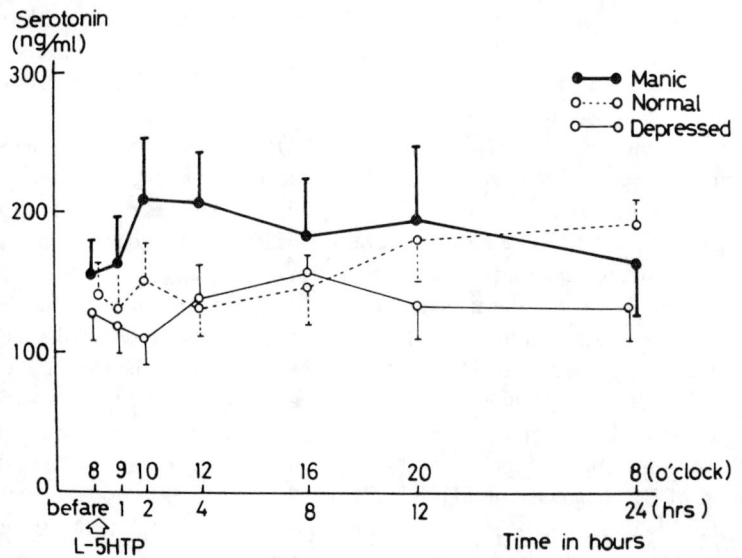

Six depressed patients, 4 manic patients and 6 normal subjects were given orally a loading dose of 3 mg/kg of body weight of L-5HTP at 8 a.m. Serum 5-HT levels were determined by Davis' method* before, 1,2,4,12, and 24 h after the loading dose. Serum 5HT levels showed different chronological changes after a load of L-5HTP among these three groups. Especially, the change in manic patients which showed a rapid and high elevation and its long duration, was a marked contrast to the changes in depressed patients with a gradual, slight elevation and it relatively short duration.

(*Davis, R.B. (1959): *Journal of Laboratory and Clinical Medicine* 54: 344-351.)

According to Tsukada et al. (1973), a marked rise in the 5HT content of various brain regions, notably such extrapyramidal regions as caudate nucleus and putamen, was observed following the administration of L-5HTP in monkeys, whereas not as much conspicuous increase in the level of 5HT was seen in the hypothalamus and inferior colliculus where 5HT is normally present at a high concentration. As for changes in CA levels of brain tissue in consequence of 5HTP administration, DA was reduced in the hindbrain and pons, while norepinephrine (NE) was diminished in the caudate nucleus and putamen. In their histochemical study Fuxe et al. (1971) suggested that 5HTP might enter DA and NE neurons, wherein it is converted to 5HT which in turn replaces DA and NE. Yunger and Harvey (1976) pointed out that the 5HT formed in CA neurons can act as a false transmitter in place of CA. According to Korf et al. (1974) however, 5HTP, when administered in large doses, is certainly converted to 5HT in neurons other than 5HT-neurons, but when small doses are given and 5HT-neurons are in a physiologically normal state, the L-5HTP administered is taken up selectively by 5HT-neurons, where it is subsequently converted to 5HT through a specific reaction catalyzed by 5HTP decarboxylase. It has been suggested that the 5HT thus formed is accumulated at nerve endings, to increase its release into the synaptic cleft (Penn and McBride, 1977). As regards the action of L-5HTP to cause the release of both DA and NE, McBride et al. (1974) maintain that small doses of L-5HTP have no influence upon CA neurons, on the basis of their observation that 1.5 mM of L-5HTP failed to cause any release of DA and NE *in vitro*. It has also been suggested that the formation in large amounts of 5HT from L-5HTP, results in an increase of the enzymatic activity of MAO (Grahame-Smith, 1971) as well as that of other metabolic pathways such as the sulfotransferase (Hidaka et al., 1969; Meck and Neff, 1973). Moir and Ecclestone (1968) reported a significant increase in 5HIAA which occurs prior to an increase in 5HT following the administration of 5HTP, a finding which suggests the existence of a metabolic shunt whereby 5HTP is quickly metabolized to 5HIAA.

From the above-mentioned results it seems possible that L-5HTP, when administered in large doses, is metabolized at least in part through unusual pathways. When given in small doses, it is supposed to be metabolized only by physiological processes. It seems likely, therefore, that in humans also the metabolic pathway for L-5HTP and hence its pharmacological actions may vary depending upon the administered dosage.

Psychopharmacological Action of L-5HTP

Euphoria that attended the use of L-5HTP may be described as one of psychopharmacological actions suggestive of its antidepressant potentiality. As already referred to in analyzing side-effects, clinical evidence indicates that euphoria is observed after 5HTP administration. According to Angst et al. (1977), during three distinct trials of L-5HTP at different dosage levels in depressive patients, euphoria occurred in 1 out of 10 cases, in 1 out of 11 cases and in 1 out of 15 cases, respectively. Euphoria has also been reported to occur in diseases other than depression after L-5HTP administration. Thus, Sano and Taniguchi (1971) noted that L-5HTP administration to patients with Parkinson's disease was associated with an elation of mood and an increased psychomotor activity; Guilleminault et al. (1973) described a case of a manic state of one hour's duration occurring in a patient with a brain stem lesion after the administration of D,L-5HTP in large doses. Trimble et al. (1975) used L-5HTP in one normal volunteer and seven neurological patients, and noted that five of them became euphoric, garrulous and uninhibited.

In a series of joint studies (Pühringer et al., 1976; Graw et al., 1976; Wirz-Justice et al., 1976; Lacoste et al., 1976) the effects of L-5HTP on normal subjects were investigated systematically from the psychopharmacological, physiological and biochemical viewpoints. L-5HTP was administered at a single intravenous injection of 200 mg after benserazide. Mood elevation as well as psychomotor agitation, changed perception and somatic side effects were observed. Particularly, mood elation, which was experienced mainly as a pleasant state of marked well-being, became conspicuous together with a tendency to dissipate 90 minutes after the administration of L-5HTP; these effects continued for two hours and then gradually decreased to disappear completely six hours after administration. During these periods the blood level of growth hormone was raised and, moreover, its time-course was well coincident with that of mood change. In addition, there was a fall (in male) or a rise (in female) in body temperature at the height of mood elation.

All these reports suggest that L-5HTP produces euphoria and it seems probable that such an action of 5HTP brings about a reduction of depressive mood with a consequent improvement of depression.

Turning to the effect of L-5HTP on sleep, the available evidence indicates that the administration of D,L-5HTP is accompanied by either an increase (Wyatt et al., 1971) or a decrease (Autret et al., 1976) of REM (rapid eye movement) sleep in healthy individuals. The effect of L-5HTP on REM sleep thus seems more than speculative. The discrepancy of finding between the two studies cited above is likely dependent on the differences in dose employed but may also be due, at least partly, to individual variations.

On the other hand, despite the fact that insomnia or disturbances of the sleep cycle are almost constantly present in depression, available evidence suggests that L-5HTP is not effective in insomnia and may even aggravate it in some cases. According to Wirz-Justice (1977), however, the effect of L-5HTP on depression bears some similarity to those induced by some Oriental ascetic practices such as sleep deprivation, fasting and Zen. Accordingly, it is also conceivable that this insomnia-aggravating effect of L-5HTP may have a favorable influence on the healing mechanism of depression. Sleep deprivation therapy has been reported to be beneficial in the treatment of depression (Pflug and Tölle, 1971) and REM deprivation (selective interruption of REM sleep) is also reported to be effective in depression (Vogel et al., 1977). Furthermore, Fujiwara et al. (1974) report that a rapid improvement of depressive mood occurs following transient worsening of insomnia in 5HTP responders. From the combined evaluation of these facts, it seems justifiable to presume that the effect of 5HTP on sleep is related to its antidepressant action.

In the above description, mention has been made of those psychopharmacological actions of L-5HTP which are thought to be related to its antidepressant property. In striking contrast to these findings, animal experiments, especially on rodents, have shown L-5HTP not exert to antidepressant but rather an opposite effect so far as food intake (Blundell and Leshem, 1975), sexual behavior (Gessa and Tagliamonte, 1974), aggressiveness (Valzelli, 1974) and conditioned behaviors (Aprison et al., 1978) are concerned. Since the pharmacological profile of 5HT varies among different animal species (Boelkins, 1973; Maas et al., 1973: Zitrin et al., 1970), it would be no surprise if the same could be said about the effect of L-5HTP.

CONCLUDING REMARKS

In this retrospective study, the pertinent literature on the antidepressant potential of L-5HTP and its mechanism of action has been reviewed. In conclusion, L-5HTP was shown to be effective in approximately half of the cases of endogenous depression and particularly beneficial in depression of the bipolar type and in involutional melancholia. L-5HTP responders were found to show anxiety, irritability, insomnia and a decreased CSF level of 5HIAA prior to treatment. After the administration of L-5HTP, depressive moods began to elevate initially, then a reduction of anxiety and irritability followed, but insomnia was adversely affected. The antidepressant action of L-5HTP was rapid in onset. As for adverse side-effects, gastrointestinal symptoms were frequently observed with L-5HTP, although these symptoms can be averted.

The fact that L-5HTP produces euphoria permits us to infer that its mechanism of action in depressive patients is to first act to elevate depressive moods. This presumed mechanism of action is mainly to increase 5HT release into the synaptic cleft of 5HT neurons. Also, the effect of CA neurons and neuroendocrine function (*e.g.*, the secretion of growth hormone) must be considered.

Critical views have recently been published as to the legitimacy of the biogenic amine hypothesis on the etiology of manic-depressive psychosis. The fact that L-5HTP proves to be beneficial in endogenous depression bespeaks the etiological importance of biogenic amines in depression. However, it is an undeniable fact that no more than half of the patients with endogenous depression improve after L-5HTP administration, which suggests the heterogenicity of depression.

Although its usefulness in depression still remains to be completely established, L-5HTP therapy not only provides a potentially useful treatment in depressive disorders, but can also be expected to serve as a useful means for the elucidation of the true etiology of this clinical entity. Further studies will be necessary to determine in what type or types of depression L-5HTP is really indicated.

REFERENCES

Alino, J.J.L.I., Gutierrenz, J.L.A., and Iglesias, M.L.M.M. (1976): 5-Hydroxytryptophan (5HTP) and a MAO (Nialamide) in the treatment of depressions. A double-blind controlled study. *International Pharmacopsychiatry 11:* 8-15.

Angst, J., Woggon, B., and Schoepf, J. (1977): The treatment of depression with L-5-hydroxytryptophan versus imipramine. Results of two open and one double-blind study. *Archiv für Psychiatrie und Nervenkrankheiten 224:* 175-186.

Aprison, M.H., Takahashi, R., and Tachiki, K. (1978): Hypersensitive serotonergic receptors involved in clinical depression–a theory. In: B. Harber and M.H. Aprison (Eds.), *Neuropharmacology and Behavior.* Plenum Publishing Corporation, New York. pp. 23-53.

Asberg, M., Bertilsson, L., Tuck, D., Cronholm, B., and Sjoqvist, F. (1973): Indoleamine metabolites in the cerebrospinal fluid of depressed patients before and during treatment with nortriptyline. *Clinical Pharmacology and Therapeutics 14:* 277-286.

Ashcroft, G.W., Crawford, T.B.B., Eccleston, D., Sharman, D.F., MacDougall, E.J., Stanton, J.B., and Binns, J.K. (1966): 5-Hydroxyindole compounds in the cerebrospinal fluid of patients with psychiatric or neurological disease. *Lancet II:* 1049-1052.

Ashcroft, G.W., Eccleston, D., Murray, L.G., Glen, A.I.M., Crawford, T.B.B., Pullar, I.A., Shields, P.J., Walter, D.S., Blackburn, I.M., Connechan, J., and Lonergan, M. (1972): Modified amine hypothesis for the aetiology of affective illness. *Lancet I:* 573-577.

Ashcroft, G.W., and Glen, A.I.M. (1974): Mood and neural functions: a modified amine hypothesis for the etiology of affective illness. *Advances in Biochemical Psychopharmacology 11:* 335-339.

Aussilloux, Ch., Castelnau, D., Chiariny, J.F., and Fraissinet, M. (1975): A propos d'une autre voie d'abord des états dépressifs les précurseurs de al sérotonine. *Journal de Medecine de Montepllier 10:* 23-25.

Autret, A., Minz, M., Bussel, B., Cathal. H.P., and Castaigne, P. (1976): Human sleep and 5-HTP. Effects of repeated high doses and of association with benserzide (Ro.04.4602). *Electroencephalography and Clinical Neurophysiology 41:* 408-413.

Baldessarini, R.J. (1975): The basis for amine hypotheses in affective disorders. *Archives of General Psychiatry 32:* 1087-1093.

Banki, C.M. (1978): 5-Hydroxytryptamine content of the whole blood in psychiatric illness and alcoholism. *Acta Psychiatrica Scandinvica 57:* 232-238.

Barlet, P., and Pailard, P. (1974): Étude clinique du 5-hydroxy-tryptophane dans les états dépressifs due troisiéme âge. *Cahiers Medicaux Lyonnais 50:* 1895-1901.

Blundell, J.E., and Leshem, M.B. (1975): The effect of 5-hydroxytrytophan on food intake and on the anorexic action of amphetamine and fenfluramine. *Journal of Pharmacy and Pharmacology 27:* 31-37.

Boelkins, R.C. (1973): Effects of parachlorophenylalanine on the behavior of monkeys. In: J. Barchas and E. Usdin (Eds.), *Serotonin and Behavior.* Academic Press, New York and London. pp. 357-364.

Bourne, H.R., Bunney, W.E., Jr., Colburn, R.W., Davis, J.M., Davis, J.N., Shaw, D.M., and Coppen, A.J. (1968): Noradrenaline, 5-hydroxytryptamine, and 5-hydroxyindoleacetic acid in hindbrains of suicidal patients. *Lancet II:* 805-808.

Bowers, M.B., Heninger, G.R., and Gerbode, F.A. (1969): Cerebrospinal fluid, 5-hydroxyindoleacetic acid and homovanillic acid in psychiatric patients. *International Journal of Neuropharmacology 8:* 255-262.

Brodie, H.K.H., Sack, R., and Siever, L. (1973): Clinical studies of L-5-hydroxytryptophan in depression. In: J. Barchas and E. Usdin (Eds.), *Serotonin and Behavior.* Academic Press, New York and London. pp. 549-559.

Bunney, W.E., Jr., Brodie, H.K.H., Murphy, D.L., and Goodwin, F.K. (1971): Studies of alpha-methyl-para-tyrosine, L-dopa, and L-trytophan in depression and mania. *American Journal of Psychiatry 127:* 872-881.

Bunney, W.E., Jr., and Davis, J.M. (1965): Norepinephrine in depressive reactions. *Archives of General Psychiatry 13:* 483-494.

Carlsson, A., Corrodi, H., Fuxe, K., and Hökfelt, T. (1969): Effect of antidepressant drugs on the depletion of intraneuronal brain 5-hydroxytryptamine stores caused by 4-methyl-α-ethyl-meta-tyramine. *European Journal of Pharmacology 5:* 357-366.

Chase, T.N., Ng, L.K.Y., and Watanabe, A.M. (1972): Parkinson's disease. Modification by 5-hydroxytryptophan. *Neurology 22:* 479-484.

Chase, T.N., Shoulson, I., and Carter, A.C. (1976): Serotonergic function in man. *Monographs of Neural Science 3:* 8-14.

Coppen, A. (1967): The biochemistry of affective disorder. *British Journal of Psychiatry 113:* 1237-1264.

Coppen, A., Eccleston, E.G., and Peet, M. (1973): Total and free tryptophan concentration in the plasma of depressive patients. *Lancet I:* 60-63.

Coppen, A., Prange, A.J., Jr., Whybrow, P.C., and Noguera, R. (1972): Abnormalities of indoleamines in affective disorders. *Archives of General Psychiatry 26:* 474-478.

Coppen, A., Shaw, D.M., and Malleson, A. (1965): Changes in 5-hydroxytryptophan metabolism in depression. *British Journal of Psychiatry 111:* 105-107.

Coppen, A., Whybrow, P.C., Noguera, R., Maggs, R., and Prange, A.J. (1972): The comparative antidepressant value of L-tryptophan and imipramine with and without attempted potentiation by liothyronine. *Archives of General Psychiatry 26:* 234-241.

Davidson, J., Sjoerdsma, A., Loomis, L.N., and Udenfriend, S. (1957): Studies with the serotonin precursor, 5-hydroxytryptophan, in experimental animals and man. *Journal of Clinical Investigation 36:* 1594-1599.

Dencker, S.J., Malm, V., Roos, B-E., and Werdinius, B. (1966): Acid monoamine metabolites of cerebrospinal fluid in mental depression and mania. *Journal of Neurochemistry 13:* 1545-1548.

Dunner, D.L., and Fieve, R.R. (1975): Affective disorder: Studies with amine precursors. *American Journal of Psychiatry 132:* 180-183.

Fujiwara, J., Ohara, Y., Hirata, J., and Otsuki, S. (1974): Four cases of indoleamine type in depression. *Japanese Journal of Clinical Psychiatry 3:* 414-420.

Fujiwara, J., and Otsuki, S. (1974): Subtypes of affective psychoses classified by response on amineprecursors and monoamine metabolism. *Folia Psychiatrica et Neurologica Japonica 28:* 93-99.

Fuxe, K., Butcher, L.L., and Engel, J. (1971): D,L-5-hydroxytryptophan-induced changes in central monoamine neurons after peripheral decarboxylase inhibition. *Journal of Pharmacy and Pharmacology 23:* 420-424.

Gaillard, J.-M., Eisenring, J.-J., and Tissot, R. (1973): Consommation cérébrale et périphérique de L-5-HTP chez les patients atteints de syndromes maniaques, dépressifs ou psychotiques. *Encephale 62:* 395-407.

Gessa, G.L., and Tagliamonte, A. (1974): Possible role of brain serotonin and dopamine in controlling male sexual behavior. *Advances in Biochemical Psychopharmacology 11:* 217-228.

Goodwin, F.K., Post, R.M., Dunner, D.L., and Gordon, E.K. (1973): Cerebrospinal fluid amine metabolites in affective illness: The probenecid technique. *American Journal of Psychiatry 130:* 73-79.

Grahame-Smith, D.G. (1971): Studies in vivo on the relationship between brain tryptophan, brain 5HT synthesis and hyperactivity in rats treated with a monoamine oxidase inhibitor and L-tryptophan. *Journal of Neurochemistry 18:* 1053-1066.

Graw, P., Pühringer, W., Lacoste, V., Wirz-Justice, A., and Gasper, M. (1976): Intravenous L-5-hydroxytryptophan in normal subjects: An interdisciplinary precursor loading study, Part II: Profile of psychotropic effects derived from protocols and psychometric investigations. *Pharmakopsychiatrie 9:* 269-276.

Growdon, J.H., Young, R.R., and Shahani, B.T. (1976): L-5-hydroxytryptophan in treatment of several different syndromes in which myoclonus is prominent. *Neurology 26:* 1135-1140.

Guilleminault, C., Cathala, J.P., and Castaigne, P. (1973): Effects of 5-hydroxytryptophan on sleep of a patient with a brain-stem lesion. *Electroencephalography and Clinical Neurophysiology 34:* 177-184.

Herrington, R.N., Bruce, A., Johnstone, E.C., and Lader, M.H. (1976): Comparative trial of L-tryptophan and amitriptyline in depressive illness. *Psychological Medicine 6:* 673-678.

Hidaka, H., Nagatsu, T., Takeya, K., Matsumoto, S., and Yagi, K. (1969): Inactivation of serotonin by sulfotransferase system. *Journal of Pharmacology and Experimental Therapeutics 166:* 272-275.

Jensen, K., Fruensgaard, K., Ahlfors, U.-G., Pihkanen, T.A., Tuomikoski, S., Ose, E., Dencker, S.J., Lindberg, D., and Nagy, A. (1975): Tryptophan/imipramine in depression. *Lancet II:* 920.

Kaneko, M. (1975): Serum 5HT level during treatment of manic-depressive illness. *Fukushima Medical Journal 25:* 7-15 (in Japanese).

Kaneko, M., Kumashiro, H., Takahashi, Y., and Hoshino, Y. (1978): L-5-HTP treatment and serum 5HT levels after L-5-HTP loading on depressed patients. *Neuropsychobiology 5:* 232-240.

Kishimoto, H. (1977): The level and circadian rhythm of plasma tryptophan, tyrosine and cortisol in manic-depressive patients and its clinical significance. *Psychiatria et Neurologia Japonica 79:* 375-392 (in Japanese).

Kline, N.S., and Sacks, W. (1963): Relief of depression within one day using an M.A.O. inhibitor and intravenous 5HTP. *American Journal of Psychiatry 120:* 274-275.

Kline, N.S., Sacks, W., and Simpson, G.M. (1964): Further studies on: One day treatment of depression with 5HTP. *American Journal of Psychiatry 121:* 379-381.

Korf, J., Venema, K., and Postema, F. (1974): Decarboxylation of exogenous L-5-hydroxytryptophan after destruction of the cerebral raphe system. *Journal of Neurochemistry 23:* 249-252.

Kumashiro, H., Aono, T., Wanatabe, K., Koizumi, S., Nakanishi, S., Kaneko, Y., Ohno, E., and Uemura, S. (1977): DC potential shifts associated with convulsive seizures and brain monoamine changes in rabbits. *Folia Psychiatrica et Neurologica Japonica 31:* 513-528.

Lacoste, V., Wirz-Justice, A., Graw, P., Pühringer, W., and Gasper, M. (1976): Intravenous L-5-hydroxytryptophan in normal subjects: An interdisciplinary precursor loading study. Part IV: Effects on body temperature and cardiovascular functions. *Pharmakopsychiatrie 9:* 289-294.

Lapin, I.P., and Oxendrug, G.F. (1969): Intensification of the central serotoninergic processes as a possible determinant of the themoleptic effect. *Lancet 1:* 132-136.

Lee, D.K., Markham, C.H., and Clark, W.G. (1968): Serotonin (5-HT) metabolism in Huntington's chorea. *Life Science 7:* 707-712.

Lloyd, K.G., Farley, I.J., Deck, J.H.N., and Hornykiewicz, O. (1974): Serotonin and 5-hydroxyindoeacetic acid in discrete areas of the brain stem of suicide victims and control patients. *Advances in Biochemical Psychopharmacology 11:* 387-397.

Luchins, D. (1976): Biogenic amines and affective disorders. A critical analysis. *International Pharmacopsychiatry 11:* 135-149.

Maas, J.W. (1975): Biogenic amines and depression. Biochemical and pharmacological separation of two types of depression. *Archives of General Psychiatry 32:* 1357-1361.
Maas, J.W., Redmond, D.E., Jr., and Gauen, R. (1973): Effects of serotonin depletion on behavior in monkeys. In: J. Barchas and E. Usdin (Eds.), *Serotonin and Behavior.* Academic Press, New York and London. pp. 351-356.
MacIndoe, J.H., and Turkington, R.W. (1973): Stimulation of human prolactin secretion by intravenous infusion of L-tryptophan. *Journal of Clinical Investigation 52:* 1972-1978.
Matussek, N., Angst, J., Benkert, O., Gmür, M., Papousek, M., Rüther, E., and Woggon, B. (1974): The effect of L-5-hydroxytryptophan alone and in combination with a decarboxylase inhibitor (Ro 4-4602) in depressive patients. *Advances in Biochemical Psychopharmacology 11:* 399-404.
McBride, W.J., Aprison, M.H., and Hingtgen (1974): Effects of 5-hydroxytryptophan on serotonin in nerve endings. *Journal of Neurochemistry 23:* 385-391.
Meek, J.L., and Neff, N.H. (1973): Biogenic amines and their metabolites as substrates for phenolsulfotransferase (EC 2.8.2.1) of brain and liver. *Journal of Neurochemistry 21:* 1-9.
Mendels, J., and Frazer, A. (1975): Reduced central serotonergic activity in mania: implications for the relationship between depression and mania. *British Journal of Psychiatry 126:* 241-248.
Mendels, J., Stinnett, J.L., Burns, D., and Frazer, A. (1975): Amine precursors and depression. *Archives of General Psychiatry 32:* 22-30.
Moir, A.T.B., and Eccleston, D. (1968): The effects of precursor loading in the cerebral metabolism of 5-hydroxyindoles. *Journal of Neurochemistry 15:* 1093-1108.
Murphy, D.L., Baker, M., Goodwin, F.K., Miller, H., Kotin, J., and Bunney, W.E., Jr. (1974): L-tryptophan in affective disorders: Indoleamine changes and differential clinical effects. *Psychopharmacologia 34:* 11-20.
Nakajima, T., Kudo, Y., and Kaneko, Z. (1978): Clinical evaluation of 5-hydroxy-L-tryptophan as an antidepressant drug. *Foria Psychiatrica et Neurologica Japonica 32:* 223-230.
Papeschi, R., and McClure, D.J. (1971): Homovanillic acid and 5-hydroxyindoleacetic acid in cerebrospinal fluid of depressed patients. *Archives of General Psychiatry 25:* 354-358.
Pare, C.M.B., and Sandler, M. (1959): A clinical and biochemical study of a trial of iproniazid in the treatment of depression. *Journal of Neurology, Neurosurgery and Psychiatry 22:* 247-251.
Pare, C.M.B., Young, D.P.H., Price, K., and Stacey, R.S. (1969): 5-hydroxytryptamine, noradrenaline, and dopamine in brainstem, hypothalamus and caudate nucleus of controls and of patients committing suicide by coal-gas poisoning. *Lancet II:* 133-135.
Penn, P.E., and McBride, W.J. (1977): The effect of injections of D,L-5-hydroxytryptophan on the efflux of endogenous serotonin and 5-hydroxyindoleacetic acid from a synaptosomal fraction. *Journal of Neurochemistry 28:* 765-769.
Persson, T., and Roos, B-E. (1967): 5-hydroxytryptophan for depression. *Lancet:* 987-988.
Pflug, B., and Tölle, R. (1971): Disturbance of the 24-hour rhythm in endogenous depression and the treatment of endogenous depression by sleep deprivation. *International Pharmacopsychiatry 6:* 187-196.
Pühringer, W., Wirz-Justice, A., Graw, P., Lacoste, V., and Gastpar, M. (1976): Intravenous L-5-hydroxytryptophan in normal subjects: An interdisciplinary precursor loading study. Part 1: Implications of reproducible mood elevation. *Pharmakopsychiatrie 9:* 260-268.
Rao, B., and Broadhurst, A.D. (1976): Tryptophan and depression. *British Medical Journal 1:* 460.
Sano, I. (1971): "Precursor therapy" with active amines. Part 1: Treatment of depression by L-5HTP (L-5-hydroxytryptophan). *Psychiatrica et Neurologica Japonica 73:* 809-815 (in Japanese).

Sano, I. (1972): L-5-hydroxytryptophan (L-5-HTP) therapie. *Folia Psychiatrica et Neurologica Japonica 26:* 7-17.
Sano, I., and Taniguchi, K. (1971): Precursor-therapy with active amines. Part II: Treatment of Parkinson's disease by L-5-HTP (L-5-hydroxytryptophan). *Psychiatria et Neurologia Japonica 73:* 835-839 (in Japanese).
Sarai, K. (1974): Clinical pharmacology of depression: 5HTP therapy. *Rinsyo Yakuri 5:* 197-202 (in Japanese).
Sarai, K., Amamoto, T., Iseki, K., Nomura, Y., Tsubokura, A., Sugimoto, S., and Nishio, Y. (1973): Studies on the tryptophanserotonin metabolism of manic-depressive illness. II. Blood 5HT, 5HIAA and urinary 5HIAA concentration after 5HTP loading on depressed patients. *Annual Report of Pharmacopsychiatric Research Foundation 5:* 74-78 (in Japanese).
Sarai, K., and Kayano, M. (1968): The level and diurnal rhythm of serum serotonin in manic-depressive patients. *Folia Psychiatrica et Neurologica Japonica 22:* 271-281.
Schildkraut, J.J. (1965): The catecholamine hypothesis of affective disorders. A review of supporting evidence. *American Journal of Psychiatry 122:* 509-522.
Shaw, D.M., Camps, F.E., and Eccleston, E.G. (1967): 5-hydroxytryptamine in the hindbrain of depressive suicides. *British Journal of Psychiatry 113:* 1407-1411.
Shopsin, B., Friedman, E., and Gershon, S. (1976): Parachlorophenylalanine reversal of tranylcypromine effects in depressed patients. *Archives of General Psychiatry 33:* 811-819.
Shopsin, B., Gershon, S., Goldstein, M., Friedman, E., and Wilk, S. (1975): The use of synthesis inhibitors in defining a role for biogenic amines during imipramine treatment in depressed patients. *Psychopharmacological Communications 1:* 239-249.
Sjöström, R., and Roos, B.-E. (1972): 5-hydroxyindoleacetic acid and homovanillic acid in cerebrospinal fluid in manic-depressive psychosis. *European Journal of Clinical Pharmacology 4:* 170-176.
Takahashi, S., and Kondo, H. (1973): Growth hormone responses to administration of L-5-hydroxytryptophan (L-5HTP) in manic-depressive psychosis. *Folia Psychiatrica et Neurologica Japonica 27:* 197-206.
Takahashi, S., Kondo, H., and Kato, N. (1975): Effect of L-5-hydroxytryptophan on brain monoamine metabolism and evaluation of its clinical effect in depressed patients. *Journal of Psychiatric Research 12:* 177-185.
Takahashi, S., Takahashi, R., Masumura, I., and Miike, A. (1976): Measurement of 5-hydroxyindole compounds during 5 HTP treatment in depressed patients. *Folia Psychiatrica et Neurologica Japonica 30:* 463-473.
Taylor, M., and Abrams, R. (1973): Manic states. A genetic study of early and late onsets affective disorders. *Archives of General Psychiatry 28:* 656-658.
Trimble, M., Chadwick, D., Reynolds, E.H., and Marsden, C.D. (1975): L-5-hydroxytryptophan and mood. *Lancet:* 583.
Tsukada, Y., Kishimoto, H., and Nagai, K. (1975): Studies on amine metabolism in the monkey brain after the administration of amine precursors. In: S. Kondo, M. Kawai, and A. Ehara (Eds.), *Contemporary Primatology.* Karger AG, Basel, pp. 56-66.
Unno, Y., Kaneko, M., Kumashiro, H., Numata, Y., Honda, K., Takahashi, Y., Hoshino, Y., and Suzuki, T. (1977): 5HT levels of brain and serum after various doses of L-5HTP administration in rabbits. *Medicine and Biology 94:* 31-33 (in Japanese).
Valzelli, L. (1974): 5-Hydroxytryptamine in aggressiveness. *Advances in Biochemical Psychopharmacology 11:* 255-263.
Van Praag, H.M., Korf, J., Dols, L.C.W., and Schut, T. (1972): A pilot study of the predictive value of the probenecid test in application of 5-hydroxytryptophan as antidepressant. *Psychopharmacologia 25:* 14-21.

Van Praag, H.M., Van den Burg, W., Bos, E.R.H., and Dols, L.C.W. (1974): 5-Hydroxytryptophan in combination with comipramine in "therapy-resistant" depressions. *Psychopharmacologia 38:* 267-269.
Van Praag, M.H. (1977): Significance of biochemical parameters in the diagnosis, treatment, and prevention of depressive disorders. *Biological Psychiatry 12:* 101-131.
Vogel, G.W., McAbee, R., Barker, K., and Thurmond, A. (1977): Endogenous depression improvement and REM pressure. *Archives of General Psychiatry 34:* 96-97.
Winokur, G., and Cadoret, R. (1977): Genetic studies in depressive disorders. In: G.D. Burrows (Ed.), *Handbook of Studies on Depression*. Excerpta Medica, Amsterdam. pp. 69-77.
Wirz-Justice, A. (1977): Theoretical and therapeutic potential of indoleamine precursors in affective disorders. *Neuropsychobiology 3:* 199-233.
Wirz-Justice, A., Pühringer, W., Lacoste, V., Graw, P., and Gasper, M. (1976): Intravenous L-5-hydroxytryptophan in normal subjects: An interdisciplinary precursor loading study. Part III: Neuroendocrinological and biochemical changes. *Pharmakopsychiatrie 9:* 277-288.
Wyatt, R.J., and Vaughan, T. (1973): 5-Hydroxytryptophan and chronic schizophrenia - a preliminary study. In: J. Barchas and E. Usdin (Eds.), *Serotonin and Behavior*. Academic Press, New York and London. pp. 487-497.
Wyatt, R.J., Zarcone, V., Engelman, K., Dement, W.C., Snyder, F., and Sjoerdsma, A. (1971): Effects of 5-hydroxytryptophan on the sleep of normal human subjects. *Electroencephalography and Clinical Neurophysiology 30:* 505-509.
Yunger, L.M., and Harvey, J.A. (1976): Behavioral effects of L-5-hydroxytryptophan after destruction of ascending serotonergic pathways in the rat: The role of catecholaminergic neurons. *Journal of Pharmacology and Experimental Therapeutics 196:* 307-315.
Zitrin, A., Beach, F.A., Barchas, J.D., and Dement, W.C. (1970): Sexual behavior of male cats after administration of parachlorophenylalanine. *Science 170:* 868-870.

ADDENDUM

Recently Oshima et al. in our laboratory presented a precursor loading study with L-5HTP which was undertaken to know the characteristic of 5HTP responder in depression.

Depressed patients (n=12) and normal subjects (n=16) were given an intravenous loading dose of L-5HTP ester (2 mg/Kg) after premedication with the peripheral decarboxylase inhibitor, venserazide (60 mg), and were investigated for subsequent changes in psychotic symptoms and blood parameters (5HT, free tryptophan, cyclic AMP, cyclic GMP, prolactin and human growth hormone). Next, the patients were treated orally with the combined administration of L-5HTP (150 mg/day) and benserazide (180 mg/day) for 2 weeks, and were divided into responders and non-responders according to their response to the treatment. The results of the loading test were compared retrospectively between responders and non-responders.

1. Eight patients were markedly or moderately improved after L-5HTP treatment (responder), but the other remained unchanged (non-responder).

2. Mood elevation was observed after an intravenous loading dose of L-5HTP ester in both normal subjects and non-responders, but not in responders. Oral temperature elevated in both normal subjects and non-responders, but not in responders.

3. After a loading dose of L-5HTP ester, blood 5-HT levels elevated with a lesser degree in responders than in normal subjects and non-responders, and prolactin secretion was delayed in non-responders.

These results suggest that the clinical and biochemical classification of 5HTP responder and non-responder in depression may be possible by a 5HTP loading test.

Since this review was submitted for publication, five papers pertinent to the clinical effects of D,L- or L-5HTP on depression have appeared.

Kline, N., and Sacks, W. (1980): Treatment of depression with an MAO inhibitor followed by 5-HTP—an unfinished research project. *Acta Psychiatrica Scandinavica 61 (Suppl. 280):* 233-241.

Laboucarie, J., Rascol, A., Guiraud-Chaumeil, B., and El-Hage, W. (1977): La place du 5-hydroxytryptophane levogyre dans les estats depressifs. *Revue de Médecine de Toulouse 13:* 519-524.

Mendlewicz, J., and Youdim, M.B.H. (1978): Anti-depressant potentiation of 5-hydroxytryptophan by L-deprenyl, and MAO "type B" inhibitor. *Journal of Neural Transmission 43:* 279-286.

Oshima, N., Kaneko, M., Numata, Y., Hoshino, Y., Yamamoto, T., Watanabe, A., Watanabe, M., and Kumashiro, H. (1981): A study of 5HTP responder in depression-psychotic symptoms and blood parameters after intravenous loading dose of L-5HTP ester in depressed patients. *Bulletin of the Japanese Neurochemical Society 20:* 52-55.

Van Hiele, L.J. (1980): L-5-hydroxytryptophan in depression: the first substitution therapy in psychiatry? The treatment of 99 out-patients with "therapy-resistant" depression. *Neuropsychobiology 6:* 230-240.

12

Long-Term Efficacy in the Treatment of Schizophrenia

Sven J. Dencker

INTRODUCTION

The term schizophrenia will in this presentation be used in the strict Bleulerian sense (Bleuler, 1911). Schizophrenia thus means a conglomerate of severely disturbing symptoms, including Schneider's first rank symptoms (Schneider, 1959), psychotic decompensation and a tendency to social regression, with a chronic course.

Chronic schizophrenia is still considered to be the most severe mental disease but the prognosis is not so dreaded as during Kraepelin's days (Kraepelin, 1913). Until the 1950s, diagnoses of schizophrenia usually meant permanent hospital care or at least social disablement. Shock treatment and psychosurgery, introduced in the Thirties and Forties, as well as intensive psychotherapy (Rosen, 1968) demonstrated that the originally malignant course could be influenced for the better. However, statistically these treatments did not prove successful although there was a tendency for the discharge figures to increase gradually in many hospitals (Lassenius et al., 1973). The introduction of the neuroleptic drugs in 1952 resulted in the first boom in psychiatry, because of the rapid improvement obtained in schizophrenic patients. For further discussion and references, see Hogarty (1977) and Romano (1977).

According to Shepherd and Watt (1977), however, the course of schizophrenia was not fundamentally altered by the psychotropic drugs. Anyhow, the consequence of the usually efficient symptom relief attained in schizophrenia by the use of neuroleptics was a patient responding to psychotherapeutic intervention and social treatment programs. We are still in this "postneuroleptic" rehabilitation phase as far as the chronic schizophrenic patient is concerned. Moreover, the treatment of the schizophrenic in the acute or relapse phase has changed during the last 25 years as a result of the knowledge gained during the "neuroleptic era."

The hospital prevalence of schizophrenia has gradually decreased (*e.g.*, Weeke and Strömgren, 1978) owing to takeover by outpatient services. However, the efficacy of aftercare programs in schizophrenia has been questioned, see *e.g.*, National Schizophrenia Fellowship, 1973 and 1974, because patients with an initially good response have fallen back in the outpatient setting to the same level of morbidity as before the treatment. Follow-up studies have thus presented the previously rehabilitated patient as a relapser returning to the hospital five years later (Watt, 1975). Other reports, however, have demonstrated good results of maintenance treatment (Freeman, 1973; Gottfries and Green, 1974; Imlah et al., 1978). All these diverging findings give a confusing impression. The long-term efficacy of the treatment of schizophrenia would evidently be increased if the patients were given more qualified attention as to details in the treatment program (Dencker, 1980).

According to many papers, the drug treatment seems to be the most important element of the total therapy program. The neuroleptics, however, only reduce the schizophrenic symptoms; they do not cure the disease. This means that there is a need for additional therapeutic measures. The gradually increased interest in structured and integrated therapeutic programs aims at obtaining optimal results in schizophrenia. However, an American group has declared in *The Advancement of Psychiatry* (1975) that the theoretical basis for combined therapy and the nature of interaction between drugs and psychotherapy still remains unclear. That may be so, but the etiology of schizophrenia is unknown and the progress in therapy is still based on eclecticism. I agree with May (1976) that drugs, psychotherapy and psycho-social methods should complement rather than compete with each other in the treatment of schizophrenia.

The purpose of this paper is to discuss the efficacy of long-term treatment programs in schizophrenia, especially with respect to: 1. details of drug treatment, and 2. the need for complementary therapy.

COMPARATIVE TREATMENT STUDIES

In his study of the efficacy of different treatments in acute schizophrenia, *viz.*, neuroleptics, ECT (*i.e.*, electroconvulsive therapy), individual psychotherapy, combination of neuroleptics and psychotherapy and "milieu treatment," May (1968) found that the group treated with neuroleptics showed the best results, followed by patients treated with ECT with respect to symptom reduction and discharge from hospital. The addition of psychotherapy to neuroleptic treatment did not markedly influence the positive response to the neuroleptic alone. Follow-up of these patients demonstrated that those treated initially with neuroleptics or ECT tended to spend less time in hospital after discharge (May et al., 1976a, b).

I presume that almost every psychiatrist will agree that neuroleptics are superior to any other treatment in the acute psychotic phase, in accordance with May's results. One special problem in the acute phase of schizophrenia is how intensive the treatment should be in terms of increased freedom from psychotic symptoms at the cost of more severe side effects (Maerz, 1976; Zavodnick, 1976). The longer the follow-up period after admission to hospital—in the sub-acute-chronic phase—the more difficult it is to evaluate the further need for neuroleptics as an alternative to other treatments, such as psychotherapy of different types and social program settings.

However, Grinspoon et al. (1972), compared two years' treatment with intensive individual psychotherapy, placebo and neuroleptics in chronic schizophrenia. A close association between symptom reduction and the use of neuroleptics was observed while psychotherapy did not give any significant improvement unless combined with neuroleptic treatment. Similar results were reported by Cowden et al. (1955, 1956), and Honigfeld et al. (1964). On the other hand, negative effects of neuroleptics on at least some subgroups of schizophrenia have been reported (Paul et al., 1972), as well as better results with "milieu treatment" than with medication (Mosher et al., 1975). When these discrepant results are considered, it must, however, be remembered that the spontaneous outcome in schizophrenia varies. Already Kraepelin reported schizophrenic patients to be socially, as well as clinically, recovered.

Many studies of the therapeutic efficacy of different modes of therapy in schizophrenia can be criticized for using biased subgroups. This risk necessitates a background description of not only the cohort but also the whole schizophrenic population from which the subgroup is taken.

CRITERIA OF OPTIMAL NEUROLEPTIC TREATMENT

High-dose phenothiazines, like chlorpromazine, are usually not used today for long-term treatment because of:
1. the risks of metabolic side effects after a total intake of .3-.5 kg of the drug with the appearance of eye changes and pigmentation of areas of the skin exposed to sunlight (Greiner and Berry, 1964; Dencker et al., 1967), and
2. their tendency to cause sedation or tiredness, at least in high doses, which is a drawback in a rehabilitation situation with great demands on the patient's concentration and attention.

These reservations do not apply to the low-dose neuroleptics. Oral administration does not satisfy the demands of intake control, which is an essential requirement in long-term treatment of schizophrenia. The patient's arbitrary change or withdrawal of the neuroleptic drug will jeopardize any total rehabilitation program (Van Putten et al., 1976).

Advantages of Depot Neuroleptics

The advantages of using depot neuroleptics are well known and widely accepted (*e.g.*, Denham and Adamson, 1971; Freeman, 1973; Ayd, 1975: Johnson, 1976a), but have been questioned (Rifkin et al., 1977; Falloon et al., 1978; Schooler et al., 1980). In my opinion it would be a mistake to refrain from using depot neuroleptics in the maintenance treatment of schizophrenia. The following main advantages may be claimed:

1. guaranteed drug delivery;
2. simple administration;
3. prolonged symptom reduction;
4. more constant plasma level with the depot form; and
5. metabolic advantages of depot preparation compared to oral forms.

Several studies have demonstrated the unreliable drug delivery when using oral products, not only in outpatients (Parkes et al., 1962; Willcox et al., 1965), but also in patients treated on the ward (Kline and Simpson, 1964; Wilson and Enoch, 1967). We must, after these reports, realize that a rather large proportion of our patients do not accept the rules and regulations of the treatment and therefore default the therapy or simply forget to take the drug (Johnson and Freeman, 1973). The depot prescription offers administrative (Platt, 1968; Lindholm and Ljungberg, 1973) as well as psychological advantages, especially for the patient who, because of poor compliance, needs repeated information and discussion on the subject of medication.

The depot principle ensures not only a long half-life, *i.e.*, prolonged therapeutic plasma concentrations of the drug, but also more constant plasma levels (Jørgensen and Fredricson Overø, 1980). Maintenance treatment with depot neuroleptics gives very low plasma concentrations, so low that they are difficult to measure with the methods available today. Perphenazine enanthate is so far the only depot neuroleptic for which there is a complete pharmacokinetic documentation. The patients studied demonstrated rather large interindividual variations as to the bioavailability of the drug (Eggert Hansen et al., 1976). Figure 1 demonstrates two perphenazine plasma curves after injection of the enanthate form. One of them shows a rather ideal, and the other one a fluctuating and unsatisfactory, curve. The ideal curve probably means a more stable concentration of the drug on the transmittor side, which theoretically seems desirable.

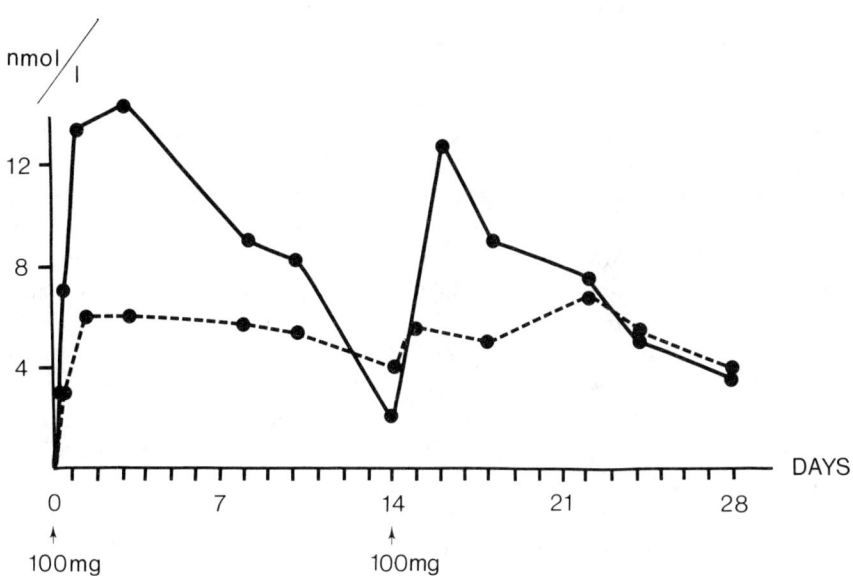

FIGURE 1. An "ideal" (dashed line) and a "nonideal" perphenazine plasma curve (solid line) in two separate subjects, receiving 100 mg of perphenazine enanthate every other week (from Eggert Hansen et al., 1976).

Metabolic Aspects

Parenteral administration of a drug means bypassing the intestinal wall and the first passage through the liver. Curry et al. (1970) demonstrated only insignificant amount of chlorpromazine in plasma in patients treated with oral chlorpromazine for years, which indicates some blockage in the intestinal wall.

Studies of the portal blood after administration of oral imipramine, however, did not reveal any signs of enzymatic breakdown in the intestine in nonpsychiatric patients (Dencker et al., 1976).

The avoidance of first pass metabolism in the liver seems especially important as imipramine is reported to be taken up very rapidly in the rat brain (Nagy, 1977). Chlorpromazine was found to reach a five time higher level in the rat brain than in the blood within one hour after intravenous injection (Gothel and Karczmar, 1963). The sulfoxide metabolite of chlorpromazine (Sakalis et al., 1973; Kolakowska et al., 1976), as well as thioridazine (Traficante et al., 1977), has been found to be present in a higher ratio to parent drug in nonresponders. Moreover, reduction of the plasma level of sulfoxide by chloroquine rapidly improved the nonresponders on thioridazine. These findings, and the need for information on the correlation between response and plasma level, create a need for methods of monitoring neuroleptic drugs, at least in nonresponsive patients.

The animal models constructed for studies of, for instance, the chemical transmission in pre- and postsynaptic parts of the receptor (Gunderson et al., 1974; Snyder et al., 1974; Carlsson, 1978), seem now to be applicable in the clinic. Cerebrospinal monoamine metabolites have thus shown to vary during neuroleptic treatment in schizophrenia (Sedvall et al., 1974; Bjerkenstedt et al., 1977, 1979). Hormones, and particularly prolactin, have claimed attention because of the neuro-anatomical and pharmacological association between neuroleptics, certain hormones and dopaminergic structures (Meltzer and Fang, 1976). The clinical studies performed of cerebrospinal fluid and blood are still preliminary. Öhman and Axelsson (1978) found, however, a correlation between the serum prolactin level and amelioration of psychiatric symptoms. Furthermore, their results suggested the possibility of monitoring the drug used, *viz.*, thioridazine, making it possible to optimize the antipsychotic medication in the individual patient.

When oral and depot neuroleptic treatment is compared as to the amount of drug given per unit time, the advantage of the depot form is clear. This factor may be of special importance in long-term treatment with respect to side effects. Moreover, the longer the duration of action of the depot neuroleptic used, the less the amount of neuroleptic drug delivered per unit time and the fewer the side effects (Dencker et al., 1973; Imlah and Murphy, 1976).

Disadvantages of Depot Neuroleptics

The disadvantages of depot neuroleptics are essentially the following:
1. ethical reservations;
2. medical risks because of prolonged action; and
3. increased frequency of extrapyramidal reactions.

The use of drugs with a prolonged action in psychotics has been considered to be unethical because of the rigid pharmacological monitoring. However, any therapeutic situation should be based on a contract between the patient and the therapist and there are no basic ethical differences between short- and long-acting drugs, only pharmacological. The problems associated with the patient's compliance will obviously be easier to solve when the patient is on depot as compared to oral medication.

The medical risks—allergy, leukopenia, ECG and EEG abnormalities and the neuroleptic malignant syndrome (Caroff, 1980), for example—must always be considered and assessed from case to case (Ayd, 1973). All other side effects, except the Parkinsonian symptoms, seem to be negligible (Imlah et al., 1978). Extensive cardiophysiological examination of patients on megadoses of chlorpromazine and thiothixene did not reveal any significant disturbances (Carlsson et al., 1971; Carlsson et al., 1976).

The dominating problem connected with the use of depot neuroleptics is the complicated association with extrapyramidal side effects. The Parkinsonian reaction is a result of the dopamine-blocking action in the nigrostriatal system of the neuroleptic drug and is both dose- and drug-related (Haase, 1978). There are no pharmacological considerations indicating any special effect caused by the form of administration of the neuroleptic drug as such. The practical depot drug situation—especially for the beginner—is, however, often characterized by severe and protracted extrapyramidal side effects.

The prolonged action of the drug means correspondingly prolonged side effects if the patient's plasma concentration has reached the level for Parkinsonian symptoms. The fluctuating plasma levels given by short-acting neuroleptics make it easier to detect the cause of side effects in comparison with the depot neuroleptics with their more constant plasma levels. The situation with long-acting neuroleptics is also complicated by spontaneous changes in the steady state plasma level, as well as other neuropharmacological and psychological factors (Dencker et al., 1978a). The following plasma level-response curve illustrates the complexity of this situation (Figure 2).

A 25-year-old woman with a manic psychosis had received one dose of 250 mg of fluphenazine enanthate (Case A). The usual result is a rapidly increasing plasma level of the drug, ending in a plateau, as demonstrated by patient B, who showed a very good symptom reduction and did not develop any Parkinsonian symptoms. In the first case (A), the plasma level increased only slowly and irregularly. That there is a lower critical dose level of the neuroleptic drugs for extrapyramidal symptoms is well known. An upper limit of the plasma concentration for Parkinsonian symptoms has also been demonstrated. These two limits are indicated in Figure 2. In this case the upper limit for Parkinsonian symptoms was 8-10 μg of fluphenazine per liter. When the plasma level of fluphenazine fell below this upper limit severe extrapyramidal side effects appeared (see Figure). A similar reaction pattern has been described for L-dopa plasma value and dystonia in Parkinson's disease (Muenter et al., 1977).

The concentration of the neuroleptic in plasma cannot alone be responsible for the Parkinsonian symptoms described, however. During the initial treatment period, with rather low but increasing fluphenazine values, no extrapyramidal side effects appeared. Thus, there seems to be some type of "incubation" period. Other mechanisms, *e.g.*, psychological factors, are apparently also involved (Van Putten, 1974a). The discovery that there are two Parkinsonian limits has taught us to use neuroleptics in high initial doses in non- and bad responders. Starting the treatment with a high dose means a rapid ascent to the upper, more or less, non-Parkinsonian range. The fear of severe Parkinsonian side effects has gradually subsided and the use of high doses of neuroleptics has become more common in patients who responded poorly or not at all to normal doses.

FIGURE 2. Separate fluphnazine plasma curves in two patients receiving 250 (A) and 750 mg (B) of fluphenazine enanthate in single doses. The dashed lines indicate the upper and lower limits for extrapyramidal side effects. The black range indicates periods of extrapyramidal side effects in case A. Note the fluctuating absorption from the muscle depot in case A.

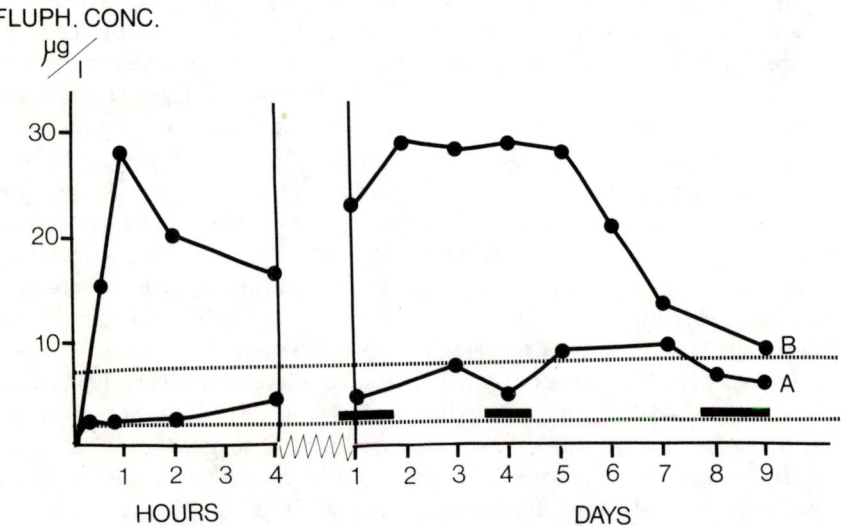

The report (Rivera-Calimlin et al., 1973) of an interaction between chlorpromazine and an anticholinergic agent, resulting in a lower plasma level of the neuroleptic, has not been confirmed when other drugs have been used (Kolakowska et al., 1976; Dencker et al., 1978a; Bolvig Hansen et al., 1979). The continuous use of anticholinergic drugs may result in postsynaptic hypersensitivity or structural brain damage and an increasing risk of permanent tardive dyskinesia (Uhrbrand and Faurbye, 1960; Kazamatsuri et al., 1972; Klawans, 1973; Tarsy and Baldessarini, 1976; Allen, 1977; Crane, 1977; Gardos et al., 1977; Gerlach, 1979). In the long-term perspective, it must be observed that an anticholinergic can give euphoria and a tendency to drug addiction especially when given parenterally or in high doses.

There are psychological components involved in the neuroleptic-induced extrapyramidal symptoms. In the treatment of Parkinsonian symptoms, anxiolytic drugs and even placebo have been shown to give the same symptom reduction as anticholinergic agents (Klett et al., 1972). Greater efficacy of anticholinergic drugs than placebo has, however, been demonstrated in a carefully designed trial (Gunby et al., 1975). Nevertheless, the anticholinergic drugs should be used with discretion and almost never routinely (Klett et al., 1972; McClelland et al., 1974; Johnson, 1978). The prolonged neuroleptic action of the depot drug may give Parkinsonian symptoms of longer duration. These symptoms are often "subclinical," without distinct extrapyramidal characteristics, *i.e.*, the akinetic syndrome. The patient feels sad and depressed and the schizophrenic symptoms may increase as a reaction to the neuroleptic-induced prolonged Parkinsonian state (Van Putten, 1974b).

The Depot Neuroleptics Used

Table I lists the injectable depot neuroleptics which are registered in Scandinavia and/or have been used by us during the last 12 years. Pharmacokinetic data are lacking for most of them. The figures for duration of action and dose are therefore based on clinical findings. Fluphenazine, perphenazine and pipothiazine are phenothiazines, flupenthixol and clopenthixol are thioxanthenes, and haloperidol and fluspirilene are butyrophenones. All depot preparations except fluspirilene are long-acting esters dissolved in oil, thus combining chemical and physical prolongation of the neuroleptic action. Fluspirilene is a microsuspension in a buffered aqueous solution.

The pharmacological actions of the depot neuroleptics are the same as with the use of the basic drugs. The esters in low amounts have been demonstrated outside the muscle depot but this finding may not have any clinical implications (Jørgensen et al., 1971; Svendsen et al., 1980). The following aspects of the use of the different depot neuroleptics listed in table I will be discussed:

1. duration of action;
2. antipsychotic efficacy;
3. other psychic effects; and
4. long-term aspects.

The ideal duration of action of a depot neuroleptic drug has been discussed for years and a drug with four-week duration is now generally used for maintenance treatment. Depot neuroleptics with a shorter duration are also widely used, however, owing to local differences in therapeutic policy as well as patients' individual needs for drugs with a shorter action. The interindividual variation in duration of effect by one and the same drug permits two alternatives:
1. titration of the individual duration of action of the drug and then use of this information for determination of the injection interval, or
2. the use of a standard dose interval, adapting the dose amount to this fixed duration.

TABLE I. The injectable depot neuroleptics used in Scandinavia. The figures give the approximate duration of action and single dose amount during maintenance treatment.

	duration in weeks	dose in mg
fluphenazine enanthate	2	6,25-50
fluphenazine decanoate	4	6,25-50
perphenazine enanthate	2	25-200
pipothiazine undecylenate	2	50-200
pipothiazine palmitate	4	50-400
pipothiazine dimethylpalmitate	8	50-400
flupenthixol decanoate	4	20-100
flupenthixol palmitate	4	20-100
clopenthixol decanoate	4	50-300
haloperidol decanoate	4	12,5-75
fluspirilene	1	1-8

All the depot neuroleptics mentioned in table I have demonstrated good antipsychotic efficacy. The usually used doses during maintenance treatment are shown in the table. At higher dose levels, and especially when megadoses are used, *i.e.*, doses about 10 times higher than a maintenance dose, the differences in neuroleptic profile are marked. Even in megadoses little sedation is usually experienced with fluphenazine and haloperidol. In higher maintenance doses the other esters give some sedation, which becomes marked when megadoses are used.

One six-month study comparing clopenthixol decanoate and perphenazine enanthate did not show any statistically significant difference in the total BPRS-score between the two drugs, but the clopenthixol-treated patients showed a better score for "hostile-suspiciousness" and "social interest" (Ahlfors et al., 1980). Flupenthixol decanoate has been reported to be effective for repressing depressive symptoms in schizophrenia (Johnson and Malik, 1975). These studies need confirmation but the results presented indicate different symptom reduction profiles of the present depot neuroleptics. It therefore seems desirable to select the right depot drug for each patient, depending on such factors as the severity of the psychotic symptoms and the presence of anxiety and a depressive personality. Floru (1977), however, has questioned the value of considering differences in the depot neuroleptic profile.

Long-Term Aspects

The requirement for optimal neuroleptic treatment in the long-term perspective relate to the following three points:
1. continuous optimal symptom control;
2. prevention of relapse; and
3. use of anti-Parkinsonian drugs.

During the long course of regressive schizophrenia the symptoms change considerably. This means, for example, that periods of turbulence alternate with periods of silent psychotic symptoms. Even during periods of quiet aftercare, there may be symptoms of anxiety, or depression (de Alarcon and Carney, 1969; Planansky and Johnston, 1978), as well as psychotic microsymptoms, necessitating the use of anxiolytic, activating and/or antidepressive drugs. The criteria of an optimal treatment program are:
1. dose flexibility of the neuroleptics used; and
2. use of the lowest effective dose.

The lack of interest for such aspects in practice is demonstrated in clinical trials, in which fixed doses of neuroleptics are often used and the follow-up period is often short, as well as in clinical practice with many patients on a constant dose for years. That usually means total overdosage as well as drug abuse. One of the most important rules of treatment with neuroleptic drugs is that the need to increase (Engelhardt et al., 1960) or decrease (Lonowski et al., 1978) the dose should be evaluated regularly, for example, every three months—which is my recommendation.

In order to ensure continuous optimal symptom control, the spontaneous changes of schizophrenic symptoms must be taken into account. The basic neuroleptic treatment should be modified periodically, as mentioned above. The question arises how to treat patients with symptoms of threatening relapse, and/or increasing anxiety and depression (Gottfries, 1971; Floru, 1977; Planansky and Johnston, 1978). There are two alternatives.

The first is to add another neuroleptic, with a different therapeutic profile, an anxiolytic or an antidepressive drug (Davis, 1975). No interaction has been demonstrated between neuroleptics and benzodiazepines or barbiturates (Freeman, 1967; Kurland and Hanlon, 1971). An interaction between neuroleptics and tricyclic antidepressants has been shown to result in a lower metabolism of the tricyclic drug (Gram and Fredricson Overø, 1972, Gram et al., 1974). From a practical point of view, this finding emphasizes the need for careful follow-up of the patient or monitoring of the plasma level.

The second alternative is to vary the basic neuroleptic according to the individual schizophrenic symptom. As discussed above, there are differences in the symptom profile between the depot neuroleptics, and these observations can be utilized to obtain better symptom reduction. The drawbacks as well as the advantages of changing the depot neuroleptic are illustrated by the results presented in Figure 3, which shows the changes in a "schizophrenic" factor during a one-year study (Dencker et al., 1978b). Two groups of patients—one treated with fluphenazine decanoate and one with pipothiazine palmitate—were compared as to this factor with high loading on *e.g.*, splitting, delusions and conceptual disorganization. All patients were in a maintenance phase and had been treated with fluphenazine decanoate and not pipothiazine palmitate. This may explain the initial deterioration in the latter group. This finding provides numerical confirmations of a frequently observed clinical phenomenon, *i.e.*, an initial deterioration following a change of drug. The pipothiazine group gradually showed a greater total improvement than the fluphenazine group, illustrating the benefits of change of medication over time.

It is not possible to give any recommendation based on controlled studies. However, it seems advisable to try changing to another depot drug after 1-2 years of continuous treatment with the same drug, provided that the patient's condition is not perfect, and discuss with the patient and his or her relatives whether or not to continue with the new drug after an adjustment period of about three-five months. The patient is usually able to state a preference. During maintenance treatment in patients well-adapted to a depot neuroleptic, additional neuroleptics, anxiolytic drugs and hypnotics are usually not necessary. In these circumstances about 40 percent of patients can be treated without

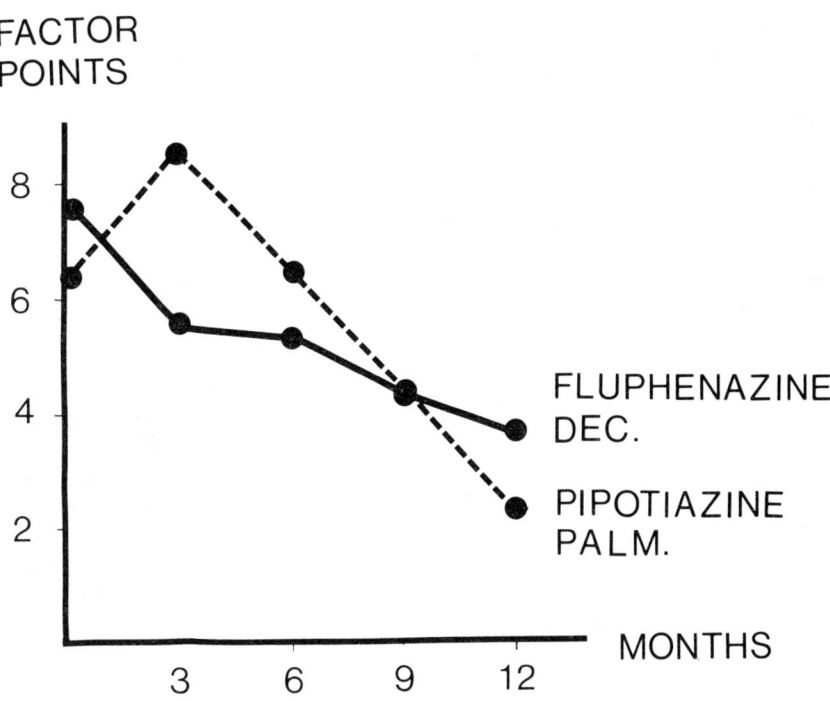

FIGURE 3. The changes in a "schizophrenic" factor during a one-year controlled study of fluphenazine decanoate and pipotiazine palmitate. The higher the value the worse the symptoms (from Dencker et al., 1978b).

any anti-Parkinsonian drugs (Dencker et al., 1973; Marriott, 1978). Anticholinergics should always be used with discretion because of the presumed increased risk of tardive dyskinesia in patients taking anticholinergic drugs for longer periods. Moreover, Andén (1972) has demonstrated a competitive action in dopaminergic structures between anticholinergic agents and neuroleptics.

The Drug Withdrawal Test

The need for neuroleptics for symptom control and/or relapse prevention will thus change during the course of the schizophrenic disease. According to a survey by Gardos and Cole (1976), the drug-placebo differences in relapse rate ranged between 12 and 59 percent when oral neuroleptics were used. They concluded that for at least 40 percent of outpatient schizophrenics, phenothiazines are essential for survival in the community.

There are only two papers presenting results of discontinuation of depot neuroleptics. Hirsch et al., (1973) carried out a controlled drug-placebo study during nine months in a cohort of schizophrenics who had been treated with fluphenazine decanoate for three months. The relapse rate was 66 percent on placebo and 8 percent in the group given active drug.

Dencker et al. (1980a) studied 32 patients in a younger age group defined as the best group with respect to psychotic symptoms out of a total schizophrenic population of about 300 patients of the chronic type. The open trial design was used because one of the inclusion criteria was the patient's wish to withdraw the depot neuroleptic. The patients had been on depot neuroleptics for at least 3 years and on the depot drug that was to be withdrawn for 15 months or more.

Follow-up of this material two years later demonstrated that only two patients had managed to live in the community without neuroleptics. Figure 4 shows the relapse figures from the two depot neuroleptic studies mentioned and two studies using oral drugs in the preceding phase (Prien et al., 1968; Hogarty et al., 1976). The figures are rather similar in spite of the different techniques used.

FIGURE 4. Cumulative relapse rate percentage curves from two materials, work numbers 1 and 4 and two "point values," work numbers 2 and 3.

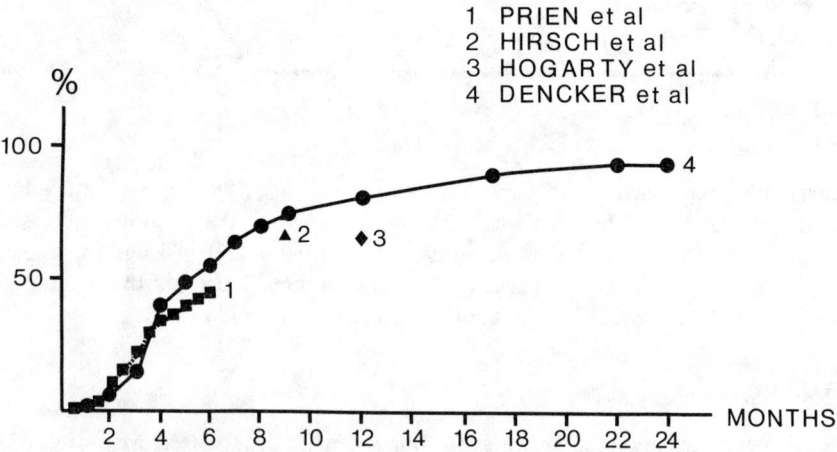

Neuroleptic withdrawal is a dangerous experiment in severe forms of schizophrenia. Relapses due to drug withdrawal are sometimes difficult to manage in spite of resumption of earlier drug treatment. Accidents during relapses are not uncommon and nor are social disasters. Moreover, repeated relapses due to drug failure may damage the schizophrenic's self-confidence, which will be a particular handicap in the continuous rehabilitation situation.

Any discontinuance of neuroleptic treatment in schizophrenia must therefore be done with respect and caution. I would suggest the following program in a procedure I prefer to call a *test of withdrawal for outpatients on depot neuroleptics:*

1. before any withdrawal test, the patient's total situation must be carefully evaluated;
2. the patient's and/or relatives' attitude must be understood. The informed consent should also include what action is to be taken if the withdrawal test results in failure;
3. slow reduction of the neuroleptic drug over a rather long period, with careful observation for any increase in schizophrenic symptoms. Rating scales might be used for checking the patient's psychiatric symptoms;
4. the patient should be followed up for at least two years during the drug discontinuation phase, with special attention to the first eight months, which are associated with the highest relapse rate; and
5. it might be prudent to try a three months' withdrawal trial, followed by automatic resumption of the neuroleptic drug. After another year's medication a new, longer withdrawal period might be tried. Carpenter (1978) has recommended a drug-free month for outpatient schizophrenics on continuous oral medication.

The withdrawal test must always be kept in mind during long-term treatment with neuroleptics. One reason is the risk of persistent side effects (Hershon et al., 1972), including tardive dyskinesia. Another reason is to reveal the placebo survivors (Hogarty and Ulrich, 1977), who cannot be identified by using any "background history form." Moreover, the evaluation of predictors for outcome of treatment in schizophrenia is difficult and has to be questioned (Goldstein et al., 1969; Goldstein, 1970; Leff and Wing, 1971; Goldberg et al., 1977; Sartorius et al., 1977; Watts and Bennett, 1977; Bland et al., 1978). Older patients, however, are known sometimes to manage better without than with neuroleptics and need lower doses (Mårtensson and Roos, 1973). In our study six one-year survivors were characterized by mild or few schizophrenic symptoms before the withdrawal test; low doses of neuroleptic drugs; and a high level of social adjustment towards work as well as towards ordinary life.

THE COMBINED TREATMENT DESIGN

The total social situation—both early and later in the course of schizophrenia—varies with respect to the content and the intensity of the treatment program. Moreover, the ultimate prognosis depends on the subtype of schizophrenia (Goldstein et al., 1969; Goldstein, 1970; Gunderson et al., 1974; Bland et al.,

1978). The different subgroups of schizophrenia associated with any treatment in the long-term perspective will therefore be presented.

Description of a Total Schizophrenic Population

Department II of Lillhagen Hospital has a defined care responsibility with a catchment area of about 100,000 persons. Our total schizophrenic population is described in Figure 5 and the figures refer to a key date in February 1978. Only chronic schizophrenics belonging to the regressive type are included. The prevalence is just under 3 per mille, which is a representative figure for a Scandinavian schizophrenic population (Strömgren, 1958). The "senile" group consists of schizophrenic patients who also have a geriatric diagnosis (7 percent of the

FIGURE 5. The schizophrenic "pyramid" from our catchment area of about 100,000 inhabitants. Only schizophrenics of regressive type are included, giving a prevalence figure of just under 3 per mille. The shaded area indicates that extramural institutions are responsible for the care of the patients. The figures present number of patients.

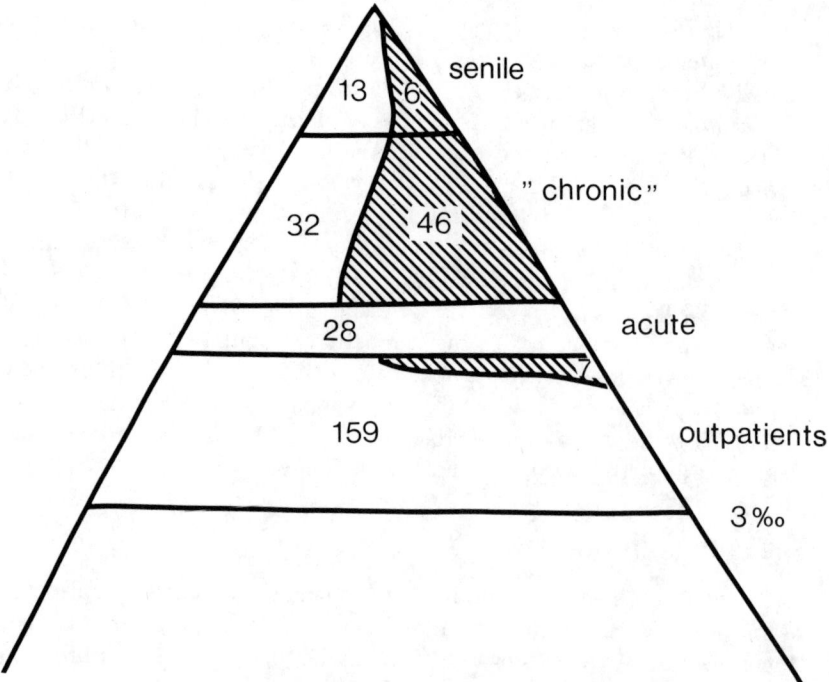

total schizophrenic population). "Chronics" (28 percent) are the remaining group—usually elderly but not senile patients who have been treated in hospital or a hostel more or less continuously for at least ten years. "Acute patients" (9 percent) are first admission cases, out-patient relapses, day patients or patients in the rehabilitation phase taken care of in a five-day-a-week ward. The "outpatients" (56 percent) are living at home, alone or with relatives. The patients nursed in hostels or living in family care are presented in the shaded area of the pyramid.

Therapy Models

A total schizophrenic population can thus be described. The subgroups presented will serve for discussion of basic aspects of treatment in the separate patient groups, mainly with respect to the long-term perspective (Figure 6).

The senile group is uninteresting from a rehabilitation point of view.

The "chronic" patients can be divided into two groups:
1. one with an acceptable social and behaviour status who remain because they prefer to stay in the ward rather than moving to a hostel (26 percent of the total material); and
2. a group who are basically refractory to treatment but usually so social that they can be treated in a ward with open doors. They are preferably cared for in hospital and not a hostel (2 percent).

Neither of these groups are permanent full-care cases. Only a few patients occasionally suffer a severe relapse necessitating total care in a ward for acute patients. In both groups it is difficult to evaluate the separate elements of the treatment—neuroleptics, other drugs, social training programs and good nursing—with respect to their importance for the final, fairly good overall result, *i.e.*, a patient living in an acceptable way in the ward and usually taking part in many activities inside, as well as outside, the hospital. With the exception of periods of severe psychotic relapse, these patients can be treated in professionally staffed hostels.

In the severely ill group—comprising altogether 78 patients—about 30 patients have been treated with megadoses of depot neuroleptics, usually fluphenazine enanthate, in a test dose of 250 mg a week for four weeks (Dencker et al., 1980b). If the patient has responded with a distinct symptom reduction, the megadose treatment has been continued off and on even up to 8 years in 14 patients. The safety as well as the efficacy of megadose treatment using, for example, chlorpromazine (Prien and Cole, 1968) peroral fluphenazine (Polvan et al., 1969; Rifkin et al., 1971), haloperidol (Oldham and Bott, 1971; Mc Creadie and MacDonald, 1977) and different depot neuroleptics (Verhaegen, 1975; Dencker, 1976) has been good.

FIGURE 6. The total schizophrenic material separated in cohorts in the in- as well as in the outpatient subgroups. The figures show percentages of the total material.

			% of total material	
inpatient group	old-senile		7	
	chronic	social	26	44
		"refractory"	2	
	acute		9	
outpatient group	relapsing		7	
	unstable		7	56
	stable		42	

In controlled studies oral (Quitkin et al., 1975), as well as depot, drugs (McClelland et al., 1976; Dencker et al., 1978c) have not demonstrated any significant tendency toward better symptom reduction on megadoses in comparison with normal doses. It must be observed, however, that only a subgroup of the patients refractory on ordinary neuroleptic doses respond satisfactorily to megadoses. Severe side effects are seldom seen on megadoses but must be anticipated. As previously stated, this subject has aroused increasing interest during the last few years and biological as well as clinical predictors might exist (Ayd, 1972; Man, 1973; Davis, 1976).

The "acute" patient usually responds to normal doses of neuroleptics. There are, however, some schizophrenics who do not respond optimally to neuroleptics. In these patients we have tried intensive individual psychotherapy for up to two to three years without any great improvement. There is much case report material but only one controlled study (Smith et al., 1967) supporting addition of ECT to neuroleptics in more or less refractory schizophrenics (see also Alexander, 1962; Weinstein and Fischer, 1971). The addition of reserpine to the neuroleptic drug has also been suggested (Bacher and Lewis, 1978). Beta-receptor blocking agents have also been reported to give symptom reduction in refractory cases, usually in high doses, in combination with neuroleptics or alone (Yorkston et al., 1974; Yorkston et al., 1976). Clozapin—a non-neuroleptic drug—has given good results in patients refractory to neuroleptics, but the risks for blood dyscrasia must be seriously considered (Simpson et al., 1978). Lithium in combination with neuroleptics has been found in a controlled study to give better symptom control than neuroleptics alone (Belmaker et al., 1978).

Only two schizophrenic patients admitted to our department during the last decade have been continuously treated in hospital for more than two years. Both patients may eventually leave the ward for alternative care at a lower treatment level. This suggests that we now have the hospital chronicism in schizophrenia under control. The "last decade patient" is therefore considered to be an "acute" patient until discharge. Some other young patients with a severe type of schizophrenia are high consumers of hospital care but they have always sooner or later been discharged to their own home, a collective home or a hostel. I agree with Gunderson (1976) that the trend toward brief hospitalization can be questioned in the more severe cases. Instead, I would suggest the non-push approach, using the necessary time to obtain optimal results. The risk of disease artefact syndrome is apparently less in the ward, with a trained staff, than when the patient is living alone in the community.

The outpatients can be divided into three subgroups:
1. patients who relapse and will be admitted to hospital from time to time (7 percent of the total material);
2. patients who seldom relapse but who have an unstable, insufficient, or rather handicapped total life situation—*i.e.,* patients who need at least some support at home or at work (7 percent); and
3. patients living their own lives without the need of support in ordinary situations (42 percent).

Our relapse rate, 7 percent of the total population, may be too high. It should, however, be noted that we adopt a very liberal policy with respect to admission to hospital. The main part of the outpatient cohort—42 percent of the total schizophrenic population—exhibited a rather stable situation in society and had few relapses. These results suggest a satisfactory long-term efficacy in the treatment of severe forms of schizophrenia. We attribute this to the following three features of our special outpatient clinic for psychotic patients:
1. the existence of a single organization with both medical and social responsibility for the patients;
2. the patients are given continuous individualized support; and
3. most patients are treated with depot neuroleptics.

Similar outpatient clinics have been described (Imlah, 1976; Imlah and Murphy, 1976; Marriott and Hiep, 1978; Marriot, 1978; Heinrich, 1978; Donlon, 1978; Imlah et al., 1978). Imlah adopts the same treatment policy as we, almost 100 percent of his patients are on depot neuroleptics. Donlon's figure is 25 percent. It also seems advisable to organize an outpatient clinic of this kind as part of the total hospital organization (Donlon et al., 1973; Byrne et al., 1974) in order to be able to take necessary action, including admission to hospital or a course of rehabilitation.

Because of the tendency to regression, it seems advisable to organize some type of standardized follow-up for most schizophrenics. After about six years' use of some pushing social training programs—with or without the token economy technique (Zimmermann and Blumhoff, 1978)—we have changed to advanced, time-unlimited and structured programs individualized with respect to drug treatment, different types of psychotherapy and training for living at home, work and leisure. In other words, an integrated treatment program (Dencker, 1980). Figure 7 shows our rehabilitation model. In the first phase after admission, the acute patient is treated with oral neuroleptics, usually finishing with depot drug treatment. If necessary, this is followed by a rehabilitation program. After this inpatient period, the patient is followed up with individualized support in a therapeutic setting at our outpatient clinic. If a nonoptimal outpatient situation is diagnozed, the patient can be referred for a new period of rehabilitation (a), followed up with intensified support. If these activities have not been successful, new rehabilitation programs with different characteristics as to duration and content (B and C) and intensified outpatient support are tried. Any escalation of the total rehabilitation process must be carefully analyzed with regard to the patient's capacity.

The relapse rate already mentioned is low in comparison with those reported by Hirsch et al. (1973) (26-29 percent during 15 months), Johnson (1976b) (41 percent during two years), and Hogarty et al. (1979) (23.4-65.5 percent in different patient groups over a 22-month period). We have been successful in reducing the relapse rate over the years but it still seems too high. Two observations can be useful when planning the further rehabilitation program:
1. schizophrenics living with highly emotional relatives are more likely to relapse (Brown et al., 1972; Leff, 1976); and
2. the demonstrated steady symptom reduction during an intensified outpatient control period is followed by a rebound increase in schizophrenic symptoms during a maintenance phase with less intensive supervision (Dencker et al., 1973, 1980c).

These observations underline the importance of different life events, the personal demands on the patient and his often frustrating and isolated situation in the community. Such schizophrenic social symptoms may be treated in a therapeutic setting, as suggested and tried by Davis et al. (1972) and Hogarty et al. (1973, 1979), who utilized advanced milieu therapy and psychotherapeutic principles (Ugelstad, 1975; Gunderson, 1976; Luborsky et al., 1976). In such a setting the problems associated with the patient's drug compliance (Johnson

FIGURE 7. Theoretical model for a schizophrenic patient in an acute as well as in a chronic period. Phase I is characterized by individualized neuroleptic therapy, usually oral, initially, and later on depot treatment. During Phase II a rehabilitation program starts, which is pursued by a support therapy program, in which depot neuroleptics are used (Phase III). In a "chronic period," when the patient does not function adequately in society, another rehabilitation period (A) can be added, followed by intensified support therapy (double lines). If this program is not sufficient, another one with a different content (B) is added, followed by a more intensive aftercare program, complemented, if necessary, with a further rehabilitation period (C).

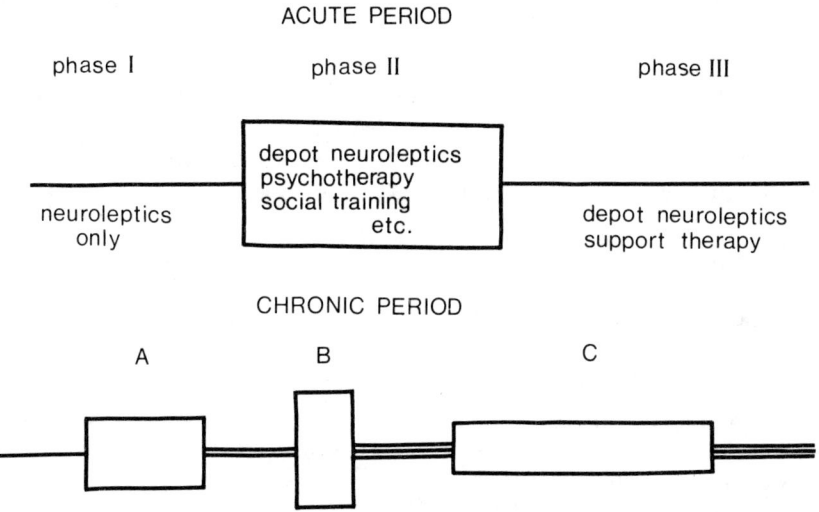

and Freeman, 1973) can be treated in a psychotherapeutic way. It has thus gradually become apparent that a multifactorial therapeutic approach can be applied (Davis, 1975; May, 1976; Cheadle et al., 1978) with promising better life situation for schizophrenic patients. The improved total situation apparently results in the use of lower doses of psychoactive drugs.

CONCLUDING REMARKS

Schizophrenia of the regressive type has traditionally been regarded as having a poor prognosis. The outcome from a symptomatological and social point of view has changed since the start of neuroleptic treatment. The introduction of injectable long-acting neuroleptics improved the total treatment situation. Two main lines of development can be recognized. An overoptimistic approach, resulting in extensive discharge of schizophrenic patients, leading in turn to their nomadic existence or a heavy burden on relatives or extramural institutions, and often total social failure in the subsequent course.

The other, more realistic approach involved preferably the use of depot neuroleptics in the first phase of the rehabilitation process and then gradually adding social training programs of varying content including long-term active support therapy. Up to now the neuroleptics seem to be the most important element of the total rehabilitation process in schizophrenia. The details of the drug treatment must be carefully scrutinized, however, in order to optimize the treatment in the long-term perspective. The long-term treatment must be individually evaluated over time with respect to type and dosage of neuroleptic drug. Interest in plasma monitoring techniques for neuroleptics must be intensified.

Schizophrenia of regressive type is a severe chronic disease. The individualized, carefully designed rehabilitation program seems to have altered the social prognosis for almost all schizophrenic patients in the long-term perspective. The regressive element of the disease, however, cannot be cured, which means a need for long-term support even in the patients who respond optimally.

REFERENCES

Ahlfors, U.G., Dencker, S.J., Gravem, A., and Remvig, J. (1980): *Acta Psychiatrica Scandinavica 61, suppl. 279:* 77-91.
deAlarcon, R., and Carney, M.W.P. (1969): *British Medical Journal 3:* 564-567.
Alexander, H.G. (1962): *Diseases of the Nervous System 23:* 526-532.
Allen, R.M. (1977): *Current Therapeutic Research 22:* 914-917.
Andén, N.-E. (1972): *Journal of Pharmacy and Pharmacology 24:* 905-906.
Ayd, F.J., Jr. (1972): *Diseases of the Nervous System 33:* 459-469.
Ayd, F.J., Jr. (1973): In: F.J. Ayd, Jr. (Ed.), *The Future of the Pharmacotherapy: New Drug Delivery Systems.* International Drug Therapy Newsletter, Baltimore. pp. 69-76.
Ayd, F.J., Jr. (1975): *American Journal of Psychiatry 132:* 491-500.
Bacher, N.M., and Lewis, H.A. (1978): *American Journal of Psychiatry 135:* 488-489.
Belmaker, R.H., Biederman, J., and Lerner, Y. (1978): *International Congress, C.I.N.P., Vienna.*
Bjerkenstedt, L., Gullberg, B., Härnryd, C., and Sedvall, G. (1977): *Archives of Psychiatry and Neurological Sciences 227:* 107-113.
Bjerkenstedt, L., Gullberg, B., Härnryd, C., and Sedvall, G. (1979): *Archives of Psychiatry and Neurological Sciences 227:* 181-192.
Bland, R.C., Parker, J.H., and Orn, H. (1978): *Archives of General Psychiatry 35:* 72-77.
Bleuler, E. (1911): *Dementia Praecox oder die Gruppe der Schizophrenien.* Franz Deuticke, Leipzig-Vienna.
Bolvig Hansen, L., Elley, J., Rosted Christensen, T., Larsen, N.E., Naestoft, J., Hvidberg, E.G. (1979): *British Journal of Clinical Pharmacology 7:* 75-80.
Brown, G.W., Birley, J.L.T., and Wing, J.K. (1972): *British Journal of Psychiatry 121:* 241-258.

Byrne, L., O'Connor, T., and Fahy, T.J. (1974): *British Journal of Psychiatry 125:* 20-24.
Carlsson, A. (1978): *American Journal of Psychiatry 135:* 164-173.
Carlsson, C., Dencker, S.J., Grimby, G., Häggendal, J., and Johnsson, G. (1971): *European Journal of Clinical Pharmacology 3:* 163-171.
Carlsson, C., Dencker, S.J., Grimby, G., Häggendal, J., and Johnsson, G. (1976): *International Journal of Clinical Pharmacology 13:* 262-268.
Caroff, S.N. (1980): *Journal of Clinical Psychiatry 41:* 79-83.
Carpenter, W.T. (1978): *Schizophrenia Bulletin 4:* 148-149.
Cheadle, A.J., Freeman, H.L., and Korer, J. (1978): *British Journal of Psychiatry 132:* 221-227.
Cowden, R.C., Zax, M., and Sproles, J.A. (1955): *American Medical Association Archives of Neurology and Psychiatry 74:* 518-522.
Cowden, R.C., Zax, M., Hague, J.R., and Finney, R.C. (1956): *American Journal of Psychiatry 112:* 898-902.
Crane, G.E. (1977): *American Journal of Psychiatry 134:* 756-789.
Curry, S.H., Marshall, J.H., Davis, M.M., et al. (1970): *Archives of General Psychiatry 22:* 209-215.
Davis, A.E., Dinitz, S., and Pasamanick, B. (1972): *American Journal of Orthopsychiatry 42:* 375-388.
Davis, J.M. (1975): *American Journal of Psychiatry 132:* 1237-1245.
Davis, J.M. (1976): *American Journal of Psychiatry 133:* 208-214.
Dencker, S.J., Enocksson, P., and Persson, P.S. (1967): *Acta Psychiatrica Scandinavica 43:* 21-31.
Dencker, S.J., Frankenberg, K., Malm, U., and Zell, B., (1973): *Acta Psychiatrica Scandinavia (Suppl.) 241:* 101-118.
Dencker, S.J. (1976): *Proceedings of the Royal Society of Medicine 69:* (Suppl. 1): 32-34.
Dencker, H., Dencker, S.J., Green, A., and Nagy, A. (1976): *Clinical Pharmacology and Therapeutics 19:* 584-586.
Dencker, S.J., Johansson, R., and Lindberg, D., (1978a): *Nordisk Psykiatrisk Tidskrift 5:* 369-373.
Dencker, S.J., Frankenberg, K., Lepp, M., Lindberg, D., and Malm, U. (1978b): *Acta Psychiatrica Scandinavica 57:* 115-123.
Dencker, S.J., Johansson, T., Lundin, L., and Malm, U. (1978c): *Acta Psychiatrica Scandinavica 57:* 405-414.
Dencker, S.J. (1980): Hospital Based Community Support Services for Recovering Chronic Schizophrenics: The Experience at Lillhagen Hospital, Göteborg, Sweden. *Monograph Number Two, World Rehabilitation Fund, New York.*
Dencker, S.J., Lepp, M., and Malm, U. (1980a): *Acta Psychiatrica Scandinavica 61:* suppl. 279: 64-76.
Dencker, S.J., Enocksson, P., Johansson, R., Lundin, L., and Malm, U. (1980b): *Acta Psychiatrica Scandinavica.* In press.
Dencker, S.J., Lepp, M., and Malm, U. (1980c): *Acta Psychiatrica Scandinavica 61,* suppl. 279: 10-28.
Denham, J., and Adamson, L. (1971): *Acta Psychiatrica Scandinavica 47:* 420-430.
Donlon, P.T., Rada, R.T., and Knight, S.W. (1973): *American Journal of Psychiatry 130:* 682-684.
Donlon, P.T. (1978): In: *Depot Fluphenazines: Twelve Years of Experience,* edited by F.J. Ayd, Jr., pp. 1-12, Waverly Press, Inc., Baltimore.
Eggert Hansen, C., Rosted Christensen, T., Elley, J., Bolvig Hansen, L., Kragh-Sørensen, P., Larsen, N.-E., Naestoft, J., and Hvidberg, E.F. (1976): *British Journal of Clinical Pharmacology 3:* 915-923.

Engelhardt, D.M., Freedman, N., Glick, B.S., Hankoff, L.D., and Mann, D. (1960): *Journal of the American Medical Association 173:* 147-149.
Falloon, I., Watt, D.C., and Shepherd, M. (1978): *Psychological Medicine 8:* 59-70.
Floru, L. (1977): *Fortschritte der Neurologie-Psychiatrie und ihre Grenzgebiete 46:* 82-104.
Freeman, H. (1967): *Psychopharmacology Bulletin 4:* 1-27.
Freeman, H. (1973): In: *Community Management of the Schizophrenic in Chemical Remission,* edited by E.H. King, pp. 10-13, Excerpta Medica, Amsterdam.
Gardos, G., and Cole, J.O. (1976): *American Journal of Psychiatry 133:* 32-36.
Gardos, G., Cole, J.O., and La Brie, R. (1977): *Archives of General Psychiatry 34:* 1206-1212.
Gerlach, J. (1979): In: Biological Psychiatry Today, vol. A., edited by A. Obiols, J. Ballús, C. Monclús, and J. Pujol, pp. 653-657, Elsevier, North Holland Biomedical Press.
Goldberg, S.C., Schooler, N.R., Hogarty, G.E., and Roper, M. (1977): *Archives of General Psychiatry 34:* 171-184.
Goldstein, M.J. (1970): *Schizophrenia Bulletin 3:* 24-37.
Goldstein, M.J., Judd, L.L., Rodnick, E.H., and LaPolla, A. (1969): *Journal of Psychiatric Research 6:* 271-287.
Gothel, B., and Karczmar, A.G. (1963): *International Journal of Neuropharmacology 2:* 39-49.
Gottfries, C.G. (1971): *British Journal of Psychiatry 119:* 547-548.
Gottfries, C.G., and Green, L. (1974): *Acta Psychiatrica Scandinavica (Suppl.) 255:* 15-24.
Gram, L.F., and Fredericson Overø, K. (1972): *British Medical Journal I:* 463-465.
Gram, L.F., Christiansen, J., and Fredricson Overø, K. (1974): *Acta Pharmacologia et Toxicologia 35:* 223-232.
Greiner, A.C., and Berry, K. (1964): *Canadian Medical Association Journal 90:* 663-665.
Grinspoon, L., Ewalt, J.R., and Shader, R.I. (1972): *Schizophrenia Pharmacotherapy and Psychotherapy.* Williams and Wilkins Co., Baltimore.
Group for the Advancement of Psychiatry (1975): *Pharmacotherapy and Psychotherapy: Paradoxes, Problems and Progress.* Vol. 9, Report No. 93.
Gunby, B., Jensen, K., Lindberg, D., Malm, U., Rossen, S., and Slinning, K. (1975): *Minor symposium II, Meda AB, Göteborg, Sweden.*
Gunderson, J.G., Autry, J.H., III, Mosher, L.R., and Buchsbaum, S. (1974): *Schizophrenia Bulletin, DHEW Publ. No. 75-145:* 16-54.
Gunderson, J.G. (1976): In: *Schizophrenia 75. Psychotherapy, Family Studies, Research.* Proceedings of the 5th International Symposium on the Psychotherapy of Schizophrenia, Oslo, Norway, August 13-17, 1975, edited by J. Jørstad and E. Ugelstad, pp. 307-326, Universitetsforlaget, Oslo.
Haase, H-J. (1978): *Acta Psychiatrica Belgica 78:* 19-36.
Heinrich, K. (1978): In: *Depot Fluphenazines: Twelve Years of Experience,* edited by F.J. Ayd, Jr., pp. 88-89, Waverly Press, Inc., Baltimore.
Hershon, H.I., Kennedy, P.F., and McGuire, R.J. (1972): *British Journal of Psychiatry 120:* 41-50.
Hirsch, S.R., Gaind, R., Rohde, P.D., Stevens, B.C., and Wing, J.K. (1973): *British Medical Journal 1:* 633-637.
Hogarty, G.E. (1977): *Schizophrenia Bulletin 3:* 587-599.
Hogarty, G.E., Goldberg, S.C., and the Collaborative Study Group (1973): *Archives of General Psychiatry 28:* 548-564.
Hogarty, G.E., Ulrich, R.F., Mussare, F., and Aristigueta, N. (1976): *Diseases of the Nervous System 37:* 494-500.
Hogarty, G.E., and Ulrich, R.F., (1977): *Archives of General Psychiatry 34:* 297-301.

Hogarty, G.E., Schooler, N.R., Ulrich, R., Mussare, F., Ferro, P., and Herron, E. (1979): *Archives of General Psychiatry 35:* 1283-1294.
Honigfeld, G., Rosenblum, M.P., Blumenthal, I.J., Lambert, H.L., and Roberts, A.J. (1964): *Journal of the American Geriatrics Society 13:* 57-72.
Imlah, N.W. (1976): *British Journal of Clinical Pharmacology 3* (Suppl. 2): 411-415.
Imlah, N.W., and Murphy, K.P. (1976): *Australian and New Zealand Journal of Psychiatry 10:* 141-145.
Imlah, N.W., Murphy, K.P., and Daniel, G.R. (1978): In: *Depot Fluphenazines: Twelve Years of Experience,* edited by F.J. Ayd, Jr., pp. 23-32, Waverly Press, Inc., Baltimore.
Johnson, D.A.W. (1976a): *Acta Psychiatrica Scandinavica 53:* 298-301.
Johnson, D.A.W. (1976b): *British Journal of Psychiatry 128:* 246-250.
Johnson, D.A.W. (1978): *British Journal of Psychiatry 132:* 27-30.
Johnson, D.A.W., and Freeman, H. (1973): *Psychological Medicine 5:* 115-119.
Johnson, D.A.W., and Malik, N.A. (1975): *Acta Psychiatrica Scandinavica 51:* 257-267.
Jørgensen, A., Fredricson Overø, K., and Hansen, V. (1971): *Acta Pharmacologia et Toxicologica 29:* 339-358.
Jørgensen, A., and Fredricson Overø, K. (1980): *Acta Psychiatrica Scandinavica 61, suppl. 279:* 41-54.
Kazamatsuri, H., Chien, C.P., and Cole, J.O. (1972): *Archives of General Psychiatry 27:* 491-499.
Klawans, H.L., Jr. (1973): *American Journal of Psychiatry 130:* 82-86.
Klett, C.J., Point, P., and Caffey, E. (1972): *Archives of General Psychiatry 26:* 374-379.
Kline, N.S., and Simpson, G.M. (1964): *American Journal of Psychiatry 120:* 1012-1014.
Kolakowska, T., Wiles, D.H., Gelder, M.G., et al. (1976): *Psychopharmacologia 49:* 101-107.
Kraepelin, E. (1913): *Psychiatrie.* Barth, Leipzig.
Kurland, A.A., and Hanlon, T.E. (1971): *Pharmakopsychiatrie-Neuropsychopharmakologie 4:* 297-307.
Lassenius, B., Ottosson, J-O., and Rapp, W. (1973): *Acta Psychiatrica Scandinavica 49:* 294-305.
Leff, J. (1976): *British Journal of Clinical Pharmacology 3. (Suppl. 2):* 385-390.
Leff, J.P., and Wing, J.K. (1971): *British Medical Journal 3:* 599-604.
Lindholm, H., and Ljungberg, L. (1973): *Acta Psychiatrica Scandinavica (Suppl.) 246:* 9-14.
Lonowski, D.J., Sterling, F.E., and Kennedy, J.C. (1978): *Acta Psychiatrica Scandinavica 57:* 97-102.
Luborsky, L., Singer, B., and Luborsky, L. (1976): *Evaluation of Psychological Therapies,* edited by R.L. Spitzer and D.L. Klein, pp. 3-22, The Johns Hopkins University Press, Baltimore-London.
Maerz, J.C. (1976): *Proceedings of the Royal Society of Medicine, Suppl. 1:* 35-39.
Man, P.L. (1973): *Diseases of the Nervous System 34:* 113-118.
Marriott, P. (1978): In: *Depot Fluphenazines: Twelve Years of Experience,* edited by F.J. Ayd, Jr., pp. 46-71, Waverly Press, Inc., Baltimore.
Marriott, P., and Hiep, A. (1978): *Journal of Clinical Psychiatry 39:* 206-212.
May, P.R.A. (1968): *Treatment of Schizophrenia. A Comparative Study of Five Treatment Methods.* Science House, New York.
May, P.R.A. (1976): *American Journal of Psychiatry 133:* 1008-1012.
May, P.R.A., Tuma, A.H., and Dixon, W.J. (1976a): *Archives of General Psychiatry 33:* 474-478.
May, P.R.A., Tuma, A.H., Yale, C., Potepan, P., and Dixon, W.J. (1976b): *Archives of General Psychiatry 33:* 481-486.

McClelland, H.A., Blessed, G., Bhate, S., Ali, N., and Clarke, P.A. (1974): *British Journal of Psychiatry 124:* 151-159.
McClelland, H.A., Farquharson, R.G., Leyburn, P., Furness, J.A., and Schiff, A.A. (1976): *Archives of General Psychiatry 33:* 1435-1439.
McCreadie, R.G., and MacDonald, I.M. (1977): *British Journal of Psychiatry 131:* 310-316.
Meltzer, H.Y., and Fang, V.S. (1976): *Archives of General Psychiatry 33:* 279-286.
Mosher, L.R., Mann, A., and Matthews, S.M. (1975): *American Journal of Orthopsychiatry 45:* 455-469.
Muenter, M.D., Sharpless, N.S., Tyce, G.M., and Darley, F.L. (1977): *Mayo Clinic Proceedings 52:* 163-174.
Mårtensson, E., and Roos, B-E. (1973): *European Journal of Clinical Pharmacology 6:* 181-186.
Nagy, A. (1977): *Journal of Pharmacy and Pharmacology 29:* 104-107.
National Schizophrenia Fellowship (1973): *Schizophrenia: The Family Burden.* National Schizophrenia Fellowship, Surbiton, Surrey.
National Schizophrenia Fellowship (1974): *Living With Schizophrenia, by the Relatives.* National Schizophrenia Fellowship, Surbiton, Surrey.
Öhman, R., and Axelsson, R. (1978): *European Journal of Clinical Pharmacology 14:* 111-116.
Oldham, A.J., and Bott, M. (1971): *Acta Psychiatrica Scandinavica 47:* 369-376.
Parkes, C.M., Brown, G.W., and Monck, E.M. (1962): *British Medical Journal 1:* 972-976.
Paul, G.L., Tobias, L.L., and Holly, B.L. (1972): *Archives of General Psychiatry 27:* 106-115.
Planansky, L., and Johnston, R. (1978): *Acta Psychiatrica Scandinavica 57:* 207-218.
Platt, R. (1968): *British Journal of Social Psychiatry 2:* 187-191.
Polvan, N., Yagcioglu, V., Itil, T.M., and Fink, M. (1969): In: *The Present Status of Psychotropic Drugs. Pharmacological and Clinical Aspects,* edited by A. Cerletti and F.J. Bové, pp. 495-497, Excerpta Medica Foundation, Amsterdam.
Prien, R.F., Cole, J.O., and Belkin, N. (1968): *British Journal of Psychiatry 115:* 679-686.
Prien, R.F., and Cole, J.O. (1968): *Archives of General Psychiatry 18:* 482-495.
Quitkin, F., Rifkin, A., and Klein, D.F. (1975): *Archives of General Psychiatry 32:* 1276-1281.
Rifkin, A., Quitkin, F., Carrillo, C., Klein, D.F., and Oaks, G. (1971): *Archives of General Psychiatry 25:* 398-403.
Rifkin, A., Quitkin, F., Rabiner, C.J., and Klein, D.F. (1977): *Archives of General Psychiatry 34:* 43-47.
Rivera-Calimlin, L., Castaneda, L., and Lasagna, L. (1973): *Clinical Pharmacology and Therapeutics 14:* 978-986.
Romano, J. (1977): *Schizophrenia Bulletin 3:* 532-559.
Rosen, J.N. (1968): *Direct Psychoanalysis.* Vol. II. Grune & Stratton, New York.
Sakalis, G., Chan, T.L., Gershon, S., et al. (1973): *Psychopharmacologia 32:* 279-284.
Sartorius, N., Jablensky, A., and Shapiro, R. (1977): *Psychological Medicine 7:* 529-541.
Schneider, K. (1959): *Psychischer Befund und psychiatrische Diagnose.* Klinische Psychopathologie, 5 Aufl., Thieme, Leipzig.
Schooler, N.R., Levine, J., Severe, J.B., Brauzer, B., DiMascio, A., Klerman, G.L., and Tuason, V.B. (1980): *Archives of General Psychiatry 37:* 16-24.
Sedvall, G., Fyrö, B., Nybäck, H., Wiesel, F.-A., and Wode-Helgodt, B. (1974): *Journal of Psychiatric Research 11:* 75-80.
Shepherd, M., and Watt, D.C. (1977): In: *Current Developments in Psychopharmacology, 4,* pp. 217-247, Spectrum, New York.

Simpson, G.M., Lee, J.H., and Shrivastava, R.K. (1978): *Psychopharmacology 56:* 75-80.
Smith, K., Surphlis, W.R.P., Günther, M.D., and Shimkunas, A.M. (1967): *Journal of Nervous and Mental Diseases 144:* 284-290.
Snyder, S.H., Banerjee, S.P., Yamamura, H.I., and Greenberg, D. (1974): *Science 184:* 1243-1253.
Strömgren, E. (1958): *Psykiatri.* 6:e ed. Munksgaard, Copenhagen, Denmark.
Svendsen, O., Dencker, S.J., Fog, R., Gravem, A.O., and Kristjansen, P. (1980): *Acta Pharmacologia et Toxicologia.* In press.
Tarsy, D., and Baldessarini, R.J. (1976): In: *Clinical Neuropharmacology, Vol. I,* edited by H.C. Klawans, chapter 2, Raven Press.
Traficante, L.J., Hine, B., Sakalis, G., et al. (1977): *Communications in Psychopharmacology 1:* 407-419.
Ugelstad, E. (1975): *British Journal of Psychiatry Spec. publ. no. 10:* 98-101.
Uhrbrand, L., and Faurbye, A. (1960): *Psychopharmacology Bulletin 1:* 408-418.
Van Putten, T.V. (1974a): *Archives of General Psychiatry 31:* 67-72.
Van Putten, T. (1974b): *Archives of General Psychiatry 30:* 102-105.
Van Putten, T., Crumptom, E., and Yale, C. (1976): *Archives of General Psychiatry 33:* 1443-1446.
Verhaegen, J.J. (1975): *Comprehensive Psychiatry 16:* 357-362.
Watt, D.C. (1975): *Psychological Medicine 5:* 222-226.
Watts, F.N., and Bennet, D.H. (1977): *Psychological Medicine 7:* 709-712.
Weeke, A., and Strömgren, E. (1978): *Acta Psychiatrica Scandinavica 57:* 129-144.
Weinstein, M.R., and Fischer, A. (1971): *Diseases of the Nervous System 32:* 801-808.
Willcox, D.R.C., Gillan, R., and Hare, E.H. (1965): *British Medical Journal 2:* 790-792.
Wilson, J.D., and Enoch, M.D. (1967): *British Journal of Psychiatry 113:* 209-211.
Yorkston, N.J., Zaki, S.A., Malik, M.K.U., Morrison, R.C., and Havard, C.W.H. (1974): *British Medical Journal 4:* 633-635.
Yorkston, N.J., Zaki, S.A., Themen, J.F.A., and Havard, C.W.H. (1976): In: *Advances in Clinical Pharmacology,* edited by H.P. Kuemmerle, G. Hitzenberger, G.M. Ling, and H. Uehleke. Vol. 12, pp. 91-104. Urban & Schwarzenberg, Müchen.
Zavodnick, S. (1976): *Diseases of the Nervous System 37:* 671-675.
Zimmerman, V., and Blumhoff, W. (1978): *Nervenarzt 49:* 228-234.

13

Central Cholinergic Mechanisms, Neuroleptic Action and Schizophrenia

Man Mohan Singh
Harbans Lal

INTRODUCTION

The discovery of neuroleptics in the early Fifties not only brought hope for the treatment of schizophrenia, but also provided a seemingly potent research tool for gaining insight into the nature of this condition. Since that time, research with this tool has led to significant advances in the neurochemical correlates of behavior, but the goal of understanding schizophrenia has proven elusive. Neuroleptics have turned out to be drugs with many and varied biochemical and behavioral effects and it remains uncertain as to which of the known actions, if any, may underly their therapeutic activity.

Much of the attention in recent years has been focused on the catecholaminergic neuronal systems in the brain stem and the limbic organization and it has been suggested that these systems are fundamentally involved in neuroleptic actions and, therefore, in schizophrenia (Van Rossum, 1967; Randrup and Munkvad, 1972; Snyder et al., 1974; Meltzer and Stahl, 1976). These views have arisen largely from experimental studies designed to find consistent relationships between neurochemical and behavioral effects in animals and therapeutic activity in humans, as well as studies on the so-called "model psychosis" experimentally induced by amphetamine.

We review here a large body of information from both animal and human studies to suggest that the so-called dopamine hypothesis tells only a part of the story and that, for understanding neuroleptic actions and the neurobiological substrate for schizophrenia, central cholinergic mechanisms seem important to consider. We then try to take this process a step further by fashioning a heuristic model that may help explain the basic adaptive difficulties which beset schizophrenics. The model incorporates the dopaminergic mechanisms within the midbrain-limbic-striatal organization, through which neuroleptics seem to act, and the cholinergic mechanisms within the same organization that seem to have direct or indirect controlling influences on the dopamine-energized processes.

INTERACTIONS BETWEEN NEUROLEPTICS, CHOLINOLYTICS AND CHOLINOMIMETICS IN EXPERIMENTAL ANIMALS

Drug-Induced Stereotypies and Excitation of Behavior

One of the most reliable properties predictive of neuroleptic efficacy in the clinic has been the antagonism of amphetamine-induced stereotypy and excitation of behavior (Janssen and Van Bever, 1975). The apomorphine effects on behavior are similar and are also consistently blocked by neuroleptics (Janssen et al., 1967). The inhibition of mouse-jumping induced by l-dopa in amphetamine-treated mice is a related test of similar importance (Lal et al., 1975, 1976). The rank order of inhibition in these tests corresponds well with clinical potency of neuroleptics.

d-Amphetamine, related stimulants such as methylphenidate, and several other stimulants such as cocaine, produce characteristic species-specific *stereotyped behaviors* which are apparently aimless and are repeated at the cost of normal adaptive function (Randrup and Munkvad, 1968). These abnormal behaviors have been seen in many vertebrate species, including the primates. In rats, they consist of continuous sniffing, licking, gnawing and biting and are grossly evident at an approximate dose of 10 mg/kg of d-amphetamine. With small doses of d-amphetamine (0.25 to 1 mg/kg), stereotypy is not evident to the naked eye but may be demonstrated through other objective tests such as T-maze or lever pressing and exploratory behaviors. Centrally-acting anticholinergic drugs such as scopolamine and benzhexol have a strong potentiating effect so that gross stereotypy is evident in animals given small amounts of amphetamines (Schelkunov, 1964; Arnfred and Randrup, 1968). Peripherally-acting anticholinergics such as methylatropine, which do not cross the blood-brain barrier, are without this effect.

With apomorphine, stereotypies similar to those with d-amphetamine are seen in rats at a dose of 1.25 mg/kg (Janssen et al., 1965, 1967). Several other species are similarly affected (Randrup and Munkvad, 1968). In mice, however, apomorphine produces only weak compulsive gnawing even at a dose of 60 mg/kg. But gross stereotypy becomes evident when scopolamine, benztropine or atropine is given 15 minutes before only 10 mg/kg of apomorphine (Ther and

Schramm, 1962; Pedersen, 1967; Scheel-Krüger, 1970). Anticholinergics, therefore, have a strong potentiating effect on apomorphine-induced stereotypy of behavior. This occurs only with centrally-active anticholinergics, as the quaternary compounds such as methylscopolamine are without significant effect.

The administration of l-dopa (400 mg/kg) to mice pretreated with d-amphetamine (4 mg/kg) results in spontaneous and aimless jumping (Lal et al., 1975) at a high rate (10 to 15 per minute). Injection of an anticholinergic agent (dexetimide) beforehand is unable to increase the rate (Colpaert et al., 1975). This is probably not surprising since there must be a limit to how often a mouse is able to jump in a minute! The general rule that central anticholinergics have a strong potentiating effect on pharmacologically-induced stereotypies of behavior is, therefore, not necessarily violated by this observation.

Central anticholinergics, when given alone, cause some but not all the perseverative behaviors seen with amphetamine or apomorphine. In rats anticholinergics produce stereotyped sniffing but not gnawing (Arnfred and Randrup, 1968; Scheel-Krüger, 1970). They also increase shaking of jiggle cages by their random movements (Meyers et al., 1964). Perseveration with anticholinergics is also evident in studies of operant behavior (Carlton, 1963).

Besides producing stereotyped behaviors, d-amphetamine, apomorphine and other stimulants also lead to *general hyperactivity or excitation.* Central anticholinergics enhance this effect (Galambos et al., 1967; Scheel-Krüger, 1970). On their own, they increase locomotion in mice and rats but to a lesser degree than amphetamine (Arnfred and Randrup, 1968; Galambos et al., 1967; Morpurgo and Theobald, 1964; Scheel-Krüger, 1970; Acquilonius, 1972).

The stereotypy and excitation of behavior seem to have different pharmacological and biochemical implications and are, therefore, distinguished (Randrup and Munkvad, 1968; Janssen et al., 1967). Sedative hypnotics, for example, can suppress behavioral stimulation without eliminating stereotypy (Munkvad and Randrup, 1966). The ability to block amphetamine and apomorphine agitation is generally considered to reflect the sedative property of a compound, while blockade of pharmacological stereotypies is much more specific in indicating the neuroleptic or antipsychotic activity of the drug. Biochemically, the behavioral stimulation is considered primarily to be due to activation of norepinephric neuronal systems in the brain, while stereotypy is thought to result from increased activity in the dopaminergic systems.

With the exception of reserpine, all the clinically effective antipsychotic agents block amphetamine stereotypy. The activity in this respect corresponds fairly closely to the neuroleptic potency of the drugs (Janssen et al., 1965; Randrup and Munkvad, 1968; Fielding and Lal, 1978). This is particularly true for the potent neuroleptics such as fluphenazine, haloperidol, perphenazine and trifluperazine which strongly block dopaminergic neurones but have little or no activity against norepinephric neurones and have minimal built-in anticholinergic activity (Fielding and Lal, 1978; Snyder et al., 1974). The rank order of less potent neuroleptics such as chlorpromazine, thioridazine and promazine on this test does not closely follow their clinical potency. Thus chlorpromazine is clinically equipotent with thioridazine but is almost 15 times more effective in blocking amphetamine stereotypy. Interestingly, chlorpormazine is less active than thioridazine both as a norepinephric blocker (Janssen et al., 1965, 1967) and as a cholinergic blocker (Snyder et al., 1974a). These biochemical differences may account for their different effects on the stereotypy tests. The reasons for the exceptional nature of reserpine have been sought in its different mode of action on the aminergic neurones (Randrup and Jonas, 1967). Unlike other neuroleptics, which probably act through synaptic blockade, this drug seems to act by depleting the neurones of monoamines. When amphetamine is given to reserpinized rats, the turnover or metabolism of dopamine, and hence its disappearance, is prevented.

The effects of neuroleptics on apomorphine stereotypy generally correspond to those on amphetamine stereotype. However, some of the less potent drugs such as thioridazine and promazine are ineffective in this test (Janssen et al., 1965; Fielding and Lal, 1978). This may be due to the fact that they have considerable anticholinergic activity which, as noted above, has strong potentiating effect on the apomorphine stereotypy (Scheel-Krüger, 1970). The neuroleptic suppression of the jumping behavior of amphetamine plus l-dopa-treated mice closely parallels their anti-amphetamine activity (Lal et al., 1976).

Sedative-hypnotic agents such as barbiturates, meprobamate and chlordiazepoxide do not antagonize pharmacological stereotypies even at high doses (Munkvad and Randrup, 1966; Van Nueten, 1962). These drugs are also ineffective as antipsychotic agents (Casey et al., 1960; Cole, 1964; Davis and Garver, 1978). Drugs with close chemical resemblance to neuroleptics but without their antipsychotic activity, such as promethazine which is a phenothiazine and (+) butaclamol which is a stereo enancomorph of active butaclamol, also do not antagonize these stereotypies (Janssen and Van Bever, 1975). Imipramine and related agents which clinically act as antidepressants, are also chemically similar to the phenothiazine neuroleptics and share with them many effects on animals. However, on the stereotypy test, they act in quite the opposite way, thus indicating the discriminative nature of this test (Halliwell et al., 1964; Goldberg and Johnson, 1964a, b; Lapin and Schelkunov, 1965; Pedersen, 1967; Randrup and Munkvad, 1965, 1968). This may be only partly due to the anticholinergic property of these compounds, for neuroleptic phenothiazines such as thioridazine also have a fair amount of anticholinergic activity but still act to block stereotypies.

The specific neuroleptic suppression of pharmacological stereotypies is reversed by centrally-active anticholinergics. In a study by Arnfred and Randrup (1968), perphenazine eliminated stereotypies induced by 10 mg/kg of d-amphetamine in rats at a dose of 0.1 mg/kg; this effect was completely antagonized by scopolamine (3 mg/kg) and benzhexol (10-30 mg/kg). In another study (Fjalland and Møller Nielsen, 1974) methylphenidate-induced gnawing in rats was terminated by haloperidol at a dose of 0.31 mg/kg, but when scopolamine (1 mg/kg) was added, this inhibition was not evident even at 1.25 mg/kg dose. Similarly, it has been shown that dexetimide (2.5 mg/kg) largely reverses the total suppression of amphetamine plus l-dopa-induced mouse jumping by pimozide (2.5 mg/kg) while the peripherally-active anticholinergic isopropamide (5.0 mg/kg) is ineffective in this respect (Colpaert et al., 1975). The gnawing in mice receiving a combination of apomorphine and a central anticholinergic is not completely abolished by a very potent neuroleptic, spiramide, even at a massive dose of 20 mg/kg (Scheel-Krüger, 1970). The inhibition of apomorphine gnawing in rats by perphenazine (0.06 mg/kg) and trifluoperazine (0.16 mg/kg) is antagonized by scopolamine (1 mg/kg) and trihexyphenidyl (5 mg/kg).

Cholinergic agents, whether acting through cholinesterase inhibition (*e.g.*, physostigmine) or through direct action on cholinergic receptors (*e.g.*, arecoline), strongly potentiate neuroleptic inhibition of stereotypies and reverse the effects of central anticholinergics noted above. In the experiment with perphenazine mentioned above (Arnfred and Randrup, 1968), physostigmine (0.4 mg/kg), oxotremorine (2 mg/kg) and arecoline (20 mg/kg), produced a strong and prolonged suppression of amphetamine stereotypy when combined with a subeffective dose of the neuroleptic. The haloperidol suppression of methylphenidate stereotypy was potentiated by physostigmine (0.5 mg/kg) so that in combination, the neuroleptic stopped gnawing at a dose of 0.08 mg/kg, while alone it did so only at a dose of 0.31 mg/kg (Fjalland and Møller Nielsen, 1974). The strong stereotypy in mice after combined treatment with an anticholinergic and apomorphine was inhibited much more effectively with physostigmine (0.10 to 1.0 mg/kg) than with the neuroleptic spiramide (up to 20 mg/kg). A combination of physostigmine (0.10 mg/kg) and spiramide (0.10 to 1.0 mg/kg) had a pronounced suppressive effect on the stereotypy (Scheel-Krüger, 1970).

In addition to inhibiting the pharmacological stereotypies, neuroleptics block the behavioral excitation produced by amphetamine and apomorphine. However, the effects on the two parameters differ. Drugs like thioridazine and chlorpromazine, which have strong antinorepinephric properties are relatively more effective against agitation than against stereotypies, while the opposite is true for potent neuroleptics such as haloperidol, fluphenazine, trifluoperazine and perphenazine, which are weak norepinephric blockers but show strong and almost selective antagonism towards dopaminergic activity (Janssen et al., 1967; Fielding and Lal, 1978). The differences on the two parameters have, therefore, been used as behavioral indices of relative antinorepinephric (agitation suppression) and antidopaminergic (stereotypy suppression) activity of neuroleptics. However, the central anticholinergics block the neuroleptic effects on agitation as well as their effects on stereotypies, thus suggesting that central cholinergic mechanisms are involved in both the phenomena. In a study by Leslie and Maxwell (1963), the suppression of dexamphetamine-induced (10 mg/kg) agitation by thioproperazine (0.5 mg/kg) was reduced by at least a factor of ten by promethazine (12.15 mg/kg) or benztropine (5 mg/kg) and over a hundredfold by hyoscine (1 mg/kg).

Recent studies with stereotyped behavior induced by chronic phenylethylamine administration have suggested that norepinephric mechanisms may be involved in addition to the dopaminergic mechanisms in the production of behavioral stereotypies (Borison and Diamond, 1978). It has, indeed, been argued that chronic phenylethylamine stereotypies may be a better model for schizophrenia than the amphetamine-induced stereotypies. One reason for this belief is that known antipsychotics such as thioridazine preferentially antagonize the phenylethylamine stereotypies (Borison et al., 1977; Borison and Diamond, 1978). It is not known if antimuscarinics are able to antagonize these stereotypies.

Brain Self-Stimulation

Animals with electrodes implanted at various sites along the medial forebrain bundle, that extends from the "limbic midbrain area" through the lateral hypothalamus to the limbic forebrain structures and neocortex, will press levers as often as 8,000 times an hour to obtain self-stimulation (Olds and Milner, 1954; Olds and Olds, 1963; Olds, 1976; Nauta, 1960, 1963, 1964). The most intense self-stimulation occurs from implants in the paramedian ("limbic") region of the midbrain and the lateral hypothalamic area. The animal can be taught to emit a predesignated response to obtain electrical stimulation. However, in its compulsive repetitiveness at the cost of normal adaptive activities, the behavior of self-stimulating animals bears a basic resemblance to the pharmacological stereotypies. Consistent with this, amphetamines considerably facilitate brain self-stimulation (Stein, 1964; Wise and Stein, 1969; Pradhan and Bowling, 1971).

From the studies of Olds (1963, 1976), Nauta (1960, 1963) and Stein (1968), the nuclei and pathways of the medial forebrain bundle system have come to be regarded as the neurobiological substrate for "pleasure," "reward" or positive reinforcement. It is a phylogenetically old system that seems to act to facilitate behaviors which produce pleasure or reward and avoid punishment. It is present in primates as well as in non-primates and its stimulation has been shown to have similar effects in many species including mouse, rat, cat, guinea pig, dog, monkey and man (Wauquier, 1977). In opposition to this is a pathway of roughly parallel distribution, the periventricular system, which contains cholinergic neurones and participates in the suppression of behaviors which are punished or unrewarded (Stein, 1968). It is termed the "punishment" system.

Neuroleptics, regardless of their chemical structure, all suppress brain self-stimulation in a dose-dependent manner (Wauquier, 1976, 1977, 1978). This suppression occurs at very small doses, which are similar to those that block amphetamine stereotypy (Fielding and Lal, 1978) and are not attended with any incapacitation of the animal. Wauquier (1977, 1978) recently found a correlation coefficient of 0.93 between the inhibition of brain self-stimulation and antagonism of amphetamine stereotypy. The effectiveness of this test, therefore, corresponds closely to the neuroleptic potency and antidopamine effect of the drugs. Both dopamine and norepinephrine have been found to play an important part in the behavior facilitation functions of the medial forebrain bundle system (Stein, 1968; Stein et al., 1972; Crow, 1976; Olds, 1976).

Centrally-active anticholinergics reverse the specific neuroleptic suppression of brain self-stimulation. Such an interaction has been demonstrated for scopolamine (0.5 mg/kg) against chlorpromazine (Olds, 1972), dexetimide (0.04 to 2.50 mg/kg) and benztropine (10 mg/kg) against 0.08 mg/kg of haloperidol (Wauquier et al., 1975), dexetimide (0.63 mg/kg) against 0.01 to 0.63 mg/kg of haloperidol and 0.04 to 2.50 mg/kg of pimozide (Wauquier and Niemegeers, 1975).

The reversal of neuroleptic action was dose-dependent. Peripherally-acting anticholinergics such as isopropamide (Wauquier et al., 1975) were ineffective even in high doses suggesting that the interactions involved were entirely central. Also, anticholinergics reversed the action principally of specific neuroleptics with mainly antidopaminergic effects; the action of sedative and strong antinorepinephric compounds such as pipamperone and clozapine (Wauquier et al., 1975, 1976) was not reversed. The effect of chlorpromazine, which is not as strong an antiadrenergic as the latter compounds but also not as strong an antidopaminergic as potent neuroleptics such as haloperidol, was reversed about 60 percent by scopolamine (Olds, 1972). This would suggest that dopamine-mediated brain self-stimulation is antagonized by cholinergic mechanisms but norepinephrine-mediated brain self-stimulation perhaps is not.

Besides neuroleptics, brain self-stimulation is suppressed by narcotics and sedative-hypnotics. Thus in the study by Wauquier et al. (1975), brain self-stimulation in rats was completely suppressed by 0.16 mg/kg of fentanyl and 2.5 mg/kg of morphine. However, this suppression was not reversed by dexetimide even in the highest dose (2.5 mg/kg) used in the study. It was noted that while the suppressant dose of the neuroleptic did not incapacitate the animal, that of the narcotics produced a general depression and catatonia. This would suggest that self-stimulation suppression by narcotics may be due mainly to a general suppressive effect on the animal, while that of neuroleptics is a more specific effect on the self-stimulation mechanisms.

The anticholinergics by themselves tend to increase brain self-stimulation but the effect and the dose-response relationships vary with the experimental conditions (Wauquier, 1976; Pradhan and Kamat, 1972, 1973). At various stimulus parameter combinations, Wauquier (1976) obtained different levels of control response rates. Expressing the results as percentage of control response rates for each stimulus parameter combination, benztropine (2.5 to 20 mg/kg), dexetimide (0.08 to 0.63 mg/kg) and scopolamine (0.63 to 40.0 mg/kg) were found to increase significantly self-stimulation responses at some of these combinations and slightly decrease the responses at others. The overall effect seemed to be one of facilitation of brain self-stimulation by these centrally-active anticholinergic drugs. In other studies, atropine and ditran have been observed to have the same effect (Pradhan and Kamat, 1972, 1973). Furthermore, these drugs have been noted to enhance facilitation of self-stimulation by drugs such as cocaine (Pradhan and Bose, 1978).

Although most anticholinergic drugs were employed in brain self-stimulation studies (*supra*) because of their known antimuscarinic properties, some of these drugs, especially benztropine, are also known to inhibit dopamine uptake by synaptosomes (Coyle and Snyder, 1969). Wauquier and his associates (Wauquier and Niemegeers, 1976; Wauquier, 1978, personal communication) tried to assess the relative importance of the two factors by determining the effects of dexetimide 0.63 mg/kg (potent antimuscarinic), benztropine 10 mg/kg (antimuscarinic and dopamine uptake blocker), trihexyphenidyl 10 mg/kg (moderate antimuscarinic), nomifensine 2.5 mg/kg (dopamine and norepinephrine uptake blocker), amphetamine 0.63 mg/kg (releaser of dopamine and norepinephrine) and apomorphine 0.31 mg/kg (dopamine agonist) on the self-stimulation suppression produced by pimozide 0.63 mg/kg (dopamine blocker), haloperidol 0.08 mg/kg (dopamine blocker) and chlorpromazine 2.5 mg/kg (dopamine and norepinephrine blocker). In the dosages used, dexetimide and nomifensine almost completely reversed the effects of pimozide and haloperidol. Benztropine and amphetamine were about half as antagonistic while trihexyphenidyl was somewhat less effective. Apomorphine, however, failed to antagonize. Against chlorpromazine, nomifensine and amphetamine produced complete reversal, benztropine was about 60 percent effective, and trihexyphenidyl produced about 17 percent reversal. However, dexetimide was without any effect, as was again the case with apomorphine. It seemed, therefore, that self-stimulation suppression through antidopamine actions may be overcome by both muscarinic blockade and an increased availability of physiological catecholamines at the synaptor site, but the simultaneous occurrences of the two is not necessarily potentiating. However, self-stimulation suppression through antinorepinephrine actions may be relatively less susceptible to muscarinic blockade.

Physostigmine, pilocarpine and arecoline—all centrally active cholinomimetics —produce a dose-dependent suppression of brain self-stimulation responses which is reversed by antimuscarinic agents such as atropine and scopolamine (Stark and Boyd, 1963; Jung and Boyd, 1966; Domino and Olds, 1968; Olds and Domino, 1969 a, b; Olds, 1972; Pradhan, 1968; Pradhan and Kamat, 1972,

1973; Pradhan, 1976). Neostigmine, with predominantly peripheral cholinergic actions, is virtually without effect (Jung and Boyd, 1966; Domino and Olds, 1968; Newman, 1972).

The suppression of self-stimulation behavior is due primarily to the central muscarinic actions of cholinomimetics (Pradhan, 1976; Wauquier, 1976). Nicotine tends to enhance self-stimulation in animals with low baseline rates (Bowling and Pradhan, 1967; Pradhan et al., 1967; Pradhan and Bowling, 1971; Newman, 1972). In animals with high baseline rates, it has the opposite effect. Physostigmine, which has both muscarinic and nicotinic effects, has overall a suppressive effect (*supra*). However, when an antimuscarinic agent is given, there is not only a reversal of this suppression but an additional enhancement which may be due to the unmasked nicotinic effects of physostigmine (Pradhan and Kamat, 1972, 1973).

Reviewing available evidence, Pradhan (1976) has suggested that there are both muscarinic and nicotinic receptors in the brain and that nicotinic receptors stimulate both the catecholaminergic neurones which facilitate self-stimulation, and the muscarinic neurones which inhibit self-stimulation. Both the adrenergic and cholinergic mechanisms, he finds, operate simultaneously and the resultant effect depends upon whether under given conditions the sum total of various influences leads to a preponderance of the adrenergic facilitation or the muscarinic suppression of self-stimulation behavior. The important point he makes is that in order to understand phenomena such as self-stimulation behavior, and its various implications, one needs to consider the indivudual neurotransmitter systems as parts of dynamically interacting and often reciprocal mechanisms, rather than in isolation of others. As an illustration of this, he cites evidence suggesting that pretreatment of animals with reserpine, which causes depletion of catecholamines (and other monoaminergic transmitters) in the brain, leads to a considerable enhancement of scopolamine-induced facilitation of self-stimulation (Pradhan, 1975, 1976). Similarly, pretreatment with antimuscarinic scopolamine often produces an enhanced facilitation of self-stimulation by nicotine (Pradhan and Kamat, 1972).

In an attempt to localize the sites of catecholaminergic-cholinergic interactions in relation to brain self-stimulation behavior, Herberg et al., (cited in Wauquier, 1977, 1978), tested the effects of intracranial injections of scopolamine or dexetimide on the neuroleptic-induced self-stimulation suppression. Injections in two dopaminergic sites, substantia nigra and the nucleus accumbens, were partially effective in reversing self-stimulation suppression by a dopamine specific neuroleptic (pimozide or spiroperidol), but those in another such site, the caudate, were without this effect. From these, rather preliminary data, it was hypothesized that a "concerted" action of the antimuscarinics on the first two (and perhaps other) sites was probably needed to completely reverse the neuroleptic-induced inhibition of brain self-stimulation.

Avoidance Behaviors

Animals trained through negative reinforcement (shock) or positive reinforcement (food) to press levers within a given time period or when exposed to a warning cue in order to avoid receiving a painful shock are said to show *active conditioned avoidance behavior*. Suppression of such behavior at doses that have no appreciable effect on escape responding (and are, therefore, not physically incapacitating or sedating) is a specific characteristic of antipsychotic drugs (Cook and Davidson, 1978). Other central nervous system depressants (*i.e.*, sedative hypnotics and anxiolytics) lack this specificity in that avoidance suppression occurs at doses which also decrease escape responding.

Antipsychotic dosages for suppression of active avoidance behaviors have been shown to correspond closely to those for inhibition of amphetamine stereotypies (Fielding and Lal, 1978). Niemegeers et al. (1969 a, b; 1970a, b), studied 20 neuroleptics concurrently in the two tests and found an almost perfect positive correlation between the ED50 values obtained. This is perhaps not surprising since the necessity to emit or repeat a motor action appears to be a common element in both the situations. Consistent with this, amphetamine has a strong facilitating effect on active avoidance behaviors (Morpurgo and Theobald, 1964; Niemgeers et al., 1972).

Passive avoidance behavior is the opposite of active avoidance in that it involves withholding a response to avoid punishment. Antipsychotics increase this behavior while anxiolytics decrease it (Geller et al., 1962; Stein, 1968).

The specific action of neuroleptics, therefore, seems to be to *withhold or suppress responses* in goal-directed activities.

Central anticholinergic drugs have been repeatedly shown to reverse the neuroleptic suppression of active avoidance behavior. This is true regardless of the chemical category of antipsychotics tested. The neuroleptics studied include: chlorpromazine, perphenazine and trifluoperazine (Morpurgo and Theobald, 1964; Hanson et al., 1970), thioridazine (Taeschler et al., 1962; Hanson et al., 1970). thiopropazate (Schaumann and Kurbjuweit, 1961), ethomoxane, chlorprothixene, reserpine, tetrabenazine (Hanson et al., 1970), spiroperidol and clozapine (Fielding and Lal, 1978). The studies were carried out in rats or monkeys and involved one or more of the following central antimuscarinic agents: benztropine, scopolamine, trihexyphenidyl and atropine. The drug dosages were similar to those in the previously reviewed (*supra*) studies of pharmacological stereotypies and brain self-stimulation.

Hanson et al. (1970), studied the effect of anticholinergic agents on the suppression of active avoidance by a number of sedative hypnotics and anxiolytics (chlordiazepoxide, pentobarbitol, meprobamate, chloral hydrate and paraldehyde) and found no effect or a slight facilitation of avoidance suppression, thus indicating that the antiavoidance effect of neuroleptics is not due to nonspecific CNS depression, nor its antagonism by anticholinergics due to nonspecific excitatory actions. *In other words, their actions have to be considered in terms of the specific facilitatory and inhibitory mechanisms involved in control of goal-directed activity.*

Cholinomimetics with central muscarinic actions such as carbaryl, pilocarpine and arecoline cause suppression of active avoidance (Pfeiffer and Jenney, 1957; Goldberg and Johnson, 1964a, b) and potentiate the antiavoidance activity of neuroleptics (Goldberg and Johnson, 1964a, b). A central anticholinergic (atropine) but not a peripheral anticholinergic (methylatropine) can block this effect (Pfeiffer and Jenney, 1957). On the other hand, anticholinergics have a stimulant effect on active avoidance (Morpurgo and Theobald, 1964) which is unrelated to their peripheral actions (Hanson et al., 1970).

Catalepsy

At dosages two to ten times those effective in blocking amphetamine stereotypies, brain self-stimulation and avoidance behaviors, neuroleptics produce a state of catalepsy in which the animal ceases all motor activity and allows itself to be placed in abnormal positions for long periods (Janssen et al., 1965; Fielding and Lal, 1978). This effect is considered an indicator of the neurological activity related to the production of Parkinsonian-like extrapyramidal reactions in patients. Potent neuroleptics, such as haloperidol, with high antidopaminergic activity and little built-in anticholinergic activity, are much more effective than the low potency neuroleptics such as chlorpromazine and thioridazine.

Central antimuscarinics such as scopolamine, benztropine, trihexyphenidyl and atropine have all been shown to reverse neuroleptic catalepsy at doses of 1 mg/kg (Morpurgo, 1962; Morpurgo and Theobald, 1964; Leslie and Maxwell, 1964) suggesting that cholinergic mechanisms are "released" by the neuroleptic blockade of dopamine receptors within the extrapyramidal system. Amphetamine and methylphenidate, which have to act through the neuroleptic-blocked dopamine receptors by increasing the dopamine concentrations at the synapse, have similar but less pronounced effects at the relatively high doses of 5 to 10 mg/kg (Morpurgo, 1962; Morpurgo and Theobald, 1964).

Intraventricular injections of 6-hydroxydopamine, which destroys the catecholamine pathways relatively selectively, produces a cataleptic state similar to that produced by high doses of neuroleptics (Schallert at al., 1978). After such a state is established, intraperitoneal injections of atropine sulphate reverse catalepsy and akinesia. However, corresponding to the development of denervation supersensitivity in the dopaminergic neurones, the walking so induced takes on an abnormal compulsive character. It would seem, therefore, that mutually antagonistic dopaminergic and cholinergic systems in the brain are involved in catalepsy and that these mechanisms are perhaps similar to those which serve pharmacological stereotypies. In summarizing, three important points should be made:

1. behavioral pharmacological effects related to the toxic extrapyramidal effects of neuroleptics occur at doses much higher than those related to their antipsychotic activity;
2. both types of effects involve similar, if not the same, mutually antagonistic dopaminergic and cholinergic systems in the brain; and
3. the anticholinergic drugs may be beneficial up to the point where the incapacitating toxic effects of neuroleptics are reversed but countertherapeutic if their effect goes beyond that into the region of therapeutic activity.

Biochemical and Neuroanatomical Considerations of Neuroleptic Actions

There is abundant and convincing evidence that antipsychotic drugs inhibit transmission in the dopaminergic neuronal system through a synaptic blockade and that, of all their *known* biochemical effects, this property correlates best with their clinical efficacy (see recent reviews by Creese et al., 1978 and Lloyd, 1978). Corresponding to animal studies, increased levels of the dopamine metabolite, homovanillic acid, that result from high turnover of dopamine following synaptic blockade, have been found in the CSF of schizophrenics receiving chronic neuroleptic therapy (Sedvall et al., 1975).

From cell bodies in the central midbrain tegmentum, one of the two principal dopaminergic pathways ascends to the caudate-putamen or neostriatum (the nigrostriatal pathway) while the other (mesolimbic pathway) goes to the so-called limbic striatum (nucleus accumbens and olfactory tubercle) and other structures in the limbic brain (Fuxe, 1965; Ungerstedt, 1971; Fuxe et al., 1974). Both the fiber systems ascend in the medial forebrain bundle that provides multisynaptic connections between midbrain, hypothalamus, striatum and limbic forebrain. Anatomically, the limbic striatum is an extension of the caudate and is considered by some to be a part of the striatal complex (Hassler, 1978). However, while the main inputs to the neostriatum come from the neocortex and somatic afferents, those into the limbic striatum come from the limbic system and visceral afferents (Hassler, 1978; Nauta et al., 1978). Both have major inputs into the pallidum (including "substantia innominata") which represents the main efferent end of the chain. Through its ascending connections to the cortex via the thalamus and the descending connections to the spinal cord via the reticular formation, the pallidum is considered to be involved in emitting programmed sequences of purposive and goal-directed behavior. At a behavioral level, therefore, the pallidum is excitatory while the striatum translates modulatory influences from various sources into selective inhibition of this activity and the directing or focusing of attention onto the intended or desired operations and goals (Hassler, 1978; Wauquier, 1977). The whole striato-pallidal system, including the limbic striatum, may therefore be regarded as a major command center for the operant end of behavior.

The dopaminergic neurones seem to energize this system so that pharmacological (*e.g.*, with amphetamine or apomorphine) or electrical stimulation of these neurones produces psychomotor arousal and an increase in operant behaviors. With increasing stimulation, the behaviors are repeatedly emitted in a stereotyped fashion, then become disorganized and, finally, tend to cease altogether with the supervention of a generalized inhibitory state (Randrup and Munkvad, 1968, 1970; Ellinwood et al., 1973; Carlton, 1968; Wauquier, 1976; Olds, 1976; Valenstein, 1976). Concomitantly, there are changes in attention with increasing responsiveness to irrelevant and distracting aspects of the internal and external environment progressing on to marked attentional perseveration (Ellinwood et al., 1973; Matthysse, 1977; Valenstein, 1976). On the other hand, damage through chemical lesions with 6-OHDA or anatomical lesions involving the cells of origin, the pathways or the sites of termination of the dopaminergic systems, leads to serious and widespread deficits in operant behaviors and sensory neglect (Randrup and Munkvad, 1970; Stein et al., 1972; Breese et al., 1973; Cooper et al., 1973, 1974; Fibiger et al., 1974: Kent and Grossman, 1973; Mitcham and Thomas, 1972; Grossman, 1976; Olmstead et al., 1976; Ungerstedt, 1974; Routtenberg, 1976; Lorens, 1976). These studies together with those involving neuroleptics (dopamine blockers), indicate that amphetamine stereotypies, brain self-stimulation behavior and active avoidance behaviors have a common neurobiological mechanism based on the dopaminergic activation of the striato-pallidal operant control system. The clinically relevant effects of neuroleptics may, therefore, be conceived as providing inhibitory control of operant behaviors and attention through actions on the dopamine-energized striato-pallidal system.

Within this system, cholinergic (muscarinic) neurones seem to be part of the mechanisms that directly or indirectly oppose the activity of dopaminergic mechanisms (Stein, 1968; Carlton, 1968; Wauquier et al., 1976; Wauquier, 1977; Lloyd, 1978).

Of the various regions of the brain, the highest concentrations of the biochemical markers of cholinergic neurones are found in the midbrain limbic area (the point of origin of the medial forebrain bundle), the striatum, various limbic structures (especially the septum, which has cholinergic connections with the hippocampus) and the habenula, which receives input from the limbic structures and sends a cholinergic habenulo-interpenducular tract to the midbrain limbic area (Kuhar, 1976; Hassler, 1978; Nauta et al., 1978). This means that the cholinergic neurones are to be found in the very structures that have dopaminergic connections and are involved in operant behaviors, attention and arousal.

In the neostriatum, and perhaps in the limbic striatum, acetylcholine appears to be a transmitter for mostly the inter-neuronal cells which are considered to be involved in the integration of different input messages (Hassler, 1978; Racagni et al., 1978; Costa and Cheney, 1978). The available information suggests that dopaminergic axons have inhibitory synapses on these interneurones which in turn have excitatory connections with GABA-nergic neurones. The latter exercise inhibitory control over pallidal neurones and also send inhibitory feedback loops to dopaminergic cells in the substantia nigra. It is postulated that there are short feedback loops in the neostriatum from cholinergic interneurones which impinge on the presynaptic areas of the dopamine terminals through enkaphlin-ergic interneurones (Costa et al., 1978). The role of these cholinergic interneurones seems to be to increase the inhibitory control over the pallidum and to regulate dopamine release. The dopamine neurones, on the other hand, inhibit this and thus release the pallidum from inhibitory restraint.

In addition to these cholinergic interneurones, there seem to be cholinergic neurones in the multi-synaptic periventricular system that runs in a roughly parallel arrangement with the medial forebrain bundle from the midbrain through the hypothalamus to the limbic forebrain and striato-pallidal complex (Stein, 1968). Stimulation of this system with cholinomimetics has an inhibitory effect on ongoing operant behavior. It has, therefore, been hypothesized to be a behavioral suppressor system which has a reciprocal relationship with the behavioral facilitatory pathways of the medial forebrain bundle, and that its activity is facilitated by input from the limbic forebrain (Stein et al., 1972).

The predominantly inhibitory control of the limbic forebrain over the striato-pallidal operant control system is suggested by the fact that the consequences of damage to limbic structures, especially the hippocampus, are in many ways similar to the effects of activation of dopaminergic neurones discussed above, *i.e.,* the animal shows stereotyped repetitiousness, failure in habituation, and disturbances in attention (Malamud, 1967; Mednick and Schulsinger, 1968; Venables, 1973; Claridge, 1978; Lorens, 1976). The similarity between these effects and the behavioral and attentional consequences of giving muscarinic blockers (Douglas, 1972; Carlton, 1968) indicate that cholinergic mechanisms may be, directly or indirectly, involved in the inhibitory control over goal-directed behavior.

Data from biochemical pharmacology studies are consistent with the view that dopaminergic and cholinergic neurones show a reciprocal antagonism within the areas of both the nigrostriatal and mesolimbic projections (see review by Lloyd, 1978, also Costa and Cheney, 1978).

In a recent review of the literature, Lloyd (1978) noted that like neuroleptics, cholinomimetics increase homovanillic acid levels in both the limbic forebrain and the striatum. Oxotremorine, a pure muscarinic agent, seems to produce a greater increase in the limbic forebrain than in the striatum, while physostigmine which has both muscarinic and nicotinic activity, has equal effects in both. Antimuscarinics counteract the neuroleptic-induced increase in homovanillic acid in both areas. Comparisons between the "limbic forebrain" as a whole and the striatum suggest that these effects are greater in the striatum. However, when the limbic striatum alone is compared with the neostriatum, the effects appear to be greater in the limbic component.

Costa and Cheney (1978) found that acute dopaminergic blockade by neuroleptics increase acetylcholine turnover in both the neostriatum and limbic striatum. With chronic administration, this effect showed an adaptation. Corresponding to this, there may also be an adaptation to the dopamine effects of neuroleptics in both areas (Waldmeier and Maitre, 1976; Carlsson, 1978). On the other hand, differential effects on the two areas have been reported. Thus Ladinsky et al. (1978), found that neuroleptics increased acetylcholine level in the neostriatum but not in the limbic striatum, leading them to postulate that the dopamine and the acetylcholine neurones may be arranged in series in the neostriatum but in parallel in the limbic striatum. At the same time, it has been suggested that, in acute experiments "classical" or "cataleptogenic" neuroleptics such as haloperidol, fluphenazine and pimozide, which have a high propensity to cause pseudoParkinsonism in patients, produce greater effects on dopamine release and homovanillic acid levels in the neostriatum than in the limbic striatum, while the "silent" or "noncataleptogenic" neuroleptics such as thioridazine and clozapine, which have a small propensity to cause pseudoParkinsonism in patients, have equal effects in the two areas (Lloyd, 1978). Similarly, in a chronic experiment (Bowers and Rozitis, 1974), homovanillic acid increase due to several neuroleptics was found to decrease with time in the "striatum" but not in the "limbic forebrain." However, more recent findings (Ohman et al., as cited by Carlsson, 1978) suggest a similar effect in the limbic system.

Based on these varied and confusing findings, several attempts have been made to suggest that the dopamine blockade by neuroleptics leading to extrapyramidal side effects has a different anatomical site and/or biochemical mechanism than that which leads to antipsychotic effect. Included are the hypotheses that the neostriatum is the site of side effects while therapeutic effects emanate from the limbic striatum, that the arrangements of dopaminergic and cholinergic neurones are different in the two areas, or that the dopaminergic-cholinergic interactions are relevant only to the extrapyramidal side effects and not the antipsychotic effects (*op.cit.*). All these speculations start with the assumption that neurobiological processes that lead to pathological extrapyramidal effects are quite different from those that produce the desired clinical changes, or, with the premise that since neuroleptics with built-in anticholinergic activity (chlorpormazine, thioridazine, clozapine) have clinical efficacy but fewer and less marked neurological effects, cholinergic mechanisms are of no relevance to the therapeutic actions of neuroleptics. These speculations ignore at once the findings reviewed above which lead one to suspect that the nigrostriatal and mesolimbic systems are both parts of an integrated operant-control system on which neuroleptics probably act to produce their therapeutic effects, and even more importantly they ignore the fact that neuroleptics with appreciable built-in anticholinergic activity (Snyder et al., 1974a) always have only a fraction of the potency of those without such an activity. No consideration has been given to the possibility that the therapeutic and toxic extrapyramidal effects of neuroleptics represent different thresholds of change within the same neurobiological system, *viz.*, the striato-pallidal operant control system.

Be as it may, the sum total of available evidence leads one to suspect at this point, that dopaminergic neurones and cholinergic neurones have reciprocal functions within the striato-pallidal system that may be of importance for the clinical effects of neuroleptics, and that central antimuscarinics may be expected to antagonize both the therapeutic and toxic neurological effects of these agents. However, the situation is by no means cut and dried. For one thing, cholinergic neurones appear to innervate both nicotinic and muscarinic receptors which may produce opposite effects (Hery et al., 1978; Pradhan, 1976) and similarly, there may be more than one type of dopaminergic receptors and these receptors may exist in different states (Costa and Cheney, 1978; Creese et al., 1978). For another, there are many other putative transmitters involved in the functioning of the striato-pallidal system. These include serotonin, GABA, glutamic acid, and endorphins (Garratini et al., 1978; Costa and Trabucchi, 1978). The observable behavior is clearly the result of complex interactions between all these neuronal systems which are far from clearly understood at present.

INTERACTIONS BETWEEN NEUROLEPTICS AND CHOLINOLYTICS IN PSYCHOTIC PATIENTS

The animal studies reviewed above strongly suggest that centrally-active antimuscarinic agents antagonize specific behavioral effects of neuroleptics which have been shown to predict both their potency and clinical efficacy as antipsychotic agents. However, one cannot extrapolate these data to patients with any assurance because not only may there be species differences but the clinicopathological relevance of the behaviors involved in empirical tests to the nature of psychotic processes is uncertain. Furthermore, most of the studies reviewed were acute tests which may or may not truly represent the clinical situation in which both neuroleptics and cholinolytics are often chronically administered. The need for such caution has been highlighted recently by a study in which the acute and chronic effects of haloperidol on the synthesis and turnover of dopamine were found to be quite different (Lerner et al., 1977). Clearly, therefore, the possibility of anticholinergic-neuroleptic antagonism suggested by the animal studies has to be demonstrated under clinical conditions before one considers the hypothesis confirmed.

Clinical Studies

Haase (1965) may have been the first person seriously to consider the possibility of a therapeutic antagonism between cholinolytics and neuroleptics in schizophrenics. On the basis of his extensive clinical psychopharmacological studies he developed the interesting hypothesis that the therapeutic activity of neuroleptics was related to certain of their extrapyramidal effects, namely, *fine extrapyramidal hypokinesia* associated with mild to moderate changes in handwriting (cramping, stiffening, miniaturization). He attempted to show that the appearance of therapeutic changes almost invariably corresponded with the development of fine extrapyramidal hypokinesia. However, the appearance of coarse extrapyramidal symptoms (rigidity, tremor, akathisia, dyskinesia, akinesia) which often corresponded to severe handwriting changes, seemed to bear no relationship to therapeutic changes and, if anything, had the opposite connotation. The anticholinergic, anti-Parkinsonism agents were beneficial, when combined, to the extent that they reduced coarse extrapyramidal symptoms. However, when they reversed the fine extrapyramidal hypokinesia, there seemed also to be a reversal of the antipsychotic effects. From these and other studies, he theorized that the antipsychotic action of neuroleptics was due to inhibition of "psychokinetic conation," that is, the process of translating drive, ideas and impulses into motor action and that this was accomplished via the extrapyramidal system through the production of fine hypokinesia, which he regarded as the *conditio sine qua non* for the antipsychotic action of these drugs. He emphasized that optimal hypokinesia was the only extrapyramidal effect of relevance to their psychiatric activity and that, essentially, it controlled the abnormal tendency of psychotic patients to act, and to repeat actions, in response to internal and external stimuli.

Haase's studies on anticholinergic-neuroleptic interactions were often nonblind and do not meet the present-day standards for controlled scientific investigations. However, his insightful hypothesis concerning the relationships between therapeutic activity of neuroleptics and their extrapyramidal actions, supported by a wealth of clinical materials, has not received the investigative attention it deserves. Indeed, based largely upon unsuccessful attempts to find a significant relationship between therapeutic change and the appearance of *coarse* extrapyramidal reactions, it has become a widely accepted belief that the therapeutic activity of neuroleptics is unrelated to their actions on the extrapyramidal system (Cole and Clyde, 1961; Goldman, 1961; Ayd, 1961; NIMH Collaborative Study Group, 1964; Bishop et al., 1965).

Shortly after Haase proposed his hypothesis, Hanlon et al. (1966), reported on a double-blind study which was designed primarily to assess the prophylactic value of benztropine against phenothiazine extrapyramidal reactions (coarse of course!) in a mixed group of acute psychotics and nonpsychotics. They made an observation in passing that psychotic manifestations such as thought disorder and perceptual dysfunctions as well as hostile behavior improved significantly better under perphenazine alone than under perphenazine-benztropine combination. The quantities of neuroleptic medication were comparable in the two groups. A little later, Allert and Schmitt (1966) reported a retrospective analysis of symptom frequencies in routinely studied patients who had received neuroleptics alone or in combination with anti-Parkinsonism drugs. They found that the addition of the latter drugs tended to delay reduction in symptom frequencies but, after four weeks of treatment, the two groups did not differ significantly. The neuroleptic dosages were not controlled. Rivera-Calimlim et al. (1973), reported five cases in which the addition of trihexyphenidyl to chlorpromazine seemed to diminish the therapeutic response.

The most systematic attempts to investigate the effects of anticholinergic anti-Parkinsonism agents on the course of therapeutic changes with neuroleptics in schizophrenia have so far been made by Singh and his associates (1971, 1973, 1975 a, b, c, 1976 a, 1978 a, b, c, 1979 a, b).

The essential strategy in these studies was to add a fixed dose of an anti-Parkinsonism agent (benztropine 4 mg a day, or trihexyphenidyl 6 mg a day) along the course of ongoing neuroleptic treatment so that a period on neuroleptic alone both preceded and followed the intervention period when the anti-Parkinsonism drug was combined with the neuroleptic. This gave an ABA' design in which each patient served as his own control. Two prototypic neuroleptics were employed. One, haloperidol, is a high potency, low-dose type neuroleptic, with little built-in anticholinergic activity, while the other, chlorpromazine, is a low potency, high-dose neuroleptic, with appreciable built-in anticholinergic activity. During an initial titration period, the neuroleptic dosages were individually determined to minimize side effects and to maximize thereputic effects and were then held constant across the periods of the interaction tests. The dosages, respectively for haloperidol and chlorpromazine, ranged from 1.5 mg to 60 mg/day and 300 mg to 1800 mg/day in these studies. Two of the three principal studies allowed for comparisons between the two neuroleptics both in terms of therapeutic activity and of interactions with an anti-Parkinsonism drug (Singh and Kay, 1975a, b). In one of these, the average haloperidol to chlorpromazine dosage ratio was 1 to 50 mg, while in the other, it was 1 to 100 mg. In one of the studies, anti-Parkinsonism medication was also given in the last two weeks of a four-week baseline placebo period.

The studies involved carefully selected schizophrenics (total N = 47) who were given prospective diagnostic and prognostic classifications according to specified criteria. Periodically along the course of the study, the patients were assessed independently by two or more raters, on up to 33 parameters of psychopathology, indices of arousal and attention (resting pulse rate, sleeplessness, span of attention) and measures of social functioning. The data were analyzed by considering the period of neuroleptic plus anticholinergic drug (B) in relation to the preceding (A) and following (A') periods on neuroleptic alone. Since neuroleptics are known to be efficacious in schizophrenia, a progressive reduction in pathology was to be expected with neuroleptic treatment. A countertherapeutic effect of a test intervention would be suggested if this therapeutic progress is interrupted or reversed during the intervention and then resumes its previous course after the intervention is ended. In other words, both periods A and A' have to be considered at once in relation to period B in order to counterbalance the order effect and therapeutic bias associated with continued neuroleptic treatment, while attempting to isolate the influence of anticholinergics on the ongoing therapeutic process. To achieve this, the ratings in outlying control periods A and A' were combined and their mean value then subtracted from the rating in period B. The patient-by-patient difference values thus obtained for each parameter were then subjected to parametric as well as nonparametric tests.

Inasmuch as the purpose was to determine the deviation in the therapeutic course produced by the test interventions, this statistical method was quite conservative, for it calculated deviation from a course much less favorable (no improvement or only a slight improvement during period B) than can reasonably be expected in neuroleptic-treated schizophrenics (Singh and Kay, 1976 c, 1979 b). As a result the calculated countertherapeutic effect was almost certainly an underestimate. However, since the true unaltered course during the intervention period could only have been guessed through extrapolation of the preintervention data, this procedure was adopted as the more cautious method. Several other factors that could have contributed to underestimates of anticholinergic-neuroleptic antagonism have been discussed by Singh and Kay (1979 b).

Despite these adverse factors, evidence from the three studies considered individually and together suggested that anti-Parkinsonism agents significantly antagonize the antipsychotic activity of neuroleptics. Recently, the authors made a comprehensive report on their studies (Singh and Kay, 1978 a, b, c, 1979 b). This included composite analyses of the 28 parameters common to the three investigations. Combining data from different studies was considered justifiable because (a) the results of individual studies were basically similar, (b) they essentially had the same research design (ABA') in terms of anticholinergic-neuroleptic interactions, and (c) the internally-controlled, patient-by-patient method of analysis obviated the significance of any differences between various studies. Since the interval qualities of psychopathology rating scales are not certain, they analyzed the $B - A+A'/2$ differences both parametrically (correlated t test, two-tailed) and nonparametrically (chi square comparing frequencies of $B>A+A'/2$ vs $B<A+A'/2$).

On parametric analyses, of the 26 psychopathology parameters plus Sleeplessness and Resting Pulse Rate measured in each study, nine had statistically significant anticholinergic effects: Thought Disorganization ($p<0.05$), Difficulty in Abstract Thinking ($p<0.05$), Bizarre and Unusual Thought Content ($p<0.01$), Delusions ($p<0.05$), Suspiciousness and Paranoid Ideas ($p<0.05$), Uncooperativeness ($p<0.10$), Disorientation ($p<0.05$), Sleeplessness ($p<0.001$) and Pulse Rate ($p<0.05$). All but one of these (Pulse Rate being the exception) were indicative of an adverse influence of anticholinergic intervention on the therapeutic course.

On nonparametric analyses, thirteen of the 28 parameters had statistically significant effects: Thought Disorganization ($p<0.02$), Bizarre and Unusual Thought Content ($p<0.01$), Suspiciousness and Paranoid Ideas ($p<0.02$), Ideas of Guilt and Worthlessness ($p<0.01$), Suicidal Ideas and Actions ($p<0.05$), Social Withdrawal ($p<0.01$), Uncooperativeness ($p<0.001$), Hostility-Belligerence ($p<0.05$), Disorientation ($p<0.01$), Disturbance of Volition ($p<0.02$), Tension ($P<0.10$), Sleeplessness ($p<0.001$) and Pulse Rate ($p<0.02$). Again, Pulse Rate was the only exception to the rule that anticholinergic intervention had a significant countertherapeutic effect.

From study-by-study analysis it was noted that the antagonistic anticholinergic effects were most likely to be apparent in the aspects of the clinical picture which are undergoing most active therapeutic change at the time of AP intervention. Thus paralleling the observations (Singh and Smith, 1973) that, longitudinally significant therapeutic changes in social dysfunctions (*e.g.*, Uncooperativeness, Social Withdrawal, Hostility) antedate by many weeks those in cognitive disturbances (*e.g.*, Thought Disorganization, Difficulty in Abstract Thinking, Bizarre and Unusual Thought Content, Delusions), the countertherapeutic anticholinergic effects were most prominent in social parameters when the anti-Parkinsonism drug was introduced early in the therapeutic course, whereas later on it was increasingly apparent in the cognitive parameters (Singh and Kay, 1976, 1979 b).

The effect of giving benztropine during the baseline, neuroleptic-free (placebo) period in one study was found generally to accentuate further the condition of patients who were already quite psychotic. This suggested that benztropine on its own was psychotogenic in such patients and did not necessarily act by pharmacologically interfering with neuroleptics in producing its countertherapeutic effects (Singh and Kay, 1975, 1979 b).

Separate analyses of data from benztropine and trihexyphenidyl interventions (Singh and Kay, 1979 b) suggested that essentially the effects of the two drugs were similar, *i.e.*, countertherapeutic, and that such differences as were apparent (less dramatic antagonism in the trihexyphenidyl study) were probably due to the fact that while 6 mg of trihexyphenidyl used was only about half as potent as 4 mg of benztropine, this drug was often employed against relatively larger amounts of antipsychotic medication and in patients (*infra*) who were less likely to show the countertherapeutic effects of anticholinergic medication.

Analyses of the combined sample data in terms of prospective diagnostic and prognostic distinctions and the post-treatment therapeutic outcome assessments revealed interesting systematic differences. The significant countertherapeutic anticholinergic effects seemed particularly to characterize the good prognosis (schizophreniform) and good outcome patients. This relationship, however, appeared to apply mainly to the non-paranoids, of whom catatonics were found to be the most susceptible to the countertherapeutic effect of anticholinergics.

Consideration of these findings together with those mentioned earlier on the symptoms most affected and the kinetic characteristics of the interaction led to the conclusion that anticholinergics acted to exacerbate the particular components of the schizophrenic process which the neuroleptics specifically improved, that is, the anticholinergics showed direct antagonism to neuroleptic actions in schizophrenia (Singh and Kay, 1978 b, c, 1979 b; Singh, 1978 a).

A comparison of these data with those from another study of similar research design in which wheat gluten was found to be another countertherapeutic factor in schizophrenia proved to be instructive (Singh and Kay, 1976 b; Singh, 1978 a). It was observed that in a group of schizophrenics maintained on a cereal grain-free, milk-free diet, and optimally treated with neuroleptic medication, a period of "blind" wheat gluten challenge was attended with a significant exacerbation of the disease process. However, the countertherapeutic gluten effects were more prominent in the *poor* outcome, nuclear types of cases and seemed particularly to involve parameters which could be expected especially to characterize the chronicity-prone, poor prognosis forms of schizophrenia. The clinical parameters to show significant gluten effects (correlated t test, one-tailed) were: Preoccupied Behavior ($p<0.01$), Hostile/Fearful Social Avoidance ($p<0.02$), Poor Rapport ($p<0.02$), Poor Judgment and Insight ($p<0.05$), Difficulty in Abstract Thinking ($p<0.02$), Stereotyped Thinking ($p<0.10$), Bizarre and Unusual Thought Content ($p<0.10$), Poor Impulse Control ($p<0.10$), Tension State ($p<0.02$), Anxiety ($p<0.05$), Depression ($p<0.10$), Elation ($p<0.10$), and Altered State of Awareness ($p<0.10$). Many of the "acute" symptoms such as Sleeplessness, Disorientation, Disorganized Thinking, Hostility and Uncooperativeness, which were all significantly worsened by anticholinergic medication were missing from this list. The suggestion, therefore, was that the schizophrenic process consists of two layers or factors; an underlying relatively drug-resistant component related to a schizoid premorbid development which can be accentuated in neuroleptic-treated patients by wheat gluten, and an acute drug-responsive component which develops with psychotic decompensation and is differentially enhanced by anticholinergics.

Support for this two-factor concept of the schizophrenic process as well as for the notion that the classical diagnostic and prognostic subtypes of the schizophrenic syndrome reflect important psychobiological differences, has come from several other studies carried out by Singh and his group. These include observations, at various stages of treatment, of cognitive dysfunctions in terms of a series of developmentally-based tests based on Piaget's theories, arousal and attention in terms of resting pulse rate, sleeplessness and a temporal measure of the ability to concentrate, and the appearance of a dysphoric state in certain patients during neuroleptic treatment (Kay and Singh, 1975 a, b, 1979; Kay et al., 1975; Singh and Kay, 1979 a). The main conclusions from these studies are that: paranoid schizophrenia may be basically different from nonparanoid schizophrenia; there are two definable prognostic subtypes in the nonparanoid category, of which one is characterized by the appearance of a dysphoric state during neuroleptic treatment along with an increase in resting pulse rate from an initially high baseline value and has poor prognosis while the other does not show these features and corresponds to the group that is most susceptible to the countertherapeutic effects of anticholinergics; the drug-responsive component of schizophrenia is essentially a disorganizational factor associated with high arousal or activation reflected in sleeplessness while the drug-resistant component shows little over-arousal of this type but may have developed during ontogenesis on the basis of abnormal reactivity of the autonomic nervous system.

None of these conclusions needs necessarily to be considered as an established fact at this point, for much more corroborative work is needed for final proof. However, they do point to the need in any pharmacological study of schizophrenia to recognize, first, that all the presently available antipsychotic agents are only partially effective in this condition and what pertains to drug effects does not represent the whole story of schizophrenia and, secondly, that carefully applied prospective diagnostic and prognostic subclassifications should be a necessary part of both the conduct and the interpretations of such studies.

The studies of Singh et al., concerning anticholinergic-neuroleptic interactions in schizophrenics have led to vigorous controversies of a technical nature (Meltzer and Stahl, 1976; Ziemba et al., 1978; Singh and Kay, 1978 c). The arguments have arisen from their use of a research design that did not include a separate control group, and therefore, did not permit the more widely recognized statistical tests such as analysis of variance, and from their use of univariate rather than a multivariate approach to analysis of data involving many dependent variables. Further criticisms have been levelled against combining the data from three separate studies which resembled each other in having the basic ABA' design but differed in some respects. The failure to observe any beneficial effects of withdrawing anticholinergic drugs from chronically-treated patients has also been put forth as a reason for doubting that anticholinergics in fact antagonize the neuroleptics. Furthermore, at a theoretical level, it has been suggested that the work of Singh et al. does not necessarily indicate the involvement of cholinergic mechanisms in schizophrenia since benztropine, which they used as the main anti-Parkinsonism agent, has not only anticholinergic effects but also has possible direct effects on dopaminergic synaptosomes. Singh and

Kay (1976 c, 1978 c) have argued against these technical and theoretical criticisms. However, only further large-scale investigations involving anti-Parkinsonism drugs with anticholinergic, anticholinergic plus dopaminergic, and mainly dopaminergic actions, against representatives of both high potency and low potency neuroleptics can really settle the basic issue of whether the anti-Parkinsonism drugs antagonize the antipsychotic activity of neuroleptics in some or all types of schizophrenics.

Electroencephalographic (EEG) Studies

The possibility of therapeutic antagonism between neuroleptics and anticholinergic agents has also been suggested by EEG investigations in humans.

It is believed that different classes of psychoactive drugs produce characteristic "signatures" on the waking EEG which can be read by a digital computer analysis and are predictive of their clinical activity (Fink, 1968; Itil et al., 1971). The neuroleptic effects consist of a general slowing and synchronization of EEG with increase in the delta and theta bands and decrease in the fast beta band. There is also a tendency for increase in alpha activity and for seizure activity. Anticholinergics, on the other hand, tend to have the opposite effects in terms of beta (increase) and alpha (decrease) bands, but they change the delta and theta bands in the same direction (increase). When combined with the neuroleptics, the anticholinergics block the EEG synchronization and slowing induced by the latter (Itil, 1973). Conversely, the EEG desynchronization associated with hallucinations and illusions caused by anticholinergic psychotogens are reversed by intravenous doses of chlorpromazine (Fink, 1960).

Pharmacokinetic Studies

Some workers have attributed the countertherapeutic effect of anticholinergic anti-Parkinsonism drugs to the lowering of plasma neuroleptic levels by these agents through absorption interference or some other peripheral effect (Rivera-Calimlim et al., 1973). Reduction in plasma levels of neuroleptics by anti-Parkinsonism medication has been reported by Rivera-Calimlim et al. (1973, 1976), Loga et al. (1975), Gautier et al. (1977), and Chouinard et al. (1977), while El-Yousef and Manier (1974), Forsman and Ohman (1977), Lee et al. (cited in Cooper, 1978) and Simpson et al. (1980) have found the anti-Parkinsonism agents to have no effect on the plasma concentrations of neuroleptics. Kolakowska et al. (1976) claimed an increase in the plasma chlorpromazine levels by concomitant anti-Parkinsonism medication!

In a recent critical review of these studies, Cooper (1978) noted that most of these studies were seriously flawed in their methodology. Except for two investigations (Lee et al., *op.cit.* and Simpson et al., *op.cit.*), they did not meet the basic requirements for controls or split crossover design. Other defects included reliance on a single blood sample for comparisons, small study samples, concomitant use of drugs other than the two drugs of interest, and pooling of data for several neuroleptics and anti-Parkinsonism drugs. The two properly done studies (*i.e.,* those of Lee et al. and Simpson et al.) had a placebo-controlled split crossover design, a minimum number of 20 patients, a period of four weeks for stabilization on medication before entering a patient into the study, multiple samples in each study period to decrease the intra-individual variations and strict prohibition against using drugs other than those being tested. The interactions studied were between benztropine and butaperazine and between trihexyphenidyl and chlorpormazine. No significant lowering of the plasma levels of antipsychotic drugs by the anti-Parkinsonism agents was found. From these, Cooper concluded that it was doubtful that anti-Parkinsonism drugs could lower plasma levels of antipsychotic drugs to the point of possible interference with treatment.

Another important conclusion reached in the same review by Cooper (1978) was that after much research effort over the past two decades, it remains quite uncertain if clinical response to antipsychotic drugs bear any predictable relationship to their concentrations in the plasma. Similar observations have been made by May and Van Putten (1978). Both the reviews have emphasized that most of the studies so far have had serious weaknesses of clinical design in terms of sample sizes, chronicity of patients, composition of study groups with regard to diagnostic types, differences of age and sex, concomitant treatments, previous drug taking, outcome criteria and longitudinal aspects of clinical responses. Probably the most crucial issue in this context may be that of heterogeneity of schizophrenia in terms of responsiveness to neuroleptics. If predominantly drug-resistant or poor prognosis patients are studied, there is no particular reason to expect that any kind of a relationship will emerge between drug levels and clinical changes, so that one is likely to falsely conclude that there exists no significant relationship between the two parameters in "schizophrenia." Therefore, to the extent that a patient group is comprised of such subjects, the overall results will be vitiated by this "nonrelationship." None of the studies in the past seems to have considered this issue. New studies based on the relationships observed by Singh et al. between anticholinergic-neuroleptic interactions and therapeutic outcome, as well as their other findings on the psychobiological significance of diagnostic and prognostic subtypes, may well provide definitive answers not only to the issue of relationships between plasma drug levels and clinical response, but also to the issue of whether these relationships are in any way altered by anti-Parkinsonism agents. Besides the possibility of basic etiological or biological differences between the drug-resistant and drug-responsive schizophrenics, one should seriously consider the possiblity that the two groups differ in the pharmacokinetics and pharmacodynamics of neuroleptics.

NEUROPHARMACOLOGICAL EXPERIMENTS IN NORMAL AND PSYCHOTIC INDIVIDUALS

Psychological and psychophysiological studies involving the intentional or accidental use of cholinergic agonists, reversible and irreversible acetylcholinesterase inhibitors, muscarinic antagonists and cholinesterase in both healthy volunteers and psychotic individuals date back to the early Fifties.

Early Treatment Studies

The earliest studies explored the possible therapeutic uses of both cholinomimetics and cholinolytics in schizophrenics. Fiamberti (1946) was the earliest to claim an improvement in schizophrenics with intravenous acetylcholine. Pfeiffer and Jenney (1957) later observed brief "lucid" periods in 17 out of 23 mute chronic schizophrenics after subcutaneous injections of muscarinic agonists, arecoline (2 to 20 mg in 22 patients) and pilocarpine (10 mg in 1 patient). Peripheral cholinolytics, methylatropine or probanthine, were used in doses of 3 to 15 mg to prevent peripheral effects. The patients became communicative and emotionally responsive. Some signs of increased attentiveness and emotionality were observed in patients who failed to show "lucid" intervals. The effects lasted 15-20 minutes.

Van Andel (1959) tried cholinergic agonist eserine in 18 chronic, mute, immobile, stuporous catatonic patients on the basis of animal data suggesting that indirect reduction of central parasympathetic activity through serotonin blockade with tryptamine caused prolonged experimental catatonia. Such catatonia in animals could be reversed with serotonin or eserine. Fourteen of the 18 patients studied were schizophrenic, three had catatonia based on chronic encephalitis, and one had hysterical catatonia. Eserine was given subcutaneously in doses of 2 to 5 mg, with probanthine being used to protect against peripheral parasympathetic effects. All of the schizophrenics showed a repeatable favorable effect beginning about 30 minutes after injection and lasting for 45 minutes. Patients began to talk and laugh and showed improved contact with the environment. Some of the patients had not spoken for many years. Their speech, however, revealed obvious schizophrenic thought disorder. No beneficial effect of eserine was seen in patients with encephalitic or hysterical catatonia, suggesting a specificity of effect for schizophrenia.

It may be noted here that these observations are consistent with the findings of Singh et al. (*supra*) that the countertherapeutic effects of cholinolytics were most evident in the catatonic schizophrenics.

Collard et al. (1965) failed to find a therapeutic effect of oxotremorine, a relatively long-acting cholinergic agonist, in five chronic schizophrenics who were given doses ranging from 0.05 mg to 5 mg. Aside from transient reduction of negativism, no improvement was noted. However, of the five cases, three were hebephrenic, one was paranoid and only one was catatonic.

Concurrent with these studies, a group of workers was obtaining therapeutic results in schizophrenics and other psychotics with the use of atropine in massive, coma-producing doses (Forrer, 1956; Grisell and Bynum, 1956; Forrer and Miller, 1958). Such comas, given three to six times a week in courses averaging 20 treatments, were found to improve psychotic patients with the diagnoses of schizophrenic, mania and involutional psychoses. Improved accessibility was noted soon after recovery from each coma. Gradually, there was reduction in psychosis and improvement in "ego-strength." The results were considered at par with those of insulin coma. The schizophrenics to benefit most were those with high manifest anxiety and an affective component in the clinical picture, *i.e.*, the schizophreniform or good prognosis patients. During the coma treatments, a biphasic response to atropine was noted in terms of many aspects, including psychological state, heart rate and respiration. Before going into the coma, patients showed increased psychotic manifestations.

Psychoses Induced by Cholinolytics and Anticholinesterases (AchE)

Anticholinergic Psychosis in Healthy Persons

Ingestion of parts of plants of the Solanaceae group which contain atropine, scopolamine and other cholinolytics, as well as of over-the-counter sleep and asthma preparations containing scopolamine and belladonna, have for long been known to be able to produce a psychotic state characterized by irritability, excitation, hallucinations, disorientation, incoherence and stupor (see Warburton, 1975, pp. 125-127 for references).

A group of synthetic anticholinergic psychotomimetic agents, the piperidyl glycolates, has been intensively studied in healthy individuals (Abood and Biel, 1962). Small groups of trained observers, including psychiatrists, psychologists, nurses and medical students, when given these compounds, experienced depersonalization, alienation and disorientation similar to those with LSD. There was general misinterpretation of the environment, with spatial and temporal disorientation. Strong illusions and hallucinations were among the most dramatic effects. Hallucinations were predominantly visual and involved clearly-defined objects, persons, animals or colors. However, frequently there were also auditory, tactile, olfactory and gustatory hallucinations. Auditory hallucinations involved musical instruments and familiar voices. As the psychosis progressed, the individuals began to respond to hallucinations and would carry on extended conversations with phantom voices. At low doses of the drugs, the subjects were able to describe their experiences coherently, but with larger doses, they talked aimlessly and incoherently, losing their train of thought many times, and progressing sometimes to complete mutism. Emotionally, they were labile, bewildered, apprehensive, panicky, and prone to angry outbursts. In addition, they showed negativism and paranoia. On psychometric testing, they showed a profile similar to that with LSD.

In attempting to find EEG correlates of behavioral changes with anticholinergic psychotogens, Fink (1960) observed that EEG desynchronization accompanied the occurrence of hallucinations, illusions, and fantasies, while predominantly slow, more synchronized activity accompanied relaxed, drowsy or euphoric states. Experimental studies have shown that atropinics decrease EEG "arousal response," *i.e.*, desynchronization, elicited either by sensory stimulation or by stimulation of the reticular formation (Rinaldi and Himwich, 1955; Bradley and Elkes, 1953). It is believed that the proper perception of a specific stimulus against the background of numerous stimuli that impinge on an organism at any time is facilitated by acetylcholine-mediated inputs along ascending reticular systems, especially the ones involved in the hippocampal circuit (Warburton, 1975; Douglas, 1975). Atropinic blockade of these inputs, therefore, tends to impair specific signal detection while allowing irrelevant, especially autistically-determined, stimuli to unduly influence behavior. This may well be the mechanism of hallucinations and would explain the occurrence of cortical desynchronization in association with hallucinations in atropinized subjects, while the general effect on EEG of cholinolytics is to produce spindle slow-wave patterns as in sleep or states of reduced reticular inputs.

It should be noted, however, that the piperidyl glycolates studied by Abood and Biel had many other effects besides their cholinolytic properties. These included increase in membrane permeability in the brain and elsewhere, antiserotonic and antihistaminic effects and a variety of metabolic effects. Not all the phenomena caused by these psychotogens may, therefore, be due to their cholinolytic actions.

Cholinolytics in Psychotic Individuals

Gershon and Olariu (1960) gave Ditran, a piperidyl glycolate, to chronic schizophrenics in doses of 5-10 mg a day orally over a period of two to four weeks. There was worsening in their psychosis with increased withdrawal, apathy, inactivity and asocial behavior. These effects were particularly seen in *paranoid* schizophrenics. Fairly rapid tolerance developed for the peripheral autonomic actions but tolerance for the central actions appeared quite slowly or not at all.

From studies of Ditran in schizophrenics, neurotics and normals, Apter and Abood (see Abood and Biel, 1962) observed that chronic schizophrenics had generally reduced responsiveness to the anticholinergic or autonomic effects of Ditran when compared to the responses of neurotic patients or normals. Schizophrenics who reacted to Ditran most like the controls, as a rule responded most effectively to psychotherapeutic agents and other therapeutic measures. The suggestion, therefore, was that the poor prognosis chronic schizophrenics had deficient or under-responsive cholinergic systems, while intact responsivity of these systems may be needed for recovery from psychosis.

Tourlentes et al. (1960) conducted an extensive triple-blind, double-placebo study of a piperazinoalkylglycolate in 32 severely chronic schizophrenics. After three months of trial, the results indicated worsening of patients with an increase in disturbed and regressed behavior, withdrawal, idleness, autism, open masturbation and other forms of sexual acting out.

Organophosphorous Anticholinesterases in Healthy Individuals

A number of organophosphorous compounds which act by inhibiting cholinesterases and thus increasing the central and peripheral cholinergic activity were studied in humans in the 1940s and 50s. These agents included therapeutic agents (DFP, TEPP, OMPA), agricultural insecticides (Parathion, Mipafox, HETP, TEPP) and nerve gases developed as warfare agents (Sarin and Tabun or GA). The symptoms produced by these agents represented both the muscarinic and nicotinic effects of acetylcholine, so that muscarinic blockers such as atropine only partially reversed their effects (Grob et al., 1947; Rowntree et al., 1950; Grob and Harvey, 1958).

Short-term exposure to these compounds (over 2-4 days) produced a clinical picture of dysphoria, inability to concentrate, slowing of intellectual and motor processes, thought blocking, difficulty in expressing their thoughts, excessive dreaming and nightmares (Grob et al., 1947; Grob and Harvey, 1958; Bowers et al., 1964). Hallucinations and delusions seldom occurred in these acute studies but the subjects appeared to have a state of altered awareness. With doses producing only mild symptoms, the EEG showed increased frequency and reduced voltage (*i.e.,* a cortical arousal pattern). However, with higher doses and more intense symptoms, bursts of high-voltage slow waves appeared and the EEG rhythms and potentials became more irregular, *i.e.,* a pattern quite similar to that associated with cholinolytic psychotomimetics (Grob and Harvey, 1958; Warburton, 1975). Psychological symptoms appeared when the whole blood cholinesterase activity levels fell below 40 percent of control.

Gershon and Shaw (1961) studied 16 cases of prolonged inadvertent exposure to organophosphorous insecticides over periods of 1.5 to 9 years. Five of these cases showed schizophrenic reactions with auditory hallucinations, persecutory and religious delusions, ideas of reference, aggression and apathy. Seven cases had a depressive picture, one showed a fugue state, while in the remaining three cases the chief problem was impaired memory and concentration. Problems of memory and concentration were present in all 16 cases. Blood cholinesterase activity measured in two cases was 50 percent and 60 percent of normal.

Organophosphorous Anticholinesterases in Psychotics

Rowntree et al. (1950) injected DFP dissolved in peanut oil over a period of several days in 17 chronic schizophrenics (five paranoid, nine hebephrenic, two catatonic, one simple), nine manic depressives (six hypomanic, one depressed, two in remission) and ten normal subjects. Thirteen schizophrenics and nine manic depressives received a total dose of 13 mg of DFP over seven days, while the remaining four schizophrenics received a mean total dose of 43 mg over an average of 37 days. Normal controls received 5 to 13 mg total doses because of their inability to tolerate higher amounts. The inhibition of true cholinesterase activity in red cells was 60-90 percent in schizophrenics, 58-84 percent in manic depressives and 43-80 percent in normals.

Physical muscarinic effects and EEG changes were quite similar in manic depressives and normals. In chronic schizophrenics, however, these effects were both less intense and less frequent suggesting an underresponsivity of their cholinergic mechanisms. This was most convincingly seen in one schizophrenic who received 63 mg of DFP over a period of 35 days! In some respects, they reacted paradoxically. Thus, while manic depressives showed a gradual fall in blood pressure, schizophrenics had a tendency for the blood pressure to rise. Only the *paranoids* among schizophrenics showed muscarinic effects comparable to those of the manic depressives.

Mentally, *three out of five paranoid schizophrenics* showed an exacerbation of their condition with DFP, but of the nonparanoids, only two out of nine hebephrenics and the lone simple schizophrenic worsened. One hebephrenic showed marked improvement which was "associated with diminution of anxiety." Depressive effects predominated in manic depressives and normals. One case of hypomania with schizophrenic symptoms (schizo-affective) improved considerably during two separate courses of DFP but relapsed each time the drug was withdrawn. Two other hypomanics improved during DFP administration and remained well afterwards. One partially recovered recurrent hypomanic became maniacal two days after withdrawal of DFP. In the only depressive patient there was a profound deepening of depression. Two remitted manic depressives and two of six hypomanics showed only slight mental changes (dysphoria, insomnia and increased dreaming) with DFP treatment.

Intraventricular Cholinesterase and Cholinergic Blockers in Chronic Catatonic Schizophrenics

Based on studies in cats in which intraventricular acetylcholine seemed to produce an akinetic stuporous state, Sherwood (1952, 1958) instilled cholinolytic enzyme cholinesterase or a cholinergic blocker, pentamethonium iodide, into the lateral ventricles of chronic schizophrenics with prolonged catatonic stupors. Of the fifteen patients treated with one or more injections of these substances, six returned to normal at one time or another. In one case the improvement lasted four years and in another two years, after the last injection. Rather large amounts of drugs were used, *e.g.,* 22.5 mg of cholinesterase. Also crystalline penicillin G was instilled in addition (in view of the recent work of Chouinard et al. (1978) suggesting that an increase of prostaglandin E_1 by penicillin may be therapeutic in schizophrenia, this may have inadvertently contributed to the therapeutic effect). The results were reminiscent of the beneficial effects of atropine coma. However, certain aspects suggested an increase rather than a decrease in central cholinergic activity, *viz.,* pupillary constriction, bradycardia and decrease in blood pressure, so that the results were perhaps much more like those obtained by Van Andel (*supra*) with a cholinomimetic than may appear to be the case at first.

Recent Investigations of the Therapeutic Effects of a Reversible Anticholinesterase Physostigmine in Psychotic Patients

In a nonblind study by Rosenthal and Bigelow (1973), five chronic schizophrenics, refractory to neuroleptic treatment for many years, were given physostigmine by mouth in increasing doses over several weeks. Total daily amounts of 4 mg to 12 mg were given in divided dosages in two cases and according to a single dose regimen in three cases. Neuroleptics were continued in all cases. Two patients were diagnosed as chronic hebephrenic, two as chronic undifferentiated and one as chronic paranoid schizophrenic. All the patients were noted to show marked clinical improvement with physostigmine, especially in terms of thought disorder. However, tolerance developed rapidly, especially on the divided dose schedule. Muscarinic peripheral effects were uncommon suggesting, as did the study of Rowntree et al. (1950), a hyporeactivity of cholinergic mechanisms.

Janowsky et al. (1973) tested the clinical effects of physostigmine over a period of one hour in patients who had been diagnosed as schizophrenic by three psychiatrists according to the DSM II criteria. By means of an infusion device, the patients received two or more doses of placebo every five minutes, then one of three active drugs (an adrenergic stimulant, methylphenidate, 0.5 mg/kg in a single dose, or a peripheral cholinomimetic, neostigmine, 0.25 mg every five minutes to reach a total of 1.25 mg, or a centrally-active cholinomimetic, physostigmine, 0.5 mg every five minutes to reach a total of 2.50 mg), followed by placebo injections every five minutes for at least 30 minutes. A nurse "blind" to the protocol rated every ten minutes for psychomotor activation-inhibition, dysphoria, irritability, unusual thought content, conceptual disorganization, blunted affect and degree of psychosis. Eight patients received physostigmine, 13 methylphenidate and 6 neostigmine.

Pre- post-treatment comparisons showed no significant effects of neostigmine. Physostigmine increased dysphoria and psychomotor inhibition, decreased psychomotor activation but had no significant effect on ratings of psychosis, unusual thought content or conceptual disorganization. Its administration was often attended with nausea and vomiting. Methylphenidate produced psychomotor activation and an increase in the level of psychosis, unusual thought content and conceptual disorganization. In a subsequent experiment, they found that physostigmine was able to reverse the methylphenidate exacerbation of schizophrenic psychosis. Similar experiments were performed in manic and depressed patients. From these data, the authors concluded that a catecholamine-acetylcholine reciprocity within the brain may be the neurobiological substrate for a continuum between and "excited-activated-euphoric" state and an "inhibited-retarded-depressed" state. The appearance of an apathetic-anergic-dysphoric state without concomitant improvement in psychosis ratings in the physostigmine-treated schizophrenics, they believed, indicated a non-specific inhibitory effect, or possibly, a consequence of concomitant physical ill-effects. Any involvement of cholinergic mechanisms in schizophrenic psychosis as such was discounted.

Davis and Berger (1978) conducted an essentially similar but "nonblind" investigation of schizophrenic and manic patients and reached the same sort of conclusions. A larger amount of physostigmine (4.0 mg) was infused slowly over a period of 60 minutes and the patients were observed for three hours. However, only three schizophrenics were studied and all of them had the poor prognosis or nuclear type of schizophrenia. No significant reduction in schizophrenic pathology was noticed. In another experiement, six schizophrenics of the same type were fed large amounts of choline chloride (up to 20 gm a day) for three to four weeks on the basis of reported studies in rats suggesting that precursor feeding may increase central cholinergic activity. Four patients had lower psychopathology scores after this treatment than in the baseline period; one patient showed dramatic improvement. After choline treatment, patients received placebo for one week and then neuroleptic treatment. One patient who showed dramatic response to choline, it seems, was not included in this part of the study. The reductions in psychopathology in the neuroleptic weeks appeared to be somewhat more than in the preceding choline treatment period. The possibility of previous choline treatment acting to potentiate subsequent neuroleptic treatment was not considered. Eight manic patients were also studied with physostigmine, but only one could be studied with choline. Euphoric manics were found to become less manic in mood and thought content and more depressed; the irritable manics, however, became more irritable. The authors concluded from these experiments that relative cholinergic imbalance may have a role in mood disorders but not in schizophrenia.

The principal reasons for rejecting the role of central cholinergic mechanisms in these studies was the lack of significant improvement with physostigmine in items such as psychosis, conceptual disorganization, unusual thought content and total BPRS scores. The main effects noted in both schizophrenics and manics over the short periods (1 to 3 hours) of the studies were psychomotor inhibition and dysphoria. These effects are not too different from what one would expect in an acute experiment with neuroleptics—the most powerful antipsychotic agents known and by some regarded as "antischizophrenic" drugs. Evidence from acute laboratory experiments (*supra*) clearly establishes that neuroleptics in general inhibit psychomotor activity and operant behavior, and have the effect of reducing excessive arousal. Dysphoria and psychomotor inhibition can be observed in schizophrenics after a single injection of neuroleptic (Van Putten and May, 1978), while significant improvements in psychosis, thought disorder and unusual thought content may take several weeks to appear (Singh and Smith, 1973 a). In a longitudinal study of acute, first-break schizophrenics (Singh and Smith, 1973 a), the earliest features to improve significantly were those reflecting overarousal (Sleeplessness) and psychomotor dyscontrol (Antisocial Behavior, Hostility, Uncooperativeness and Disturbance of Volition), while significant improvement in cognitive-integrative dysfunctions (Unusual Thought Content, Delusions, Thought Disorder) took four to seven weeks to appear. Ward activities requiring mostly motor interactions improved earlier than those requiring verbal interactions. Thus any expectation of seeing an improvement in areas of psychopathology other than those related to overarousal and psychomotor dysfunction in a one to three hour experiment in schizophrenics has to be regarded as unrealistic.

Physostigmine reversal of the acute accentuation in psychosis by the arousing and psychomotor stimulant effects of methylphenidate was not only consistent with this but provided a direct support for the hypothesis suggested by the studies of Singh et al. (*supra*) that is, a cholinergic mechanism may be directly or indirectly involved in an arousal-related, drug-responsive, disorganizational component of the schizophrenic process. The extended observations that were possible in the choline-feeding experiment of Davis and Berger were also supportive of this idea. Despite the fact that only poor prognosis schizophrenics were included, four of the six patients studied improved over the 3-4 week period of choline treatment. Subsequent treatment with neuroleptics seemed to be slightly more effective but the order effect of treatments was not controlled. If the notion that choline feeding increases central cholinergic activity is correct, then these observations suggest, as do those of Singh et al., *that decreased activity or effectiveness* of some central cholinergic mechanisms is involved in at least some aspects of schizophrenic psychosis.

The Many Paradoxes of the Psychiatric Consequences of Cholinolytics and Cholinomimetics

The data reviewed above could be used to support all three possibilities concerning involvement of central cholinergic mechanisms in schizophrenia, *viz.*, there is underactivity, overactivity or no particular abnormality of such mechanisms in schizophrenia! Quite possibly, all three explanations are correct, if one recognizes that schizophrenia is a heterogenous, longitudinally-evolving, chronicity-prone condition.

Collectively considered, the aforementioned studies seem to suggest that catatonic and acute schizophrenics may have inhibited, but responsive cholinergic mechanisms which when directly or indirectly stimulated within a physiological range, lead to clinical improvement.

On the other hand, the chronic hebephrenic or undifferentiated types of schizophrenics may have both under-reactive and under-active central cholinergic mechanisms. Inasmuch as central cholinergic mechanisms seem to be involved in cortical arousal (*infra*), one of the consequences of a cholinergic deficit in chronic schizophrenics may be impaired arousability of neo-cortical mechanisms. This is, to some extent, borne out by the interesting observations of Ingvar and Franzén (1974) and Franzén and Ingvar (1975) indicating that highly deteriorated, mostly nonparanoid, chronic schizophrenics showed relatively decreased blood flows in the frontal areas, relatively high flows occipito-temporally and an abnormal absence of flow changes in the frontal areas when performing psychological tasks. This pattern was the reverse of one seen in normal persons. There was no reduction of mean blood flow in the brain as a whole. Younger, relatively preserved patients did not show these abnormalities. The suggestion, therefore, was that in the advanced stages of illness in the nonparanoid patients, the environmental inputs had abnormal access to the posterior perceptual areas of the cortex but that there was a decreased access of these inputs to the neural programs of actions and thoughts, or an impoverishment of such programs, in the frontal motor areas. A state of nonspecific generalized or transmarginal inhibition seemed to exist in the latter areas. Douglas (1975) regards such an inhibition to be a primitive or immature function of the hippocampal formation which in the course of normal maturation gives way to more adaptive selective inhibitory functions involving cholinergic neurones of the midbrain-septal-hippocampal circuit. As will be discussed later, a failure of the latter functions may be an important factor in the pathogenesis of schizophrenia.

One of the implications of certain schizophrenics having inactive or under-active cholinergic mechanisms is that drugs such as physostigmine which act indirectly by cholinesterase inhibition may be much less effective in facilitating cholinergic functions than the direct cholinergic agonists such as arecoline and pilocarpine (Matthysse and Sugarman, 1978).

In contrast to nonparanoids, the paranoid schizophrenics may have quite normally active and reactive cholinergic mechanisms. Correspondingly, Ingvar and Franzén (*op.cit.*) found that, among the schizophrenics they investigated, the paranoids had normal or even increased frontal blood flow patterns.

What is the explanation for both the cholinergics and cholinolytics producing psychotic symptoms and also for both of them producing therapeutic changes in schizophrenics? The answer to these puzzles seems to lie in the knowledge that at high doses, these drugs, especially, it seems, the cholinomimetics, often have effects opposite to those at lesser doses, and that the gap between an optimal and an overdose of these substances can be quite small (Feldberg, 1964; Russell, 1966; Warburton, 1972, 1975; Douglas, 1975). At dosages that lower the cholinesterase activity level to below 70 percent of normal, anticholinesterases begin to behave like cholinergic blockers because the excess acetylcholine so produced is believed to produce a *depolarization block* of cholinergic receptors. Beyond this critical point, test performances facilitated by cholinergic activity are impaired as they are with atropinics and the propensity for psychotic manifestations such as hallucinations is increased (Warburton, 1975). The problem would be expected to be greater with irreversible anticholinesterases, as they would produce prolonged depolarization blocks. So it can be seen as to how and why, in the studies reviewed earlier, the potent and usually irreversible anticholinesterases, given in doses producing profound cholinesterase inhibition, produced results quite similar to those with cholinolytics. Understandably also, the results were most serious in cases exposed for long periods to these agents.

For somewhat similar reasons, it can be understood why coma-producing doses of atropinics or large intraventricular instillations of cholinolytics had the same sort of therapeutic effects in schizophrenics as did the small, non-toxic doses of cholinergic agents. The appearance of parasympathetic effects in the intraventricular instillation experiments was pointed out earlier. The possibility is that the desired clinical effect (*i.e.,* reduction of psychosis) resulted from a cholinergic rebound or release following profound receptor block by cholinolytics. Results might have been the opposite with cholinolytics acting through inhibition of the production of acetylcholine.

Another issue of importance in considering the effects of cholinergic agents is that they act on two types of receptors—muscarinic and nicotinic—which are both present in the brain and, when activated, appear to have opposite effects on the activity of catecholaminergic and serotonergic systems and may, therefore, lead to different psychophysiological and behavioral consequences (Frankenhaeuser et al., 1971; Pradhan, 1976; Hery et al. 1978). As was discussed before, the nicotinic effects in some respect resemble those of catecholamines in being facilitatory to behaviors such as brain self-stimulation, while the muscarinic actions, like those of neuroleptics, are strongly inhibitory. Anticholinesterases such as physostigmine and organophosphates have, like acetylcholine, both types of effects, *i.e.,* they act as agonist-antagonist mixtures by simultaneously stimulating opposing systems. On the other hand, cholinergic agonists such as arecoline, pilocarpine and oxotremorine have mostly muscarinic effects, so that studies with two classes of drugs may produce different results. In ordinary circumstances, and at doses which are perhaps nonpsychotogenic, the muscarinic effects of anticholinesterases predominate over their nicotinic effects. The biphasic action of these drugs suggests that this relationship may well change at high doses. Furthermore, the two types of receptors may have different thresholds or they may be differentially affected in disease states. Thus the paradoxical increase in blood pressure with DFP noted in chronic schizophrenics (Rowntree et al., 1950) may suggest a muscarinic deficit or a relative nicotinic preponderance in these cases, for only the nicotinic receptors, through enhancement of sympathetic activity, could in such an experiment account for the blood pressure rise; the effect of muscarinic stimulation would be in the opposite direction (Grob and Harvey, 1958).

In these dualistic actions of acetycholine may lie at least a part of the explanation for the paradox of cholinergic agents both relieving and producing psychosis. If one looks at the relevant studies carefully, the pattern that seems to emerge is that antipsychotic activity perhaps occurs with mild to moderate stimulation of muscarinic receptors, while a dysphoric psychotic state is the consequence when both muscarinic and nicotinic receptors are simultaneously subjected to strong and prolonged stimulation. In this context, it may be of interest to note that LSD, which also produces a dysphoric psychotic state, has dualistic angonist-antagonist actions on serotonergic as well as on acetylcholaminergic neurones (Warburton, 1975; Creese et al., 1978). Similarly dysphoric psychotic states have been noted to occur with nalorphine and cyclazocine which have both agonistic and antagonistic actions on receptors on which morphine acts to produce its euphoriant and analgesic effects (Jaffe and Martin, 1975). Polypeptides with similar mixed actions have been found in digestates of wheat gluten (Klee et al., 1978), which in turn has been observed to exacerbate schizophrenia (Dohan et al., 1969; Singh and Kay, 1976 b, c). One wonders if there might be a general principle in all this.

IMPAIRED SELECTIVE INHIBITORY CONTROL FUNCTIONS IN SCHIZOPHRENIA AND THE CHOLINERGIC MECHANISMS IN MESO-DIENCEPHALIC-LIMBIC ORGANIZATION

It has for long been suspected that some crucial discriminative inhibitory control mechanisms in the brain organization are defective in schizophrenia (Elkes, 1961). Information in recent years from psychological and psychophysiological studies indicating disturbances in the processes of orienting or selective attention, attentional sets, habituation, extinction, specific and nonspecific arousal and coping with new and changing circumstances in schizophrenics have put this idea on a rather firm footing (*infra*). At the same time, neuropharmacological, lesioning and stimulation studies in animals have led to the conclusion that acetylcholine-mediated neuronal mechanisms are part of the meso-diencephalic-limbic circuitry that seems to serve the internal inhibitory mechanisms involved in such processes (*infra*).

On the interoceptive visceromotive side, (for reviews see Shakow, 1971, 1977; Venables, 1973, 1977; Zahn, 1977; Garmezy, 1978; Gruzelier and Hammond, 1978), the schizophrenics usually fall on opposite sides of the normal—absent or exaggerated—for autonomic orienting responses (GSRs) to stimuli, and their adaptation to repeated neutral or unreinforced stimuli (habituation) is generally impaired. The basal autonomic arousal as indicated by nonspecific GSRs and heart rate is frequently elevated (Cohen and Patterson, 1937; Zahn et al., 1968; Shakow, 1971). Autonomic functioning in terms of both anticipatory preparation and the separation of the more important or meaningful aspects of the environment from those of lesser significance is impaired in schizophrenics (Zahn et al., 1981). Differences have been noted between paranoid and nonparanoid schizophrenics as well as between acute and chronic patients. Thus in a study with chronic patients, Zahn et al. (1968) found the paranoid schizophrenics showed greater responsivity and hebephrenics lower than normal responsivity of GSR to stimuli. In a more recent study with acute patients, Horvath and Meares (1979) noted that habituation failure was mostly a characteristic of the nonparanoids while the paranoids seemed to have difficulty with dishabituation or switching of attention.

At least some of these autonomic nervous system abnormalities have been shown to antedate overt schizophrenia, suggesting that defective autonomic reactivity in relation to input regulation may be a basic biological defect in schizophrenia (Zahn, 1977).

On the exteroceptive somatomotive side (see reviews by Shakow, 1971; Zahn and Carpenter, 1978; Garmezy, 1978), schizophrenics show a number of adaptive difficulties in Reaction Time studies. Their reaction times are generally slower and much more variable than normal, and except at very short preparatory intervals, they do not benefit from the regularity of preparatory periods, even when they know what to expect and are allowed to pace themselves (Zahn et al., 1961 a, b, 1963). They are, therefore, an inefficient biological system and have difficulty in maintaining an attentional set or a state of preparedness. Impairment in their performance is particularly marked when there is a demand quality in the environment and the stimulus load is increased. They are disproportionately impaired in situations of uncertainty, *e.g.*, in short preparatory interval trials in series with irregular presentations of stimuli. Furthermore, previous experimental conditions interfere with performance in current trials and earlier, presumably helpful, cues tend to impair their reaction time performance. This suggests that schizophrenics have problems in shifting sets and that the past tends to interfere with the present in these patients. In studies measuring GSRs to the preparatory and imperative signals in Reaction Time tasks, the reactions to the more meaningful or demanding signals are impaired as compared to the less demanding ready signals suggesting difficulty in selecting relevant stimuli (Zahn et al., 1981). Again at least some of these abnormalities seem to antedate overt schizophrenia and can be demonstrated in remitted as well as in drug-treated patients.

In experiments designed to study nonspecific arousal and the capacity to sustain attention, *e.g.,* with the Continuous Performance Test (for reviews see Garmezy, 1978; Kornetsky and Orzack, 1978), about half of the schizophrenics do poorly. This seems to be related to high nonspecific arousal, high frequency choppy activity in EEG, and loss of slow wave sleep. Neuroleptics, which have a synchronizing effect on EEG, significantly but not completely improve this impairment. Patients with more high frequency fast activity (arousal) and lesser degrees of alpha and slow waves have much better outcome with neuroleptics than others (Itil et al., 1975). It would seem, therefore, that neuroleptic-responsive components of schizophrenia may be related to increased nonspecific arousal and heightened distractibility. At the same time, schizophrenics may have decreased specific arousal (selective attention) which is probably not improved much by neuroleptics (Zahn, 1975). Problems in sustaining attention may antedate overt schizophrenia, as it seems do those in selective attention.

Schizophrenics, therefore, seem to have severe problems both in selectively focusing attention on relevant aspects of a situation while ignoring the myriad irrelevant aspects, and in reducing the arousal strength of stimuli as they become familiar on repeated exposure. In other words, they have failure of discriminative inhibitory control mechanisms leading to both unsteadiness of attention and rigid attachment of attention. From observations such as these, and others with a variety of psychological tests, in the course of many years of longitudinal investigations of carefully selected schizophrenics, Shakow (1971) came to the conclusion that poor adaptation to stimuli (nonhabituation) and/or a tendency to repeat behaviors well past the need (perseveration) are the rule rather than exception in schizophrenics. They have neophobia or aversion of the new and they cling to the past, repeating the preprogrammed and the automatic rather than developing new behaviors. They respond in bipolar fashion: too much or too little, often both in succession. Failure to extinguish old patterns characterizes adult schizophrenics as well as children destined to develop overt schizophrenia.

Data from many lines of investigation in experimental animals, suggest that at least some of the discriminative inhibitory functions impaired in schizophrenia are probably served by the meso-diencephalic-limbic circuits centered at the hippocampus in which the ascending limbs contain cholinergic neurones (see reviews by Carlton, 1968; Douglas, 1972, 1975; Warburton, 1972, 1975; Warburton and Brown, 1972; Isaacson, 1972, 1974; Pribram and McGuiness, 1975; Pribram and Isaacson, 1975; Karczmar, 1978).

From the classical studies of Shute and Lewis (1967) and Lewis and Shute (1967), at least three cholinergic projection systems originating in the midbrain tegmentum have been recognized—two ascending reticular systems and a hippocampal circuit. Of the ascending reticular systems, the dorsal tegmental system projects to the thalamic regions and corresponds to the thalamic reticular activating system that connects to the cortex through noncholinergic neurones and includes neurones of the strio-pallidal chain (Hassler, 1978). The second ascending system originates in the ventral tegmental area and connects with the striatum, hypothalamus and the neocortex. The ventral tegmental area is also the origin of projections that reach the hippocampus via medial septal nuclei and are part of the limbic or hippocampal cholinergic circuit. From the hippocampus, efferents which are noncholinergic pass via the fornix to the hypothalamus and the midbrain tegmental nuclei, thus completing the limbic-midbrain circuit of Nauta. Weak electrical stimulation or cholinergic stimulation with small amounts of carbachol or physostigmine along the ventral tegmental systems, especially the hippocampal circuit, produce electrocortical arousal, enhancement of late components of evoked potentials considered necessary for perception of specific stimuli, facilitation of discrimination of stimuli in object discrimination tasks and of the cortical resolution of two flashes, and improvement in reaction times. Cholinolytics, large doses of anticholinesterases or cholinomimetics producing depolarization blocks, strong electrical stimulations and lesions in the same areas have essentially opposite effects (see Warburton, 1972, 1975; Douglas, 1972, 1975). The electrocortical arousal produced by cholinergic stimulation is associated with general inhibition of somatomotor activity ("Alert Non-Motile Behavior," Karczmar, 1978). This is believed to reflect mobilization of networks related to selective inhibition and formation of new stimulus-response connections (Douglas, 1975).

The crucial role of the hippocampus in all this is suggested by the observations that there is a strong correlation between hippocampal activity and neocortical activity and that bilateral lesions of the hippocampus result in abnormal GSRs (increased responses with more rapid recovery, as seen in many schizophrenics and children at risk for schizophrenia), impaired habituation to stimuli as well as problems in dishabituation in some circumstances, and deficits in extinction, discrimination reversal (which require extinction of previously-learned behavior and acquisition of newly correct responses), passive avoidance (which requires withholding of response to avoid shock), complex maze learning, spontaneous alternation and go-no go alternation behaviors (Douglas, 1975; Pribram and McGuiness, 1975; Pribram and Isaacson, 1975). Almost all these deficits, which are believed to reflect failure of discriminative inhibitory functions in the brain, are reproduced by anticholinergics given systemically or locally along the cholinergic pathways originating in the midbrain reticular formation.

In view of such observations, it has been concluded that ascending cholinergic pathways play an important role in the selection of relevant stimuli from internal and external environments by exercising inhibitory stimulus control. They seem to do so by producing cortical arousal (desynchronization) which increases the probability of detection of larger evoked potentials induced by specific stimuli while masking the smaller ones from the background noises. This occurs, however, mainly with modest increases in activation, for high levels of reticular activation tend to block the specific evoked potentials producing impairment in responding and disruption of behavior. The anticholinergics, by blocking the cortical arousal by the ascending reticular systems, will reduce signal to noise ratios and allow irrelevant stimuli to influence behavior. As the cholinergic and anticholinergic effects on stimulus selection are most specifically reproduced by modifications of hippocampal functions, the cholinergic hippocampal circuit seems to be of crucial importance in these processes.

It is believed (Pribram and McGuiness, 1975; Pribram and Isaacson, 1975) that in many circumstances the orienting to stimuli and activation of "go" mechanisms centered on the basal ganglia which allow preprogrammed and semi-automatic behaviors to be emitted are yoked. Hippocampal circuits become important in situation of uncertainty or novelty where there is a mismatch between the present and what went before or the existing strategies are not up to the demands of the environment. They serve to uncouple the stimulus-response connections and thus allow new central representations to be formed and new response strategies to be developed. Since dealing with new circumstances and situations of uncertainty is precisely the adaptive function that seems to be impaired in schizophrenia, it is not unreasonable to implicate defective hippocampus-centered circuits in at least some forms of schizophrenia and to suspect that cholinolytics will tend to worsen the basic adaptive difficulties of the schizophrenics.

It must be recognized, however, that the inhibitory output from the hippocampus is noncholinergic so that a cholinergic deficit does not necessarily have to be postulated in considering hippocampal failure as a factor in schizophrenia. Nevertheless, since cholinergic input from the reticular formation seems to be an important factor in mobilizing hippocampal circuits, impairment of schizophrenic processes may be expected with cholinolytics without there being anything wrong with cholinergic neurones *per se*. On the other hand, cholinergic deficits may well be a factor in some cases or at some stages of the illness. Some support for this possibility has come from the studies of Bird et al. (1977) in which significant reduction in the cholinergic marker enzyme CAT was found in the nucleus accumbens and hippocampus in the post-mortem schizophrenic brain. The concentrations of dopamine, the transmitter of the "go" mechanisms of basal ganglia (*supra*), were increased in the nucleus accumbens—the limbic striatum.

In view of the important role that ascending cholinergic systems seem to play in discriminative inhibitory functions in the brain, it is unfortunate that systematic studies of cholinergic and anticholinergic effects on adaptive dysfunctions in schizophrenia have not been carried out. However, studies in healthy volunteers do suggest that cholinolytics produce attentional difficulties (*e.g.*, in maintaining attentive set) of the type associated with schizophrenic psychoses (Callaway and Band, 1958; Ostfeld et al., 1960; Ostfeld and Aruguete, 1962).

REFERENCES

Abood, L.G., and Biel, J.H. (1962): Anticholinergic psychotomimetic agents. *International Review of Neurobiology 6,* 218-273.

Acquilonius, S.M., Lundholm, B., and Winbladh, B. (1972): Effects of some anti-cholinergic drugs on cortical acetylcholine release and motor activity in rats. *European Journal of Pharmacology 20,* 224-230.

Allert, M.L., and Schmitt, W. (1966): Zur Frage des Einflusses von Anti-Parkinsonmitteln auf den neuroleptischen Behandlungseffect. In: *Proceedings of the 4th International Congress of the Collegium International Neuropsychopharmacologicum,* H. Brill, Ed., 1075-1079, New York, Excerpta Medical Foundation.

Arnfred, T., and Randrup, A. (1968): Cholinergic mechanisms in brain inhibiting amphetamine-induced stereotypy of behavior. *Acta Pharmacologica et Toxicologica 26,* 384-394.

Ayd, F.J. (1961): Neuroleptic and extrapyramidal reactions in psychiatric patients. In: *Extrapyramidal System,* Jean-March Bordeleau, Ed., 355-365, Montreal, Editions Psychiatrique.

Bird, E.D., Spokes, E.G., Barnes, J., Mackay, A.V.P., Iversen, L.L., and Shepherd, M. (1977): Increased brain dopamine and reduced glutamic acid decarboxylase and choline acetyltransferase activity in schizophrenia and related psychoses. *Lancet II,* 1157-1159.

Bishop M., Gallant, D., and Sykes, T. (1965): Extrapyramidal side effects and therapeutic response. *Archives of General Psychiatry 13,* 155-162.

Borison, R.L., and Diamond, B.L. (1978): A new animal model for schizophrenia: interactions with adrenergic mechanisms. *Biological Psychiatry 13,* 217-225.

Borison, R.L., Havdala, H.S., and Diamond, B.L. (1977): Chronic phenylethylamine-induced stereotypy: A new animal model for schizophrenia. *Life Sciences 21,* 117-122.

Bowers, M.B., Jr., Goodman, E., and Sim, Van N. (1964): Some behavioral changes in man following anticholinesterase administration. *Journal of Nervous and Mental Disease 138,* 383-389.

Bowers, M.B., Jr. and Rozitis, A. (1974): Regional differences in homovanillic acid concentrations after acute and chronic administration of antipsychotic drugs. *Journal of Pharmacy and Pharmacology 26,* 743-745.

Bowling, C., and Pradhan, S.N. (1967): Interaction of some drugs on nicotine-induced facilitation of self-stimulation in rats. *Pharmacologist 9:* 201.

Bradley, P.B., and Elkes, J. (1953): The effect of atropine, hyoscyamine, physostigmine and neostigmine on the electrical activity of the conscious cat. *Journal of Physiology 120,* 14P-15P.

Breese, G.R., Cooper, B.R., Smith, R.D. (1973): Biochemical and behavioral alternations following 6-hydroxydopamine administration into brain. In:*Frontiers in Catecholamine Research,* E. Usdin and S.H. Snyder, Eds., 701-706, New York, Pergamon Press.

Callaway, E., and Band, R.J. (1958): Some psychopharmacological effects of atropine. *Archives of Neurology and Psychiatry 79*, 91-102.
Carlsson, A. (1978): Mechanism of action of neuroleptics. In: *Psychopharmacology: A Generation of Progress*, M.A. Lipton, A. DiMascio and K.F. Killam, Eds., 1057-1070, New York, Raven Press.
Carlton, P.L. (1963): Cholinergic mechanisms in the control of behavior by the brain. *Psychological Review 70*, 19-39.
Carlton, P.L. (1968): Cholinergic mechanisms in the control of behavior. In: *Psychopharmacology: A Review of Progress 1957-1967*, D.H. Efron, J.O. Cole, J. Levine, and J.E. Wittenborn, Eds., 125-135, Washington, D.C.: U.S. Government Printing Office.
Casey, J.F., Lasky, J., Klett, J.C., and Hollister, L.E. (1960): Treatment of schizophrenic reactions with phenothiazine derivatives. *American Journal of Psychiatry 117*, 97-105.
Chouinard, G., Annable, L., and Cooper, S. (1977): Antiparkinsonism drug administration and plasma levels of penfluridol, a new long-acting neuroleptic. *Communications in Psychopharmacology 1*, 325-331.
Chouinard, G., Annable, L., and Horrobin, D.F. (1978): An antipsychotic action of penicillin in schizophrenia. *IRCS Medical Science 6*, 187.
Claridge, C. (1978): Animal models of schizophrenia. The case for LSD-25. *Schizophrenia Bulletin 4*, 186-209.
Cohen, L.H., and Patterson, M. (1937): Effect of pain on the heart rate of normal and schizophrenic individuals. *Journal of General Psychology 17*, 273-289.
Cole, J.O. (1964): Phenothiazine treatment in acute schizophrenia. *Archives of General Psychiatry 10*, 246-261.
Cole, J.O., and Clyde, D.J. (1961): Extrapyramidal side effects and clinical response to the phenothiazines. In: *Extrapyramidal System*, Jean-March Bordeleau, Ed., 469-478, Montreal, Editions Psychiatrique.
Collard, J., Lecoq, R., and Demaret, A. (1965): Un essai de therapeutique pathogenique de la schizophrenie par un acetylcholinique: l'oxotremorine. *Acta Neurologica Belgica 65*, 122-126.
Colpaert, F.C., Wauquier, A., Niemegeers, C.J.E., and Lal, H. (1975): Reversal by a central anticholinergic drug of pimozide-induced inhibition of mouse jumping in amphetamine dopa-treated mice. *Journal of Pharmacy and Pharmacology 27*, 536-537.
Cook, L., and Davidson, A.B. (1978): Behavioral pharmacology: animal models involving aversive control of behavior. In: *Psychopharmacology. A Generation of Progress*, M.A. Lipton, A. DiMascio, and K.F. Killam, Eds., 563-567, New York. Raven Press.
Cooper, B.R., Breese, G.R., Grant, L.D., and Howard, J.L. (1973): Effects of 6-hydroxydopamine treatment on active avoidance responding: evidence for involvement of brain dopamine. *Journal of Pharmacology and Experimental Therapeutics 185*, 358-370.
Cooper, B.R., Howard, J.L., Grant, L.D., Smith, R.D., and Breese, G.R. (1974): Alteration of avoidance and ingestive behavior after destruction of catecholamine pathways with 6-hydroxydopamine. *Pharmacology, Biochemistry and Behavior 2*, 639-649.
Cooper, T.B. (1978): Plasma level monitoring of antipsychotic drugs. *Clinical Pharmacokinetics 3*, 14-38.
Costa, E., and Cheney, D.L. (1978): Regulation of cholinergic neurons by dopaminergic terminals; influence of cataleptogenic and noncataleptogenic antipsychotics. In: *Interactions Between Putative Neurotransmitters in the Brain*, S. Garattini, J.F. Pujol, and R. Samanin, Eds., 23-38, New York, Raven Press.
Costa, E., Fratta, W., Hong, J.S., Moroni, F. and Yang, H.-Y.T. (1978): Interactions between enkaphlinergic and other neuronal systems. *Advances in Biochemical Pharmacology 18*, 217-226.

Costa, E., and Trabucchi, M. (1978): *Advances in Biochemical Psychopharmacology, Vol. 18.* New York, Raven Press.

Coyle, J.R., and Snyder, S.H. (1969): Antiparkinsonian drugs: inhibition of dopamine uptake in the corpus striatum as a possible mechanism of action. *Science 166,* 899-901.

Creese, I., Burt, D.R., and Snyder, S.H. (1978): Biochemical actions of neuroleptic drugs; focus on the dopamine receptor. In: *Handbook of Psychopharmacology, Vol. 10, Neuroleptics and Schizophrenia,* L.L. Iversen, S.D. Iversen, and S.H. Snyder, Eds., 37-89, New York, Plenum Press.

Crow, T.J. (1976): Specific monoamine systems as reward pathways: evidence for the hypothesis that activation of the ventral mesencephalic dopaminergic neurones and noradrenergic neurones of the locus coeruleus complex will support self-stimulation responding. In: *Brain-Stimulation Reward,* A. Wauquier, and E.T. Rolls, Eds., 211-237, Amsterdam, North-Holland Publishing Company.

Davis, K.L., and Berger, P.A. (1978): Pharmacological investigations of the cholinergic imbalance hypotheses of movement disorders and psychosis. *Biological Psychiatry 13,* 23-49.

Davis, J.M. and Garver, D.L. (1978): Neuroleptics: Clinical use in psychiatry. In: *Handbook of Psychopharmacology, Vol. 10, Neuroleptics and Schizophrenia,* L.L. Iversen, S.D. Iversen, and S.H. Snyder, Eds., 129-164, New York, Plenum Press.

Dohan, F.C., Grasberger, J.C., Lowell, F.M., Johnston, H.T., Jr., and Arbegast, A.W. (1969): Relapsed schizophrenics: more rapid improvement on milk- and cereal-free diet. *British Journal of Psychiatry 115,* 595-596.

Domino, E.F., and Olds, M.E. (1968): Cholinergic inhibition of self-stimulation behavior. *Journal of Pharmacology and Experimental Therapeutics 164,* 202-211.

Douglas, R.J. (1972): Pavlovian conditioning and the brain. In: *Inhibition and Learning,* R.A. Boakes, and M.S. Halliday, Eds., 529-553, London, Academic Press.

Douglas, R.J. (1975): The development of the hippocampal function: Implications for theory and for therapy. In: *The Hippocampus, Vol. 2,* R.L. Isaacson and K.H. Pribram, Eds., 327-361, New York, Plenum Press.

Elkes, J. (1961): Schizophrenic disorder in relation to levels of neural organization. The need for some conceptual points of reference. In: *Clinical Pathology of the Nervous System,* J. Folch-Pi,, Ed., 648-665, London, Pergamon Press.

Ellinwood, E.H. Jr., Sudilovsky, A., and Nelson, L.M. (1973): Evolving behavior in the clinical and experimental amphetamine (model) psychoses. *American Journal of Psychiatry 130,* 1088-1093.

El-Yousef, M.K., and Manier, D.H. (1974): The effect of benztropine mesylate on plasma levels of butaperazine maleate. *American Journal of Psychiatry 131,* 471-472.

Feldberg, W. (1964): Discussion on extrapolation from animals to man: catatonia. In: *Animal Behavior and Drug Action,* H. Steinberg, Ed., 429-439, London, Churchill.

Fiamberti, A. (1946): L'aceticolina nelle sindromi schizofreniche. *Riv. Pat. Nerv. Ment. 66,* 1. As cited in Gershon and Shaw (1961).

Fibiger, H.C., Philips, A.G., and Zis, A.P. (1974): Deficits in instrumental responding after 6-hydroxydopamine lesions of the nigro-neostriatal dopaminergic projections. *Pharmacology, Biochemistry and Behavior 2,* 87-96.

Fielding, S., and Lal, H. (1978): Behavioral actions of neuroleptics. In: *Handbook of Psychopharmacology, Vol. 10, Neuroleptics and Schizophrenia,* L.L. Iversen, S.D. Iversen, and S.H. Snyder, Eds., 91-128, New York, Plenum Press.

Fink, M. (1968): EEG classification of psychoactive compounds in man: A review and theory of behavioral associations. In: *Psychopharmacology – A Review of Progress 1957-1967,* D. Efron, J.O. Cole, J. Levine, and J.R. Wittenborn, Eds., 497-507, Washington, D.C., Government Printing Office.

Fink, M. (1960: Effect of anticholinergic compounds on post-convulsive EEG and behavior of psychiatric patients. *Electroencephalography and Clinical Neurophysiology 12*, 359-369.

Fjalland, B., and Møller-Nielsen, I. (1974): Methylphenidate antagonism of haloperidol: interaction with cholinergic and anticholinergic drugs. *Psychopharmacology 34*, 111-118.

Forrer, G.R. (1956): Symposium on atropine toxicity therapy. *Journal of Nervous and Mental Disease 124*, 257-283.

Forrer, G.R., and Miller, J.J. (1958): Atropine coma: a somatic therapy in psychiatry. *American Journal of Psychiatry 155*, 455-458.

Forsman, A., and Ohman, R. (1977): Applied pharmacokinetics of haloperidol in man. *Current Therapeutic Research 21*, 396-408.

Frankenhaeuser, M., Myrsten, A.L., Johansson, G., and Post, B. (1971): Behavioral and physiological effects of cigarette smoking in a monotonous situation. *Psychopharmacologia 22*, 1-7.

Franzén, G., and Ingvar, D.J. (1975): Absence of activation in frontal structures during psychological testing of chronic schizophrenics. *Journal of Neurology, Neurosurgery, and Psychiatry 38*, 1027-1032.

Fuxe, K. (1965): Evidence for the existence of monoamine neurons in the central nervous system. IV. Distribution of monoamine nerve terminals in the central nervous system. *Acta Physiologica Scandinavica 64*, Supplementum 247.

Fuxe, K., Hokfelt, T., Johansson, O., Jonsson, G., Lidbrink, P., and Ljungdahl, A. (1974): The origin of dopamine nerve terminals in limbic and frontal cortex. Evidence for mesocortical dopamine neurons. *Brain Research 82*, 349-355.

Galambos, E.A., Pfeiffer, K., Györgi, L., and Milnar, J. (1967): Study on the excitation induced by amphetamine, cocaine and alphamethyltryptamine. *Psychopharmacology 11*, 122-129.

Garattini, S., Pujol, J.F., and Samanin, R. (1978): *Interactions Between Putative Neurotransmitters in the Brain*. New York, Raven Press.

Garmezy, N. (1978): Attentional processes in adult schizophrenics and in children at risk. *Journal of Psychiatric Research 14*, 3-34.

Gautier, J., Jus, A., Villeneuve, A., Jus, K., Peires, P., and Villeneuve, R. (1977): Influence of the antiparkinsonian drugs on the plasma levels of neuroleptics. *Biological Psychiatry 12*, 389-399.

Geller, I., Kulak, J.T., Jr., and Seifter, J. (1962); The effects of chlordiazepoxide and chlorpromazine on a punishment discrimination. *Psychopharmacology 3*, 374-385.

Gershon, S., and Olariu, J. (1960): J.B. 329° — a new psychotomimetic, its antagonism by tetrahydroaminocrin and its comparison with LSD, mescaline and sernyl. *Journal of Neuropsychiatry 1*, 283-292.

Gershon, S., and Shaw, F.H. (1961): Psychiatric sequelae of chronic exposure to organophosphorous insecticides. *Lancet, 1*, 1371-1374.

Goldberg, M.E., and Johnson, H.E. (1964a): Behavior effects of a cholinergic stimulation in combination with various psychotherapeutic agents. *Journal of Pharmacology and Experimental Therapeutics 145*, 367-372.

Goldberg, M.E., and Johnson, H.E. (1964b): Potentiation of chlorpromazine-induced behavior changes by anti-cholinesterase agents. *Journal of Pharmacy and Pharmacology 16*, 60-61.

Goldman, D. (1961): Parkinsonism and related phenomena from the administration of drugs, their production and control under clinical conditions and possible relation to therapeutic effect. In: *Extrapyramidal System*, Jean-March Bordeleau, Ed., 453-464, Montreal, Editions Psychiatrique.

Grissell, J.L., and Bynum, H.J. (1956): Symposium on atropine toxicity therapy. A study of the relationship between anxiety level, ego strength and response to atropine toxicity therapy. *Journal of Nervous and Mental Disease 124*, 265-268.

Grob, D. and Harvey, A.M. (1958): Effects on man of anticholinesterase compound sarin (isopropyl methyl phosphorafluoridate). *Journal of Clinical Investigation 37*, 350-368.

Grob, D., Harvey, A.M., Langworthy, O.R., and Lilienthal, J.L. Jr. (1947): The administration of di-isopropylfluorophosphate (DFP) to man. III — The effect on the central nervous system, with special reference to the electrical activity of the brain. *Bulletin of Johns Hopkins Hospital 81*, 257-266.

Grossman, S.P. (1976): A loss of complex learned behavior following transection of the lateral connections of the hypothalamus: Are pathways essential for "reward" interrupted? In: *Brain-Stimulation Reward*, A. Wauquier and E.T. Rolls, Eds., 385-396, Amsterdam, North-Holland Publishing Company.

Gruzelier, J.H., and Hammond, N.V. (1978): The effect of chlorpromazine upon psychophysiological, endocrine and information processing measures in schizophrenia. *Journal of Psychiatric Research 14*, 167-182.

Haase, H.-J. (1965): Clinical observations on the actions of neuroleptics. In: *Actions of Neuroleptics. A Psychiatric, Neurologic and Pharmacological Investigation*, H.-J. Haase and P.A.J. Janssen, Eds., 1-118, Amsterdam, North-Holland Publishing Company.

Halliwell, G., Quinton, R.M., and Williams, F.E. (1964): A comparison of imipramine, chlorpromazine and related drugs in various tests involving autonomic functions and antagonism of reserpine. *British Journal of Pharmacology 23*, 330-350.

Hanlon, T.E., Schoenrich, C., Freinek, W., Turek, I., and Kurland, A.A. (1966): Perphenazine-benztropine mesylate treatment of newly-admitted psychiatric patients. *Psychopharmacologia 9*, 328-339.

Hanson, H.M., Stone, C.A., and Witoslawski, J.J. (1970): Antagonism of the anti-avoidance effects of various agents by anticholinergic drugs. *Journal of Pharmacology and Experimental Therapeutics 173*, 117-124.

Hassler, R. (1978): Striatal control of locomotion, intentional actions and of integrating and perceptive activity. *Journal of the Neurological Science 36*, 187-224.

Herberg, L.J. and co-workers—Personal communication cited in Wauquier, A. (1977, 1978).

Hery, F., Giorguieff, M.F., Hamon, M., Besson, M.J., and Glowinski, J. (1978): Role of cholinergic receptors in the release of newly synthesized amines from the serotonergic and dopaminergic terminals. In: *Interactions Between Putative Neurotransmitters in the Brain*, S. Garattini, J.F. Pujol, and R. Samanin, Eds., 39-51, New York, Raven Press.

Horvath, T., and Meares, R. (1979): The sensory filter in schizophrenia: a study of habituation, arousal and dopamine hypothesis. *British Journal of Psychiatry 134*, 39-45.

Ingvar, D.H., and Franzén, G. (1974): Abnormalities of cerebral blood flow distribution in patients with chronic schizophrenia. *Acta Psychiatrica Scandinavica 50*, 425-462.

Isaacson, R.L. (1972): Neural systems of the limbic brain and behavioral inhibition. In: *Inhibition and Learning*, R.A. Boakes and M.S. Halliday, Eds., 41-71, New York, Academic Press.

Isaacson, R.L. (1974): *The Limbic System*. New York, Plenum Press.

Itil, T.M. (1973): *Electroencephalographic Studies in Endogenous Psychoses And Their Treatment with Psychotropic Drugs with Special Consideration of the Thiopental (Pentothal) Electroencephalogram*. St. Louis, Psychiatric Research Foundation of Missouri, 44-45.

Itil, T.M., Güven, F., Cora, R., Hsu, W., Polvan, N., Ucok, A., Sanseigne, A., and Ulett, G.A. (1971): Quantitative pharmacoelectroencephalography using frequency analyzer and digital computer methods in early drug evaluations. In: *Drugs, Development, and Brain Functions*, W.L. Smith, Ed., 145-166, Springfield, Illinois, Charles C. Thomas.

Itil, T.M., Morasa, J., Saletu, B., Davis, S., and Mucciardi, A.M. (1975): Computerized EEG: Prediction of outcome in schizophrenia. *Journal of Nervous and Mental Disease 160*, 188-203.

Jaffe, J.J., and Martin, W.R. (1975): Narcotic analgesics and antagonists. In: *The Pharmacological Basis of Therapeutics, 5th Edition*, L.S. Goodman and A. Gilman, Eds., 245-283, New Jersey, Macmillan.

Janowsky, D.S., El-Yousef, M.K., Davis, J.M., and Sekerke, H.J. (1973): Antagonistic effects of physostigmine and methylphenidate in man. *American Journal of Psychiatry 130*, 1370-1376.

Janssen, P.A.J., Niemegeers, C.J.E., and Schellekens, K.A.L. (1965): Is it possible to predict the clinical effect of neuroleptic drugs (major tranquillizers) from animal data. Part I. Neuroleptic activity spectra for rats. Arzneim Forsch. (Drug Research) *15*, 104-117, 1965. Part II. Neuroleptic activity spectra in dogs. *Arzneim Forsch 15*, 1196-1206.

Janssen, P.A.J., Niemegeers, C.J.E., Schellekens, K.A.L., and Lenaerts, F.M. (1967): Is it possible to predict the clinical effects of neuroleptic drugs (major tranquillizers) from animal data. Part IV. An improved experimental design for measuring the inhibitory effects of neuroleptic drugs on amphetamine- or apomorphine-induced "chewing" and "agitation" in rats. *Arzneim Forsch 17*, 841-854.

Janssen, P.A.J., and Van Bever, F.M. (1975): Advances in the search for improved neuroleptic drugs. In: *Current Developments in Psychopharmacology, Vol. 2*, W.B. Essman and L. Valzelli, Eds., 165-184, New York, Spectrum Publications.

Jung, O.H., and Boyd, E.S. (1966): Effects of cholinergic drugs on self-stimulation response rates in rats. *American Journal of Physiology 210*, 432-434.

Karczmar, A.G. (1978): Exploitable aspects of central cholinergic functions, particularly with respect to the EEG, motor, analgesic and mental functions. In: *Cholinergic Mechanisms and Psychopharmacology*, D.J. Jenden, Ed., 679-708, New York, Plenum Press.

Kay, S.R., and Singh, M.M. (1975a): A developmental approach to delineate components of cognitive dysfunctions in schizophrenia. *British Journal of Social and Clinical Psychology 14*, 387-399.

Kay, S.R., and Singh, M.M. (1979): Cognitive abnormality in schizophrenia. A dual process model. *Biological Psychiatry 14*, 155-176.

Kay, S.R., and Singh, M.M. (1975b): Pulse rate and sleeplessness in relation to nosological distinctions in schizophrenia. *Perceptual Motor Skills 40*, 178.

Kay, S.R., Singh, M.M., and Smith, J.M. (1975): Colour Form Representation Test: A developmental method for the study of cognition in schizophrenia. *British Journal of Social and Clinical Psychology 14*, 401-411.

Kent, E.M., and Grossman, S.P. (1973): Elimination of learned behaviors after trans-section of fibers crossing the lateral border of the hypothalamus. *Physiology and Behavior 10*, 953-963.

Khavari, K.A., and Russell, R.W. (1966): Acquisition, retention and extinction under conditions of water deprivation and of central cholinergic stimulation. *Journal of Comprehensive Physiology and Psychology 61*, 339-345.

Klee, W.A., Zioudrou, C., and Steaty, R.A. (1978): Exorphins – peptides with opioid activity isolated from wheat gluten, and their possible role in the etiology of schizophrenia. In: *Endorphins in Mental Health Research*, E. Usdin, Ed., 209-218, New Jersey, Macmillan.

Kolakowska, T., Wiles, D.H., Gilder, M.G., and McNeilly, A.S. (1976): Clinical significance of plasma chlorpromazine levels. *Psychopharmacology 49*, 101-107.

Kornetsky, C., and Orzack, M.H. (1978): Physiological and behavioral correlates of attention dysfunction in schizophrenic patients. *Journal of Psychiatric Research 14*, 69-79.

Kuhar, M.J. (1976): The anatomy of cholinergic neurons. In: *Biology of Cholinergic Functions,* A.M. Goldberg and I. Hanin, Eds., 3-27, New York, Raven Press.

Ladinsky, H., Consolo, S., Bianchi, S., Ghezzi, D., and Samanin, R. (1978): Link between dopaminergic and cholinergic neurons in the striatum as evidenced by pharmacological, biochemical and lesion studies. In: *Interactions Between Putative Neurotransmitters in the Brain,* S. Garattini, J.F. Pujol, and R. Samanin, Eds., 3-21, New York, Raven Press.

Lal, H., Colpaert, F.C., and Laduron, P. (1975): Narcotic withdrawal-like mouse jumping produced by amphetamine and L-DOPA. *European Journal of Pharmacology 30,* 113-116.

Lal, H., Marky, M., and Fielding, S. (1976): Effects of neuroleptic drugs on mouse jumping induced by L-DOPA in amphetamine-treated mice. *Neuropharmacology 15,* 669-671.

Lapin, I.P., and Schelkunov, E.L. (1965): Amphetamine-induced changes in behavior of small laboratory animals as simple tests for evaluation of central effects of new drugs. In: *Pharmacology of Conditioning, Learning and Retention.* Oxford, Pergamon Press.

Lee, J.H., Cooper, T.B., Srivastava, R.K., and Simpson, G.M.: A study of butaperazine plasma levels with or without anti-parkinsonism agents. Cited in Cooper, 1978.

Lerner, P., Nose, P., Gordon, E.K., and Lovenberg, W. (1977): Haloperidol: effect of long-term treatment on rat striatal dopamine synthesis and turnover. *Science 197,* 181-183.

Leslie, G.B., and Maxwell, D.R. (1964): Some pharmacological properties of thioproperazine and their modification by anti-Parkinsonism drugs. *British Journal of Pharmacology 22,* 301-317.

Lewis, P.R., and Shute, C.C.D. (1967): The cholinergic limbic system: projections to hippocampal formation, medial cortex, nuclei of the ascending cholinergic reticular system and the subfornical organ and supra-optic crest. *Brain 90,* 521-540.

Lloyd, K.G. (1978): The biochemical pharmacology of the limbic system: neuroleptic drugs. In: *Limbic Mechanisms,* K.E. Livingston and O. Hornykiewicz, Eds., 263-305, New York, Plenum Press.

Loga, S., Curry, S., and Lader, M. (1975): Interaction of orphenadrine and phenobarbitone with chlorpromazine plasma concentrations and effects in man. *British Journal of Clinical Pharmacology 2,* 197-208.

Lorens, S.A. (1976): Anatomical substrate of intracranial self-stimulation: contribution of lesion studies. In: *Brain-Stimulation Reward,* A.Wauquier and E.T. Rolls, Eds., 41-50, Amsterdam, North-Holland Publishing Company.

Malamud, N. (1967): Psychiatric disorders with intracranial tumors of the limbic system. *Archives of Neurology 17,* 113-123.

Manto, P.G. (1967): Blockade of epinephrine-induced decrement in activity by scopolamine. *Psychonomic Sciences 7,* 203-204.

Matthysse, S. (1977): The biology of attention. *Schizophrenia Bulletin 3,* No. 3, 370-372.

Matthysse, S., and Sugarman, J. (1978): Neurotransmitter theories of schizophrenia. In: *Handbook of Psychopharmacology Vol. 10. Neuroleptics and Schizophrenia,* L.L. Iversen, S.D. Iversen, and S.H. Snyder, Eds., 221-242, New York, Plenum Press.

May, P.R.A., and Van Putten, T. (1978): Plasma levels of chlorpromazine in schizophrenia. A critical review of the literature. *Archives of General Psychiatry 35,* 1081-1087.

Mednick, S.A., and Schulsinger, F. (1968): Some premorbid characteristics related to breakdown in children with schizophrenic mothers. *Journal of Psychiatric Research 6,* 354-362.

Meltzer, H.Y., and Stahl, S.M. (1976): The dopamine hypothesis of schizophrenia: A review. *Schizophrenia Bulletin 2,* 19-76.

Meyers, B.K., Roberts, G., Riciputi, H., and Domino, E.F. (1964): Some effects of muscarinic cholinergic-blocking drugs on behavior and the electrocardiogram. *Psychopharmacology 5,* 289-300.

Mitcham, J.C., and Thomas R.K. (1972): Effects of substantia nigra and caudate nucleus lesions on avoidance learning in rats. *Journal of Comparative and Physiological Psychology 81*, 101-107.

Morpurgo, C. (1962): Effects of antiparkinson drugs on a phenothiazine-induced catatonic reaction. *Archives Internationales de Pharmacodynamie et de Therapie 137*, 84-90.

Morpurgo, C., and Theobald, W. (1964): Influence of anti-Parkinsonism drugs and amphetamine on some pharmacological effects of phenothiazine derivatives used as neuroleptics. *Psychopharmacology 6*, 178-191.

Munkvad, I., and Randrup, A. (1976): The persistence of amphetamine sterotypies of rats in spite of strong sedation. *Acta Psychiatrica Scandanavica Suppl. 191*, 178.

Nauta, W.J.H. (1963): Central nervous organization and the endocrine motor system. In: *Advances in Neuroendrocrinology*, A.V. Albandor, Ed., 5-21, Urbana, Illinois, University of Illinois Press.

Nauta, W.J.H. (1964): Some efferent connections of the prefrontal cortex in monkey. In: *The Frontal Cortex and Behavior*, J. M. Warren and K. Akert, Eds., 397-409, New York, McGraw Hill.

Nauta, W.J.H. (1960): Some neural pathways related to the limbic system. In: *Electrical Studies on the Unanaesthetized Brain*, E.R. Rainey and D.S. O'Doherty, Eds., 1-16, New York, Hoeber.

Nauta, W.J.H., Smith, G.P., Faull, R.L.M., and Domesick, V.B. (1978): Efferent connections and nigral afferents of the nucleus accumbens septi in the rat. *Neuroscience 3*, 385-401.

Newman, L.M. (1972): Effects of cholinergic agonists and antagonists on self-stimulation behavior in the rat. *Journal of Comprehensive Physiology and Psychology 79*, 394-413.

Niemegeers, C.J.E., Verbruggen, F.J., and Janssen, P.A.J. (1970b): The influence of various neuroleptic drugs on noise escape response in rats. *Psychopharmacology 18*, 249-259.

Niemegeers, C.J.E., Verbruggen, F.J., and Janssen, P.A. J. (1969a): The influence of various neuroleptic drugs on shock avoidance responding in rats. Part I. Non-discriminated Sidman Avoidance Procedure. *Psychopharmacology 16*, 161-174.

Niemegeers, C.J.E., Verbruggen, F.J., and Janssen, P.A.J. (1969b): The influence of various neuroleptic drugs on shock avoidance responding in rats. Part II. Non-discriminated Sidman Avoidance Procedure with alternate reinforcement and extinction periods and analysis of the inter response time (IRT). *Psychopharmacology 16*, 175-182.

Niemegeers, C.J.E., Verbruggen, F.J., and Janssen, P.A.J. (1970a): The influence of various neuroleptic drugs on shock avoidance responding in rats. Part III, Amphetamine antagonism in the discrimination Sidman Avoidance Procedure. *Psychopharmacology 17*, 151-159.

Niemegeers, C.J.E., Verbruggen, F.J., Wauquier, A., and Janssen, P.A.J. (1972): The influence of haloperidol and amphetamine in two different noise-escape situations in rats. *Psychopharmacology 25*, 22-31.

NIMH Collaborative Study Group (1964): Phenothiazine treatment in acute schizophrenia. *Archives of General Psychiatry 10*, 246-261.

Olds, J. (1976): Reward and drive neurons. In: *Brain-Stimulated Reward*, A. Wauquier and E.T. Rolls, Eds., 1-27, Amsterdam, North-Holland Publishing Company.

Olds, J., and Milner, P. (1954): Positive reinforcement produced by electrical stimulation of septal area and other regions of rat brain. *Journal of Comparative Physiology and Psychology 47*, 419-417.

Olds, J., and Olds, M.E. (1963): Approach-avoidance analysis of rat diencephalon. *Journal of Comparative Neurology 120*, 259-295.

Olds, M.E. (1972): Alterations by centrally-acting drugs of the suppression of self-stimulation behavior in the rat by tetrabenzine, physostigmine, chlorpromazine and pentobarbital. *Psychopharmacology 25*, 299-314.

Olds, M.E., and Domino, E.F. (1969a): Comparison of muscarinic and nicotinic cholinergic agonists on self-stimulation behavior. *Journal of Pharmacology and Experimental Therapeutics 166*, 189-204.

Olds, M.E., and Domino, E.F. (1969b): Differential effects of cholinergic agonists on self-stimulation and escape behavior. *Journal of Pharmacology and Experimental Therapeutics 170*, 157-167.

Olmstead, C.E., Villablanca, J.R., Marcus, R.J., and Avery, D.L. (1976): Effects of caudate nuclei or frontal cortex ablations in cats. IV. Bar pressing. maze learning and performance. *Experimental Neurology 53*, 670-693.

Ostfeld, A.M., and Aruguete, A. (1962): Central nervous system effects of hyoscine in man. *Journal of Pharmacology 137*, 133-139.

Ostfeld, A.M., Machne, X., Unna, K.R. (1960): The effects of atropine on the electroencephalogram and behavior in man. *Journal of Pharmacology 128*, 265-272.

Pedersen, V. (1967): Potentiation of apomorphine effect (compulsive gnawing behavior) in mice. *Acta Pharmacologica et Toxicologie 25*, 63.

Pfeiffer, C.C., and Jenney, E.H. (1957): The inhibition of conditional response and counteraction of schizophrenia by muscarinic stimulation of the brain. *Annals of New York Academy of Sciences 66*, 753-764.

Pradhan, S.N. (1976): Balance of central neurotransmitter actions in self-stimulation behavior. In: *Brain-Stimulation Reward,* A. Wauquier and E.T. Rolls, Eds., 171-185, Amsterdam, North-Holland Publishing Company.

Pradhan, S.N. (1975): Balances among central neurotransmitters in self-stimulation behavior. In: *Neurotransmitters, Balances and Behavior,* E.F. Domino and J.M. Davis, Eds., 75-97, Ann Arbor, Michigan, Edward Brothers, Inc.

Pradhan, S.N. (1968): Effects of cholinergic and anticholinergic agents on self-stimulation. *Pharmacologist 10*, 204.

Pradhan, S.N., and Bose, S. (1978): Interactions among central neurotransmitters. In: *Psychopharmacology: A Generation of Progress,* M.A. Lipton, A. DiMascio, and K.F. Killam, Eds., 271-281, New York, Raven Press.

Pradhan, S.N., and Bowling, C. (1971): Effects of nicotine on self-stimulation in rats. *Journal of Pharmacology and Experimental Therapeutics 176*, 229-243.

Pradhan, S.N., and Kamat, K.A. (1972): Action and interaction of cholinergic agonists and antagonists on self-stimulation. *Archives Internationales de Pharmacodynamie et de Therapie 196*, 321-329.

Pradhan, S.N., and Kamat, K.A. (1973): Effects of anticholinergic agents on self-stimulation. *Archives Internationales de Pharmacodynamie et de Therapie 201*, 16-24.

Pribram, K.H., and Isaacson, R.L. (1975): *The Hippocampus, Vol. II.* 429-441, New York, Plenum Press.

Pribram, K.H. and McGuiness, D. (1975): Arousal, activation and effort in the control of attention. *Psychological Review 82*, 116-140.

Racagni, G., Bruno, F., Cattabeni, F., Maggi, A., DiGiulio, A.M., and Gropetti, A. (1978): Interactions among dopamine, acetylcholine, and GABA in the nigrostriatal system. In: *Interactions Between Putative Neurotransmitters in the Brain,* S. Garattini, J.F. Pujol, and R. Samanin, Eds., 61-72, New York, Raven Press.

Randrup, A., and Jonas, W. (1967): Brain dopamine and the amphetamine-reserpine interaction. *Journal of Pharmacy and Pharmacology 19*, 483-484.

Randrup, A., and Munkvad, I. (1968): Behavioral stereotypies induced by pharmacological agents. *Pharmacopsychiatry 1*, 18-26.

Randrup, A., and Munkvad, I. (1970): Biochemical, anatomical and psychological investigations of stereotyped behavior induced by amphetamines. In: *Amphetamines and Related Compounds,* E. Costa and S. Garratini, Eds., 695-713, New York, Raven Press.

Randrup, A., and Munkvad, I. (1972): Evidence indicating an association between schizophrenia and dopaminergic hyperactivity in the brain. *Orthomolecular Psychiatry 1,* 2-7.

Randrup, A., and Munkvad, I. (1965): Pharmacological and biochemical investigations of amphetamine-induced abnormal behavior. *Neuro-psychopharmacology 4,* 301.

Rinaldi, R., and Himwich, H.E. (1955): A cholinergic mechanism involved in the function of mesodiencephalic activating system. *Archives of Neurology and Psychiatry 173,* 396-402.

Rivera-Calimlim, L., Castaneda, L., and Lasagna, L. (1973): Effects of mode of management on plasma chlorpromazine in psychiatric patients. *Clinical Pharmacology and Therapeutics 14,* 978-986.

Rivera-Calimlim, L., Nasrallah, H., Strauss, J., and Lasagna, L. (1976): Clinical response and plasma levels: Effect of dose, dosage schedules and drug interactions of plasma chlorpromazine levels. *American Journal of Psychiatry 133,* 646-652.

Rosenthal, R., and Bigelow, L.B. (1973): The effects of physostigmine in phenothiazine resistant chronic schizophrenic patients: preliminary observations. *Comprehensive Psychiatry 14,* 489-494.

Routtenberg, A. (1976): Self-stimulation pathways: Origins and terminations – a three-stage technique. In: *Brain-Stimulation Reward,* A. Wauquier and E.T. Rolls, Eds., 31-39, Amsterdam, North-Holland Publishing Company.

Rowntree, D.W., Nevin, S., and Wilson, A. (1950): The effects of diisopropylfluorophosphonate in schizophrenia and manic depressive psychosis. *Journal of Neurology, Neurosurgery and Psychiatry 13,* 47-62.

Russell, R.W. (1966): Biochemical substrates of behavior. In: *Frontiers in Physiological Psychology,* R.W. Russell, Ed., 185-246, New York, Academic Press.

Schallert, T., Whishaw, I.Q., Ramirez, V.D., and Teitelbaum, P. (1978): Compulsive, abnormal walking caused by anticholinergics in akinetic, 6-hydroxydopamine-treated rats. *Science 199,* 1461-1463.

Schaumann, W., and Kurbjuweit, H.-G. (1961): Beeinflussung verschiedener Wirkungen von Thiopropazat durch ein zentrales Stimulans. *Arzneimittel-Forsch. 11,* 353-350.

Scheel-Krüger, J. (1970): Central effects of anticholinergic drugs measured by the apomorphine gnawing test in mice. *Acta Pharmacologica et Toxicologica 28,* 1-16.

Schelkunov, E.L. (1964): The technique of phenamine sterotypy for evaluating the effect produced by remedial agents on the central adrenergic processes. *Pharmacol. Toxicol.* (Russ.) *27,* 628-633.

Sedvall, G., Fyro, B., Nyback, H., and Wiesel, F.A. (1975): Actions of dopaminergic antagonists in the striatum. In: *Advances in Neurology Vol. 9,* D.B. Calne, T.N. Chase, and A. Barbeau, Eds., 131-140, New York, Raven Press.

Shakow, D. (1977): *Schizophrenia, Selected Papers. Psychology Issues 10, No. 2.* Monograph No. 38. New York, International Universities Press.

Shakow, D. (1971): Some observations on the psychology (and some fewer on the biology) of schizophrenia. *Journal of Nervous and Mental Disease 153,* 300-316.

Sherwood, S.L. (1958): Consciousness, adaptive behavior and schizophrenia. In: *Schizophrenia: Somatic Aspects,* D. Richter, Ed., 131-146, London, Pergamon.

Sherwood, S.L. (1952): Intraventricular medication in catatonic stupor. *Brain 75,* 68-75.

Shute, C.C., and Lewis, P.R. (1967): The ascending cholinergic reticular system: neocortical, olfactory and subcortical projections. *Brain 90,* 497-520.

Simpson, G.M., Cooper, T.B., Bark, N., Sud, I., and Lee, J.H. (1980): Effect of antiparkinsonian medication on plasma levels of chlorpromazine. *Archives of General Psychiatry 37*, 205-208.

Singh, M.M. (1978a): Some insights into the pathogenesis of schizophrenia. In: *The Biological Basis of Schizophrenia*, Gwynneth Hemmings and W.A. Hemmings, Eds. 179-195, Baltimore, University Park Press.

Singh, M.M., and Kay, S.R. (1975a): A comparative study of haloperidol and chlorpromazine in terms of clinical effects on therapeutic reversal with benztropine in schizophrenia Theoretical implications for potency differences among neuroleptics. *Psychopharmacologia 43*, 103-113.

Singh, M.M., and Kay, S.R. (1975b): A longitudinal therapeutic comparison between two prototypic neuroleptics (haloperidol and chlorpromazine) in matched groups of schizophrenics. Nontherapeutic interactions with trihexyphenidyl. Theoretical implications for potency differences. *Psychopharmacologia 43*, 115-223.

Singh, M.M., and Kay, S.R. (1976a): Cholinergic processes in schizophrenia. *World Journal of Psychosynthesis 8*, 34-41.

Singh, M.M., and Kay, S.R. (1979a): Dysphoric response to neuroleptic treatment in schizophrenia, its relationship to automonic arousal and prognosis. *Biological Psychiatry 14*, 275-292.

Singh, M.M., and Kay, S.R. (1978b): Nosological and prognostic classification of schizophrenia: Pharmacological validation in terms of therapeutic antagonism between anticholinergic anti-Parkinsonism agents and neuroleptics. *Neuropsychobiology 4*, 288-304.

Singh, M.M., and Kay, S.R. (1979b): Therapeutic antagonism between anticholinergic anti-Parkinsonism agents and neuroleptics in schizophrenia. Implications for a neuropharmacological model. *Neuropsychobiology 5*, 74-78.

Singh, M.M., and Kay, S.R. (1978c): Therapeutic antagonism between anticholinergics and neuroleptics. Possible involvement of anticholinergic mechanisms in schizophrenia. *Schizophrenia Bulletin 4*, 3-6.

Singh, M.M., and Kay, S.R. (1975c): Therapeutic reversal with benztropine in schizophrenics. Practical and theoretical significance. *Journal of Nervous and Mental Disease 160*, 258-266.

Singh, M.M., and Kay, S.R. (1976b): Wheat gluten as a pathogenic factor in schizophrenia. *Science 191*, 401-402.

Singh, M.M., and Kay, S.R. (1976c): Wheat gluten – schizophrenia findings. *Science 194*, 448-450.

Singh, M.M., and Smith, J.M. (1973a): Kinetics and dynamics of response to haloperidol in acute schizophrenia – A longitudinal study of the therapeutic process. *Comprehensive Psychiatry 14*, 393-414.

Singh, M.M., and Smith, J.M. (1973b): Reversal of some therapeutic effects of an antipsychotic agent by an anti-Parkinsonism agent. *Journal of Nervous and Mental Disease 157*, 50-58.

Singh, M.M., and Smith, J.M. (1971): Reversal of some therapeutic effects of an antipsychotic agent by an anti-Parkinsonism agent. *Pharmacologist 13*, 287.

Snyder, S.H. (1973): Amphetamine psychosis: A "model" schizophrenia mediated by catecholamines. *American Journal of Psychiatry 130*, 61-67.

Snyder, S.H., Banerjee, S.P., and Yamamura, H.I. (1974): Drugs, neurotransmitters and schizophrenia. *Science 184*, 1243-1253.

Snyder, S., Greenberg, D., and Yamamura, H.I. (1974): Antischizophrenic drugs and brain cholinergic receptors. Affinity for muscarinic sites predicts extrapyramidal effects. *Archives of General Psychiatry 31*, 58-61.

Stark, P., and Boyd, E.S. (1963): Effects of cholinergic drugs on hypothalamic self-stimulation response in dogs. *American Journal of Physiology 205*, 745-748.
Stein, L. (1964): Amphetamine and neural reward mechanisms. In: *Ciba Foundation Symposium on Animal Behavior and Drug Action*, H. Steinberg, A.V.S. de Reuch and J. Knight, (Eds.), 91-113, J&A Churchill, London.
Stein, L. (1968): Chemistry of reward and punishment. In: *Psychopharmacology: A Review of Progress 1957-1967*, D.H. Efron, J.O. Cole, J. Levine, and J.R. Wittenborn, Eds., 105-123, Washington, D.C., U.S. Government Printing Office.
Stein, L., Wise, C.D., and Berger, B.D. (1972): Neuroadrenergic reward mechanisms, recovery and function in schizophrenia. In: *The Chemistry of Mood, Motivation and Memory*, J.L. McGaugh, Ed., 81-103, New York, Plenum Press.
Taeschler, M., Weidmann, H., and Cerletti, A. (1962): Zur Pharmakologie von Ponalid, einem neuen zentralen Anticholinergicum. *Schweizerische Medizinische Wochenscrift 92*, 1542-1545.
Ther, L., and Schramm, H. (1962): Apomorphin-synergismus (Zwangsnagen bei Mäusen) als Test zue Differenzierung psychotroper Substanzen. *Archives Internationales de Pharmacodynamie et de Therapie 138*, 302-310.
Tourlentes, T., Axiotis, A., Hunsicker, A., Hurd, D., Vassilon, G., and Abood, L.C. (1960): Effects of new piperazinoglycolate on chronic schizophrenics. *Journal of Neuropsychiatry 2*, 49-53.
Ungerstedt, U. (1971): Stereotaxic mapping of monoamine paths in the rat brain. *Acta Physiologica Scandinavica, Supplementum 367*.
Ungerstedt, U. (1974): Brain dopamine neurons and behavior. In: *Neurosciences, Third Study Program*, F.O. Schmitt and F.G. Worden, Eds., 695-703, Cambridge, The M.I.T. Press.
Valenstein, E.S.. (1976): The interpretation of behavior evoked by brain stimulation. In: *Brain-Stimulation Reward*, A. Wauquier and E.T. Rolls, Eds., 557-575, Amsterdam, North-Holland Publishing Company.
Van Andel, H. (1959): Neuropharmacological studies in catatonic phenomena. In: *Neuropharmacology*, P.B. Bradley et al. Eds., 701-703, Amsterdam, Elsevier.
Van Nuetan, J.-M. (1962): Etude des effets de derives phenothiaziniques et butyrophenoniques sur l'action de l'amphetamine chez le rat. Dissertation, Paris.
Van Putten, T., and May, P.R.A. (1978): Subjective response as a predictor of outcome in pharmacotherapy: the consumer has a point. *Archives of General Psychiatry 35*, 477-480.
Van Rossum, J.M. (1967): The significance of dopamine-receptor blockage for the action of neuroleptic drugs. In: *Neuropsychopharmacology*, H. Brill, Ed., 321-329. The Hague, Excerpta Medica Foundation.
Venables, P. (1973): Input regulation and psychopathology. In: *Psychopathology – Contributions from the Social, Behavioral and Biological Sciences*, M. Hammer, K. Salzinger, and S. Sutton, Eds., 261-284, New York, John Wiley and Sons.
Venables, P.H. (1977): The electrodermal psychophysiology of schizophrenics and children at risk for schizophrenia: controversies and developments. *Schizophrenia Bulletin 3*, 28-48.
Waldmeier, P.C., and Maitre, L. (1976): Clozapine: reduction of the initial dopamine turnover increase by repeated treatment. *European Journal of Pharmacology 38*, 197-203.
Warburton, D.M. (1975): *Brain, Behavior and Drugs. Introduction to the Neurochemistry of Behavior*. Chapters 1, 3, 4 and 7. London, John Wiley.
Warburton, D.M. (1972): The cholinergic control of internal inhibition. In: *Inhibition and Learning*, R. Boakes and M.S. Halliday, Eds., 431-460, London, Academic Press.

Warburton, D.M., and Brown, K. (1972): The facilitation of discrimination performance by physostigmine sulphate. *Psychopharmacology 27*, 275-284.

Wauquier, A. (1977): Basal ganglia, control functions of instrumental behavior. In: *Symposium on Basal Ganglia — Cellular and Functional Aspects.* July 10-13. Frankfurt, Germany.

Wauquier, A. (1978): Neuroleptics and brain self-stimulation behavior. *International Review of Neurobiology 21*, in press.

Wauquier, A. (1976): The influence of psychoactive drugs on brain self-stimulation in rats: a review. In: *Brain-Stimulation Reward,* A. Wauquier and E.T. Rolls, Eds., 123-170, Amsterdam, North-Holland Publishing Company.

Wauquier, A. (1978): Personal Communication.

Wauquier, A., and Niemegeers, C.J.E. (1976): Restoration of self-stimulation inhibited by neuroleptics. *European Journal of Pharmacology 40*, 191-194.

Wauquier, A., and Niemegeers, C.J.E. (1975): The effects of dexetimide on pimozide-haloperidol- and pipamperine-induced inhibition of brain self-stimulation in rats. *Archives Internationales de Pharmacodynamie et de Therapie 217*, 280-292.

Wauquier, A., Neimegeers, C.J.E., and Lal, H. (1975): Differential antagonism by dexetimide of inhibitory effects of haloperidol and fentanyl on brain self-stimulation. *Psychopharmacology 41*, 229-235.

Wauquier, A., Niemegeers, C.J.E., and Lal, H. (1976): Selective reversal of haloperidol-induced inhibition of self-stimulation by the anticholinergic dexetimide. In: *Drugs and Central Synaptic Transmission,* P.B. Bradley and B.N. Dhawan, Eds., 201-209, London, MacMillan Press.

Zahn, T.P. (1977): Autonomic nervous system characteristics possibly related to a genetic pre-disposition to schizophrenia. *Schizophrenia Bulletin 3,* No. 1, 49-60.

Zahn, T.P. (1975): Psychophysiological concomitants of task performance in schizophrenia. In: *Experimental Approach to Psychopathology,* M.L. Kietzman, S. Sutton, and J. Zubin, Eds., 109-131, New York, Academic Press.

Zahn, T.P., and Carpenter, W.T. Jr. (1978): Effects of short-term outcome and clinical improvement on reaction time in acute schizophrenia. *Journal of Psychiatric Research 14,* 59-68.

Zahn, T.P., Carpenter, W.T. Jr., and McGlashan, T.H. (1981): Automonic nervous system activity in acute schizophrenia. I. Method and comparison with normal controls. II. Relationships to short-term prognosis and clinical state. *Archives of General Psychiatry, 38,* 251-266.

Zahn, T.P., Rosenthal, D., and Lawlor, W.G. (1968): Electrodermal and heart rate orienting reactions in chronic schizophrenia. *Journal of Psychiatric Research 6,* 117-134.

Zahn, T.P., Rosenthal, D., and Shakow, D. (1963): Effects of irregular preparatory intervals on reaction time in schizophrenia. *Journal of Abnormal Social Psychiatry 67,* 44-52.

Zahn, T.P., Rosenthal, D., and Shakow, D. (1961a): Reaction time in schizophrenic and normal subjects in relation to the sequence of a series of regular preparatory intervals. *Journal of Abnormal Social Psychiatry 63,* 161-168.

Zahn, T.P., Shakow, D., and Rosenthal, D. (1961b): Reaction time in schizophrenic and normal subjects as a function of preparatory and inter-trial intervals. *Journal of Nervous and Mental Diseases 133,* 283-287.

Ziemba, T., Meltzer, H.Y., and Davis, J.M. (1978): Do anticholinergics antagonize antipsychotic drug action? *Schizophrenia Bulletin 4,* 7-12.

ACKNOWLEDGEMENTS

For research, literary assistance and final preparation of the manuscript we owe deep gratitude to Barbara Mason.

Stanley R. Kay, M.A. provided valuable collaboration in the early stages of this work. Jeannie Nations, B.Sc. and Roger K. Pitman, M.D. were also generous with their help.

INDEX

Abstinence syndrome, *See* Withdrawal
Aceperone, 223
Acetic acid, 241
Acetylcholine, 46, 47, 72, 73, 76, 77, 133, 140, 145, 146, 178, 179, 241, 350, 351, 361, 363, 364, 365, 367, 370, 371
Acetylcholineesterase inhibitors, 361, 364, 365, 369–70, 374
    physostigmine, *See* Physostigmine
ACH, *See* Acetylcholine
ACTH, *See* Adrenocorticotropic hormone
Acupuncture, 52, 54
Adrenalectomy, 10–11
Adrenaline, nicotine and, 41, 44, 45, 46, 48
Adrenergic receptor sites, 55, 345
Adrenocorticotropic hormone (ACTH), 50, 51–52, 53, 54, 55, 147
Addiction:
    alcohol, *See* Alcoholism
    drugs, 317
    nicotine, 41–60, 67–97
Advertising, 32
Affectional bonds, formation of, 20–21
Afferent stimulation, 28
Aggression, clonidine and, 231–32

Aging, 108, 143–47
Akathisia, 214
Akynesia, 214
Alcohol, 32, 69, 243
    abuse, *See* Alcoholism
    drugs and, 53, 243
    memory impairment, 128–29
Alcoholism, 19, 21, 22, 30–34, 167–68
    Korsakoff's syndrome, 129, 166–72, 181, 234
Allergies, 315
Allopurinal, 137
Alpha-bungarotoxin, 77
Alpha-methyl paratyrosine, 78, 140, 222, 223, 227, 229, 232
Altruism, 29
Alzheimer's disease, 145, 176–78, 179
Aminergic neurones, 340
Amino acids, 12, 13
Amitriptyline, 120, 121, 232, 281, 283
Amnesia, 106, 112, 114, 117, 120–29, 132, 136, 137, 140, 146, 163–82
Amphetamines, 53, 69, 76, 106, 110, 120, 123, 130–31, 212, 222, 223, 225, 229, 230, 232, 234, 236, 243, 337, 338, 339, 340, 341–42, 343, 344, 346, 347, 349

INDEX

Amygdala, 52, 214
Analeptics, 7, 131–32
Analgesia, 126, 188, 233–42, 371
Anesthetics, 125–28
Anomie, 22, 30
Antibiotics, 112
Anticholinesterases, 365
Anticholinergic drugs, 44–45, 339–45, 346–47, 350, 352, 354–59, 361–63, 374–76
Anticipation stress, 8
Anticonvulsants, 295
Antidepressants, 110, 141, 142, 213, 264, 266, 267, 271, 281, 319, 320, 340
   amitriptylene, 120, 121, 232, 281, 283
   imipramine, 120, 121, 245, 261, 266, 267–68, 279, 281, 282, 283, 291, 314, 340
   L-5-hydroxytryptophan, 279–301, 307–8
   monoamine oxidase inhibitors, 113, 114, 141–43, 280, 281, 285, 291, 292
   tricyclic compounds, 120–21
Antidopaminergics, 347, 348
Anti-euphoric drugs, 261, 265, 270
Antihistamines, 363
Antimuscarinics, *See* Anticholinergics
Anti-Parkinsonism agents, 351, 353, 354–55, 358, 360
Antipsychotic drugs, 261, 265, 270, 271, 339, 340, 351, 352, 353
   Neuroleptic drugs, *See* Neuropletics
Antiserotonins, 363
Anxiety, 211, 259, 260, 267, 319, 362
   withdrawal, 243
Anxiogenic drugs, 261, 267
Anxiolytic drugs, 258, 259, 261, 268–69, 270, 272, 317, 319, 320, 346
Apomorphine, 223, 225, 227, 229, 232, 234, 237, 246, 338, 339, 340, 341, 344, 349
Appetite, 243–45
Arecoline, 341, 344, 347, 361, 370
Aspirin, 28
Asthma, 109

Ataxia, 167
ATPase, 12
Atropine, 72, 77, 78, 108, 109, 139, 224, 228, 231–32, 236, 238, 244–46, 344, 346, 347, 362, 363, 364, 366, 370
Authoritarianism, 28, 30
Autism, 364
Avoidance responses, 73, 75, 346–47, 349, 374

Barbital, 23
Barbiturates, 106, 108, 110, 114, 116, 118–20, 320, 340
BE, *See* Beta-endorphin
Belladonna, 362
Benserazide, 287, 288, 291, 292, 293, 294, 300, 307
Benzhexol, 338, 340
Benzodiazepines, 114, 118, 119–20, 121, 126, 320
Benztropine, 342, 343, 344, 346, 347, 353, 354, 356, 358, 360
Beta-adrenergic blockers, 44
Beta-endorphin, 25, 26, 41, 51–55, 57, 58, 188
Beta-lipotropic hormone (BLPH), 51–52
Bhang, *See* Marijuana
Blackouts, 128, 129
Blood pressure, *See* Hypertension; Hypotension
BLPH, *See* Beta-lipotropic hormone
Bradycardia, 366
Brain, 51, 164, 165, 167–70
   development, 19
   minimal brain damage, 106
   nicotine and, 44–45, 46
   self-stimulation, 76, 229–30, 342–45, 349, 370
Breast feeding, 31
Bunitrolol, 245
Butaclamol, 340
Butaperazine, 360
Butyrophenones, 317

CA, *See* Catecholamines

INDEX

Caffeine, 134–35, 223, 232
Cannon's Law of Denervation
  Supersensitivity, 24
Carbachol, 374
Carbaryl, 347
Carbidopa, 286, 287, 292, 293
Carbonic anhydrase inhibitors, 114
Carboxyhaemoglobin, 82–83
Catalepsy, 226, 347–48
Catatonia, 343, 361, 365
Catechol, 78
Catecholamines, 72, 95, 140, 141, 178, 180, 227, 229, 231, 246, 280, 292, 295, 298, 337, 345, 367, 370
  nicotine and, 44, 47–49
Chewing gum, nicotine, 83, 85–87
Child abuse, 21
Childrearing practices, 28, 30
Choline chloride, 367–68
Cholinergic mechanisms, 337–39, 340, 341–42, 345–48, 349–51, 361, 364, 365–71, 374–76
Cholinesterase, 364, 366
Cholinolytics, 352, 353, 361, 362, 363, 364, 368–70, 374
Cholinomimetics, 346, 350, 361, 366, 368–70, 374
Chloral hydrate, 23, 110, 236, 346
Chlordiazepoxide, 119, 266, 340, 346
Chlorimipramine, 213, 215
Chlorpromazine, 23, 28, 73, 229–30, 232, 237, 261, 268, 269, 270, 271, 311, 313, 315, 317, 325, 340, 341, 343, 344, 346, 351, 354, 360
  profile, 265–66
Chlorprothixine, 346
Choice of drug, social factors in, 32
Cholesterol, 49
Cholineacetyltransferase, 176, 177, 180
Cholinergic agents, 123, 145–46, 178, 344, 345
Cholinergic mechanism, 44–47, 60, 78, 139, 145
Cholinomimetics, 344, 345
Cigarettes, *See* Nicotine; Smoking
Clomipramine, 281, 292

Clonazepam, 213, 215
Clonidine, 54, 171, 221–47
Clopenthixol, 317, 318, 319
Clozapin, 327, 343, 346, 351
CNS Augmenters, 27, 28
CNS Reducers, 27–28
Cocaine, 69, 70, 338, 344
Cognition:
  dysfunction, *See* Learning dysfunction
  nicotine and, 55–57
Colchicine, 137
Compensatory behaviors, 21
Compulsive behavior, 210, 211
Concentration, 364
Consciousness, state of, 20, 21
Convulsions, 7, 80, 133, 294, 295
Coprolalia, 208, 209, 210
Copropraxia, 208
Coronary heart disease, 49
Corticosteroids, 11, 49–50, 51, 55, 75
Cortisol, 49, 50, 51, 57
Curare, 77
Cyclazocine, 371
Cytosine, 113
Cytospectrophotometry, 5, 6, 7, 9, 10

D-tubocurarine, 45
DALA (D-Ala^2-Me 1-enkephalinamide), 23
Deafferetation, 24
Decamethonium, 77
Delirium, 294
Dementia, 143–47
Denervation sensitivity, 28
Dependence:
  alcohol, *See* Alcoholism
  nicotine, 42–43
Depot neuroleptics, *See* Neuroleptics
Depressants (generally), 24
  barbiturates, *See* Barbiturates
  tranquilizers, 73–74, 264
Depression, 120, 212, 258, 259, 261, 265–66
  nicotine and, 73–74, 78
  schizophrenia and, 279–301, 307–8, 319, 343, 364, 365, 367

Desipramine, 229
Destructive behavior, 20
Dexamphetamine, 215
Dexetimide, 339, 341, 343, 344, 345
Dextroamphetamine, 261, 266–67, 268
Diabetes, 109
Diamphetamine, 130
Diazepam, 8, 119, 121–23, 124, 127–28, 260, 261, 266, 268–69, 270, 271, 272, 285, 289
Dibenamine, 78, 235, 236, 243, 245
Dicter's neurons, 3, 4, 5
Diencephalon, 163, 168
Diethyl ether, 125–26, 127, 128
Digestive system, 95
Disulfiram, 230, 232
Ditran, 344, 363–64
Diuretics, 108
Dopamine, 72, 76, 78, 171, 179, 180, 212, 213, 214, 215, 222, 223, 224, 225, 228, 229, 231, 232, 286, 287, 292, 293, 321, 337, 338, 340, 344, 348–52, 375
Dopaminergic receptors, 47, 222, 234, 339, 342, 343
Down's syndrome, 109
Drug abuse, 30–34
Drug administration methods, 312
Drunkenness, *See* Alcoholism
Dyskinesia, 214, 259, 321, 323, 353
Dysmnesia, 163–82

Echolalia, 208, 209, 210
Echopraxia, 208, 209, 210
Egalitarianism, 29
Electroconvulsive shock therapy (ECS), 114–15, 223, 309, 310–11, 326
Electroencephalographs, 175
Electropuncture, 53
Encephalopathy, 108
Endogenous opiates, 58
Endorphins, 22, 23, 24, 25, 26–27, 52, 54, 59–60, 188–89
  Beta-, *See* Beta-endorphin
Endotoxin hypotension, 52–53

Enkephalins, 52, 187, 188, 189, 190, 198, 204
Epilepsy, 172, 295
Epinephrine, 176
Ergot alkaloids, 144
Ergotamine, 222
Eserine, 176, 361
Estradiol, 11
Ethanol, *See* Alcohol
Ethomoxane, 346
Euphoria, 258, 259, 261, 267, 279, 294, 299, 301, 317, 357, 363, 367, 371
Evolution of Chastity, The, 30
Exploitive behavior, 20, 28
Extrapyramidal drugs, 258, 259, 261, 265, 270, 272
Extrapyramidal reactions, 347–48, 351, 352, 353
  Parkinsonism, 347, 351, 353, 354, 359

Family psychopathology, 28, 30, 31, 212
Fathers, role of, 31
Fentanyl, 235, 343
Fetal conditioning, 31
Filters, nicotine and, 91
5HIAA, *See* 5-hydroxyindoleacetic acid
5HT, *See* Serotonin
5-hydroxyindoleacetic acid, 280–81, 295, 296, 299
5-hydroxytryptophan, 279–301, 307–8
  side effects, 293–95
Flupenthixol, 317, 318
Fluphenazine, 315–16, 317, 318, 319, 320, 322, 325, 339, 341, 351
Fluroxene, 127
Fluspirilene, 317, 318
Forane, 126
Fornix, 164, 167, 169, 170, 172, 181

GABA, *See* Gamma amino butyric acid
Gamma amino butyric acid (GABA), 147, 176, 179, 350
  receptors, 132, 133
Gas chromatography, 81

INDEX

Gilles De la Tourette's syndrome, *See* Tourette's syndrome
Glutamic acid, 133
Glycine, 232
Growth hormones, 95
Guanethidine, 110

Hallucinations, 362–63, 364, 370
Hallucinogens, 22, 69
Haloperidol, 223, 226, 234, 235, 245, 246, 269–70
    schizophrenia, in, 317, 318, 319, 325, 339, 341, 343, 344, 347, 351, 352, 354
    Tourette's syndrome, in, 213, 214, 215
Halothane, 126, 127, 128
Hand preference, 112–13
Harlow monkeys, 21
Heart action:
    bradycardia, 366
    nicotine and, 49, 82, 83, 85, 90
    tachycardia, 260
Hebephrenia, 365, 366, 369, 372
Hepatic diseases, *See* Liver disease
Heroin, 32, 243
    addiction, 47–48, 49
Herpes simplex, 172
Hexamethonium, 71, 78
Hexobarbital, 23
Hippocampal syndrome, 172–78, 181
Holograms, 181
Homesickness, 45
Hormones, growth, 95
Huntington's chorea, 146, 209, 295
Hydergine, 144
Hydrotherapies, 33
Hydroxycorticoids, 10, 50
Hyoscine, 122, 123, 342
Hyperactivity, 258, 259–60
Hyperendorphinism, 27
Hyperoxy, 7
Hypertension, 221, 260, 365
Hypnotics, 69, 264, 269, 272, 339, 343, 346
Hypoglycemia, 109

Hypokynesia, 9, 215, 353
Hypotension, 222, 243, 260, 365, 366
Hypothermia, 4, 245–46
Hypoxia, 4–5, 9

ICSS, *See* Intracranial self-stimulation
Illusions, 362
Imidazoline, 222, 231, 239
Imipramine, 120, 121, 245, 261, 266, 267–68, 279, 281, 282, 283, 291, 314, 340
Imubacco, 209
Indoleamine, 78, 279, 280, 292
Infancy, social isolation during, 20, 21
Inflammation, 241
Insecticides, 364
Insomnia, 258, 259, 267, 270
    depression and, 292, 293, 294, 300, 301
    schizophrenia and, 356, 357, 358, 368
Institutionalization, 31
Insulin, 108, 109, 362
Intimacy, 20–21
Intracranial self-stimulation (ICSS), 76, 229–30, 342–45, 349, 370
Involutional melancholia, 291, 293, 301
Involutional psychoses, 362
Iproniazid, 142
Isopropamide, 341, 343

Korsakoff's syndrome, 129, 166, 167–72, 181, 234

L-dopa, 338, 340, 341
L-5-hydroxytryptophan (L-5HTP), 279–301, 307–8,
    side effects, 293–95
Labetalol, 235
Lactate dehydrogenase, 5
Latah, 209
Learning:
    clonidine and, 234
    dysfunction, 105–49, 259, 362–63, 364–65, 366–68
    nicotine and, 71, 73
Lecithin, 145, 178

Left-handedness, 208
Lidocaine hydrochloride, 114–15, 133
Limbic arousal mechanisms, 75
Lithium, 327
Lithium carbonate, 125
Lithium chloride, 232
Liver disease, 108
Lorazepam, 124
LSD, *See* Lysergic acid diethylamide
Lysergic acid diethylamide (LSD), 236, 362–63, 371

Magnesium pemoline, 137–38
Malizia, 54
Malnutrition, 167–68
Malonitrile, 112, 113–14, 115
Mania, 294, 299
Manic-depressive psychosis, 279–80, 365, 367
MAO, *See* Monamine oxidase
Maphensin, 232
Marchiafava-Bignami syndrome, 167
Marijuana, 22, 23, 32
Massage, 33
Mecamylamine, 44, 46, 47, 70, 71, 72, 74, 76, 77, 78, 89–90, 244, 245
Meclofenoxate, 145
Meclofexate, 145
Memory, 111–12
  clonidine and, 234
  dysfunction, 105–49, 163–82, 364
Meprobamate, 340, 346
Metabolism, 1, 3, 8, 11–13
Metamphetamine, 130
Metatyrosine, 223
Methadone, 32, 243
Methylatropine, 338, 347, 361
Methylphenidate, 215, 234, 338, 341, 347, 366, 367, 368
Methyl xanthine, 137
Methysergide, 236, 246
Metoclopramide, 286, 287, 289, 293
Metrazol, 7
Minimal brain damage, 106
Monoamine oxidase, 108, 109, 180

Monoamine oxidase inhibitor, 113, 114, 141–43, 280, 281, 285, 291, 292
Mood altering drugs (generally), 33, 120, 140–141, 257–72
  See also: individual drugs
Morphine, 11, 73, 117, 123, 124, 188, 189, 191, 195, 202, 204, 227, 233, 234, 238, 240, 242, 246, 343
Mothers' role in substance abuse, 31
MSH, 147
Muscarine, 76
Muscarinic receptors, 46, 47
Muscle, tension, 80
Myriachit, 209

NA, *See* Noradrenaline
Naja naja toxin, 77
NAL, *See* Nalaxone
Nalorphine, 232, 371
Naloxone, 23, 24, 25–27, 52–55, 57–60, 188
  clonidine and, 227, 228, 239, 240, 241, 242, 243, 246
Naltrexone, 25, 188
Naphazoline, 231, 246
Narcissism, 28
Narcotics, 343
Neocortex, 47
Neostigmine, 345, 366
Nerve gases, 364
Neuroleptics, 11, 309–20, 337–76
  depot, 312–20, 325–29, 330
  side effects, 314–17, 351
  withdrawal, 322–23
Neurotransmitter density, 27
Nialamide, 288, 291
Nicotine, 41–60, 67–97, 138–41
  blood level of, 43, 48–49, 50, 51, 81–82, 83–84
  urine in, 43, 48, 88–89
  withdrawal, 69, 71, 80–81
Nicotine receptors, 47, 60, 72, 77, 345, 350, 352, 364, 370–71
Nitrous oxide, 53, 126–27, 128
Nomifensine, 344

INDEX

Noradrenaline, 44, 45, 47–49, 54, 55, 72, 75, 76, 78, 79, 95
  depression and, 292
Noradrenergic receptors, 222, 223, 224, 229, 230, 234, 235
Norepinephrine, 110, 142, 147, 171, 172, 175, 176, 179, 180, 213, 222, 225, 227, 228, 229, 230, 231, 234, 235, 237, 241, 243, 246, 298, 339, 340, 341, 342, 343, 344
Nucleotide metabolites, 111
Nurturance, 20, 21, 29, 30
Nystagmus, 167

Obesity, 53
Obsessive behavior, 210, 211
Olfaction, 20
Ophthalmoplegia, 167
Opiate receptors, 23, 24, 27, 187, 188–89, 202, 242, 243
Opiates, endogenous, *See* Enkephalins; Substance P
Opioid antagonists, 23
Orfenadrine, 261
Organophosphorus compounds, 364–65, 370
Oxotremorine, 341, 350, 361, 370
Oxprenolol, 44, 49
Oxygen deficiency, 4–5, 9
Oxymetazoline, 231, 241, 246
Oxymorphone, 23

Pain perception, 25, 27–28, 187–204, 238–39
Pantolinium, 44
Papaverine, 143–44
Papez circuit, 169, 174, 175
Para-chlorophenylalanine, 78, 116, 117, 232, 281
Paraldehyde, 346
Paranoia, 212, 358, 363, 365, 366, 369, 372
Parasympathicolytic drugs, 261, 265, 268, 270
Parasymathicomimetic drugs, 261

Parkinsonism, 213, 214, 295, 299, 315–17, 321, 347, 351, 352, 354, 359
PCPA, *See* Para-chlorophenylalanine
Peer friendships and substance abuse, 31–32
Pelizaeus-Merzbacher disease, 209
Penicillin, 366
Pentobarbital, 118–19, 346
Pentolinium, 89–90
Pentamethonium iodide, 365
Pentamethylenetetrazol, 7
Pentapeptides, 188
Pentylene tetrazol, 131, 132, 133
Peptides, 51, 52, 111, 147–48
  pain perception and, 187–204
Perineuronal tissue, 3, 4, 5, 8, 11
Perphenazine, 312–13, 317, 318, 319, 339, 341, 346, 354
Pethidine, 122, 125
Pharmaceutical industry, 32
Phenelzine, 229
Phenobarbital, 23, 107, 114, 119
Phenothiazines, 311, 321, 340, 353
  chlropromazine, *See* Chlorpromazine
Phenotolamine, 49,
Phenoxybenzamine, 222, 223, 228, 230, 232, 234, 235, 236, 238–39, 240, 241, 243, 244, 245
Phentolamine, 231–32, 234, 235, 236, 237, 240, 241, 243, 244, 245, 246
Phenylepherine, 241
Phenylethylamine, 342
Phenytoin, 107, 114
Phobias, 210
Phospholipids, 4
Physical intimacy in infancy, 20–21
Physostigmine, 123, 180, 236, 261, 341, 344, 345, 350, 366–69, 374
Piblokto, 209
Picrotoxin, 7, 131, 132
Pilocarpine, 344, 347, 361, 370
Pimozide, 215, 223, 246, 270–71, 341, 343–45, 351
Pindolol, 245

Pineal gland, 187
Pipamperone, 343
Piperazinoalkylglycolates, 364
Piperidyl glycolates, 362, 363
Piperoxane, 228, 230, 233, 235–37, 241, 242, 243, 244, 245
Pipothiazine, 317, 318, 320
Piracetam, 145
Piribedil, 223, 225
Pituitary, beta-endorphin synthesized by, 51
Pole-jump avoidance, 73
Polypeptides, 371
Pregnancy, chemical ingestion during, 29, 31
Premarital sexuality, 20
Probanthine, 361
Procaine, 141–43
Progesterone, 11
Prolactin, 314
Promazine, 340
Promethazine, 340, 342
Propranol, 49, 78, 240, 245
Prostaglandin, 366
Protein, 4, 5, 7, 11, 111, 112
Psychosis, 259, 267
Psychosurgery, 309
Psychotherapy, 309, 310, 326, 328–29
Psychotogenic drugs, 261, 267, 268–69, 270
Psychotropic drugs (generally), 33, 120, 140–41, 257–72
  primary and secondary effects distinguished, 263
Punishment system (cholinergic), 342
Purkinje cell, 5, 10, 26–27
Puromycin, 112

Quillen, 48

REM sleep, 300
Renal function, drug-excretion and, 107–8
Renshaw cells, 47, 77
Reserpine, 76, 116, 117–18, 222, 223, 232, 236, 237, 261, 280, 326, 339, 340, 345, 346

Ribonucleic acids (RNA), 4–11, 110–15, 136

SAD, *See* Somatosensory Affectional Deprivation (SAD)
St. Vito's dance, 209
Salivation, nicotine and, 95
Schizophrenia, 309–30, 337–76
  electroshock therapy, 309, 310–11, 326
  paranoid, 358, 363, 365, 366, 369, 372
  pyschotherapy, 309, 310, 326, 328–29
Scopolamine, 47, 122–23, 146, 180, 224, 338, 341, 343, 344, 345, 346, 347, 362
Sedatives (generally), 69, 118–20, 259, 264, 269, 270, 271, 339, 343
Self-stimulation, intracranial, *See* Intracranial self-stimulation
Senile dementia, 144, 177–78
  schizophrenics, 325
Senses, emotional deprivation of, 20
Serotonin, 47, 72, 76, 79, 116–17, 118, 120, 128, 129, 130, 136, 140, 142, 147, 171, 176, 178, 179, 213, 215, 231, 246, 280–81, 298, 299, 361, 370, 371
Sexual behavior, 20–25, 28
  adolescence, 31–32
  maloxone and, 25, 53
Shock treatment, *See* Electroconvulsive therapy
Shuttle box avoidance, 73
Six-hydroxy dopamine, 347
Sleep, 235–37, 300
  disorders, *See* Insomnia
Smoking, 41–60
  withdrawal, 45, 53–55, 60, 69, 71, 80–81
Smoking and Health: A Report of the Surgeon General, 41, 45
Social isolation, 20–23, 27
Socioreligious controls, 28, 32
Somatosensory Affectional Deprivation (SAD), 19–34
Somesthesis, 20, 22, 28, 31, 33–34
Spatial perception dysfunction in, 172, 176

INDEX

Spiramide, 341
Spiroperidol, 222, 223, 345, 346
Steroids, 107
Stereotypy, 338–39, 340–41, 342, 343, 346, 347, 349, 357
Stimulants, 24, 130–38, 259, 267, 270, 271
   amphetamines, *See* Amphetamines
   nicotine, 73–74, 78, 79
Stress, 1, 4–5, 6, 8–11, 75, 78
Strychnine, 131–32
Substance abuse, 19
   alcohol, *See* Alcoholism
   endorphins and, 22–26
   Naloxone and, *See* Naloxone
   premarital and extramarital sex and, 21
   types of abusers, 22
Substance P, 187–88, 189, 190, 191, 195, 198, 201–4
Suicide, 280
Sydenham's chorea, 209
Sympatholytic drugs, 261, 265, 268, 270, 271
Sympathicomimetic drugs, 261, 267

Tachycardia, 260
Tars, 42, 43, 95
TCAP, *See* Tricyanoamino propene
Teilhard de Chardin, P., S.J., 22, 30
Temperature, nicotine abstinence and, 45
Tetrabenazine, 346
Tetrabenzine, 227
Tetracyano propene, 115–16
Tetrahydrocannabinol, 73
Tetryzoline, 246
Thalamus, 164, 165, 170
   memory and, 167–69
Thermal stimulation, 188, 201
Theophylline, 232
Thiamine deficiency, 167
Thiopental, 119, 126
Thiopentone, 127
Thiopropazate, 346
Thioproperazine, 342
Thioridazine, 144, 314, 340, 341, 342, 346, 351

Thioxanthenes, 317
Thiothixine, 315
Thymoxamine, 235
Thyroid, 11, 109
Tics, 207–11, 212, 215
Time perception, dysfunction in, 166–67
Tobacco, *See* Nicotine; Smoking
Tolazoline, 223, 235, 236, 243, 244, 245
Tolerance to nicotine, 42, 44, 58, 78–80
Tourette's syndrome, 207–15
Tranquilizers, 264
   nicotine, 73–74
Transketolase, 167
Tranylcypromine, 142–43
Trichloroethylene, 127
Tricyanoaminopropene (TCAP), 113–15
Tricyclic compounds, 120–21
Trifluoperazine, 271–72, 339, 341, 346
Trihexyphenidyl, 289, 293, 344, 346, 347, 354, 356, 360
Tryptamine, 361
Tryptophan, 381–84

Uric acid, 135–36
Urinalysis, 43, 48, 50, 88–89

Vasopressin, 170–72, 175
Venserazide, 307
Vestibular, 20, 22, 31, 33–34
Violence, 20, 21, 24, 30, 214, 231–32

Warfarin, 110
Weight, nicotine abstinence and, 80
Wernicke's disease, 129, 167
Wheat gluten, 357, 371
Withdrawal
   alcohol, 243
   barbiturates, 80
   clonidine and, 233–34, 242–43
   nicotine, 45, 53–55, 60, 69, 71, 80–81
   schizophrenia, 322–23, 364
Women, role of, 29–30

Yohimbine, 223, 228, 235, 236, 243

Zuckerhandl's bundle, 175

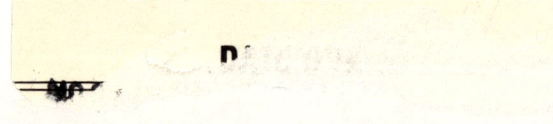